ONE Touch Pediatrics

For NEET/NEXT/FMGE/INI-CET

ONE Touch Pediatrics

For NEET/NEXT/FMGE/INI-CET

Anand Bhatia MBBS, MD (Pediatrics)
Assistant Professor
North DMC Medical College & Hindu Rao Hospital, New Delhi
Senior Residency
Lady Hardinge Medical College and North DMC Medical College & Hindu Rao Hospital, New Delhi

CBSPD
Dedicated to Education
CBS

CBS Publishers & Distributors Pvt Ltd

• New Delhi • Bengaluru • Chennai • Kochi • Kolkata • Lucknow • Mumbai
• Hyderabad • Jharkhand • Nagpur • Patna • Pune • Uttarakhand

ONE Touch Pediatrics

For NEET/NEXT/FMGE/INI-CET

ISBN: 978-93-94525-35-1

First Edition: 2024

Published by **Satish Kumar Jain** and produced by **Varun Jain** for

CBS Publishers & Distributors Pvt Ltd
4819/XI Prahlad Street, 24 Ansari Road, Daryaganj, New Delhi 110 002, India.
Ph: +91-11-23289259, 23266861, 23266867 Website: www.cbspd.com
Fax: 011-23243014
e-mail: delhi@cbspd.com; cbspubs@airtelmail.in.

Corporate Office: 204 FIE, Industrial Area, Patparganj, Delhi 110 092
Ph: +91-11-4934 4934 Fax: 4934 4935
e-mail: feedback@cbspd.com; bhupesharora@cbspd.com

Branches

- **Bengaluru:** Seema House 2975, 17th Cross, K.R. Road, Banasankari 2nd Stage, Bengaluru-560 070, Karnataka
  Ph: +91-80-26771678/79 Fax: +91-80-26771680 e-mail: bangalore@cbspd.com
- **Chennai:** 7, Subbaraya Street, Shenoy Nagar, Chennai-600 030, Tamil Nadu
  Ph: +91-44-26680620, 26681266 Fax: +91-44-42032115 e-mail: chennai@cbspd.com
- **Kochi:** 68/1534, 35, 36-Power House Road, Opp. KSEB, Cochin-682018, Kochi, Kerala
  Ph: +91-484-4059061-65 Fax: +91-484-4059065 e-mail: kochi@cbspd.com
- **Kolkata:** Hind Ceramics Compound, 1st Floor, 147, Nilganj Road, Belghoria, Kolkata-700056, West Bengal
  Ph: +033-2563-3055/56 e-mail: kolkata@cbspd.com
- **Lucknow:** Basement, Khushnuma Complex, 7-Meerabai Marg (Behind Jawahar Bhawan), Lucknow-226001, Uttar Pradesh
  Ph: +0522-4000032 e-mail: tiwari.lucknow@cbspd.com
- **Mumbai:** PWD Shed, Gala No. 25/26, Ramchandra Bhatt Marg, Next to J.J. Hospital Gate No. 2, Opp. Union Bank of India, Noor Baug, Mumbai-400009, Maharashtra
  Ph: +91-22-66661880/89 Fax: +91-22-24902342 e-mail: mumbai@cbspd.com

Representatives

- **Hyderabad** +91-9885175004
- **Jharkhand** +91-9811541605
- **Nagpur** +91-9421945513
- **Patna** +91-9334159340
- **Pune** +91-9623451994
- **Uttarakhand** +91-9716462459

Printed at : Goyal Offset Works Pvt. Ltd. Haryana (INDIA)

Preface

Hello friends!

First of all, I would like to extend my heartfelt thanks to all of you for reading my book and giving your blessings. I still remember, when I was doing MBBS, I faced huge difficulty in covering my syllabus. I had no idea how to study in a proper way and how to crack exams. That day, I promised myself that one day I will change the whole thought process of teaching and will introduce a different way of learning.

So, here is the result of my day and night efforts. I am introducing to you this book which covers all the theories and clinical topics for your UG and PG exams. There is one precious message I would like to convey to all of you: "Never stop believing in your dreams, they were given to you for a reason. Just find the purpose of your existence in this life and once you find it, spend your whole life cherishing it; because once you follow your passion, life becomes beautiful."

Who Can Use This Book?

Anyone Who is Preparing for UG and PG Exams.

How Should I Read This Book?

- If you are a final year student then develop the habit of finishing one chapter in a day. By the end of the same day, call one of your close friends and just teach him/her whatever you read. (You will never forget that topic in your life).
- If you are appearing for PG entrance exam—you must finish this book in 5 days.
- Time for first reading: 5 days
- Time for second reading: 3 days
- Time for third reading: 2 days

  (Try to focus on the images and tables)

Always Remember:

"10 किताबों को एक बार नहीं, एक किताब को 10 बार पढ़ो।"

"Instead of reading 10 books one time, Read one book 10 times."

"Life is a one-time offer—use it well."

Anand Bhatia

Contents

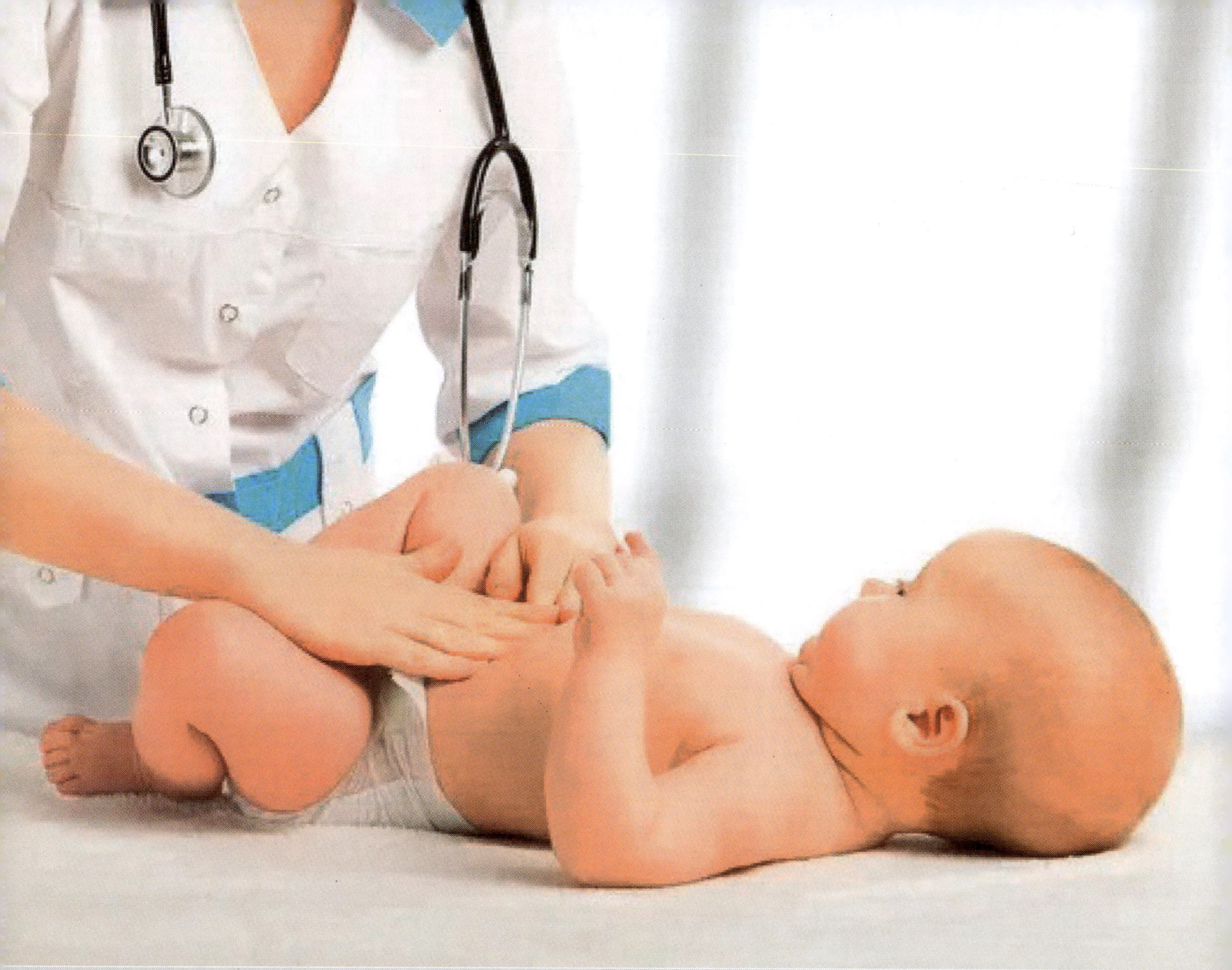

THEORY

1. GROWTH AND DEVELOPMENT

"If the world was blind, how many people you would have impressed."

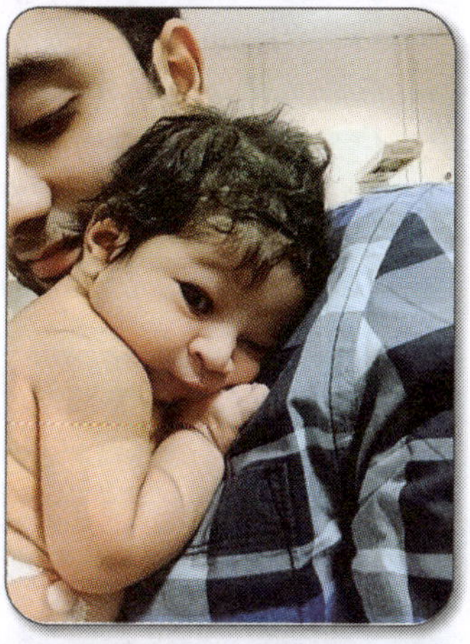

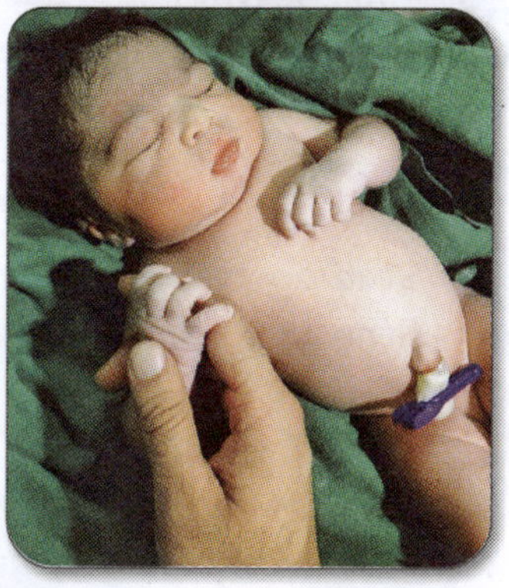

Greek Meaning of Pediatrics

Pedia = child
Latrics = healer

Periods of Growth

Ovum: 0–2 weeks
Embryo: 3–8 weeks
Fetus: 9 weeks—birth

IMPORTANT DEFINITIONS

- Neonate: 0–28 days of life
- Early neonate: 0–7 days
- Late neonate: 7–28 days
- Infant: 29 days till 1 year
- Toddler: 1–3 years
- Preschool: 3–6 years
- School: 6–12 years
- Adolescent period:
  - Early: 10–13 years
  - Middle: 14–16 years
  - Late: 17–19 years
  - Normal head circumference (HC) at birth: 33–35 cm
  - Rate of increment:
    - 0–3 months: 2 cm/month
    - 3–6 months: 1 cm/month
    - 6–12 months: 0.5 cm/month
- Normal weight of a newborn: 2.5–4 kg
- Average Indian baby weight: 3 kg
- Weight doubles by 5 months and triples by 1 year

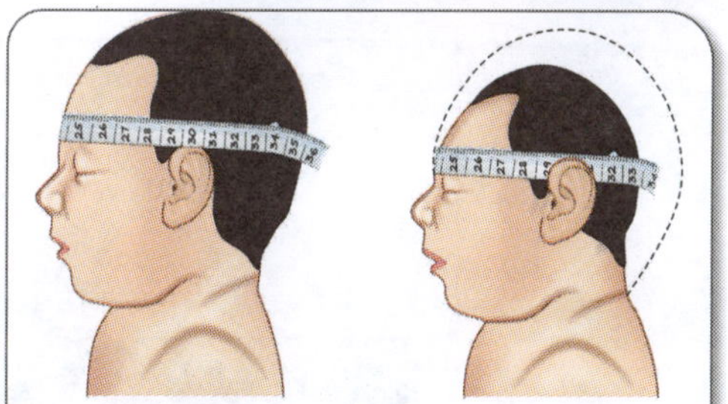

Baby with typical head size | Baby with microcephaly

RATE OF INCREMENT OF WEIGHT

1. **0–2 months:** 20–40 g/day
2. **3–12 months:** 400 grams every month till 1 year
3. 2 kg/year for next 7 years
4. After 7 years—3 kg/year

Remember

Weight of a 1-year-old is 10 kg

As the age increases, weight increases in even number, that means

Wt. of a 2-year-old will be 12 kg

3-year-old: 14 kg **4-year-old:** 16 kg **5-year-old:** 18 kg **6-year-old:** 20 kg

Weech's Formula for calculating expected weight

1. 3–12 months = $\frac{9 + x}{2}$ $x \Rightarrow$ age in months
2. 1–6 years = $2x + 8$ $x \Rightarrow$ age in years
3. 7–12 years = $\frac{7x - 5}{2}$ $x \Rightarrow$ age in years

Note: * Repeated question
** Multiple times repeated question

Golden Points

- Length of a newborn: 48–50 cm (19–21 inches)
- Length doubles by 4 years and triples by 12 years
- Length of a 4-year-old will be 100 cm and 12-year-old will be 150 cm
- After 4 years, child gains 6 cm/year height every year till 12 years
- Length of a 1-year-old is 75 cm (means from birth till 1 year there is an increment of 25 cm)
- Expected height formula: Age (in years) multiply by 6 + 77
- <2 years we take the length of baby
- >2 years we take the height

Legal Age Definitions	
Definition of child	<18 years
Minimum age of marriage	Boy <21 years, Girl <18 years
Responsibility of crime	12 years
Juvenile criminal	12–18 years
Compulsory free education	6–14 years

Infantometer: To Measure the Length of 0–2 years

- Stadiometer: To measure the height of >2 years
- Standing height is about 0.7 cm less than the recumbent length

Harpenden Caliper

1. To know the caloric reserve of the body
2. Measured to the nearest of 1 cm

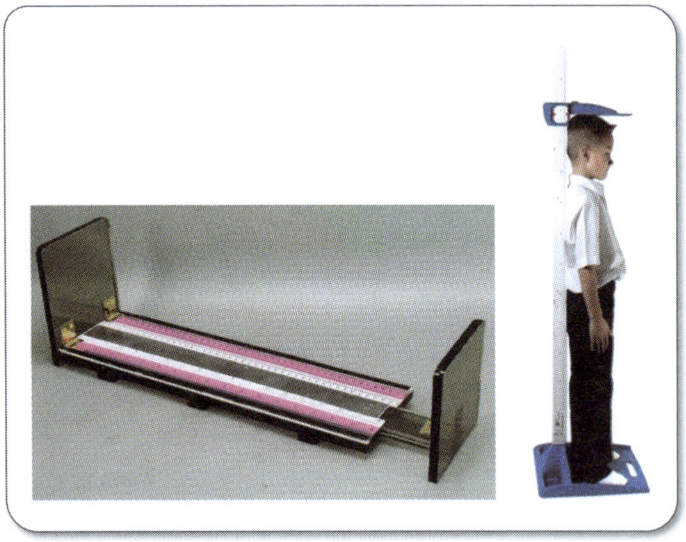

Infantometer

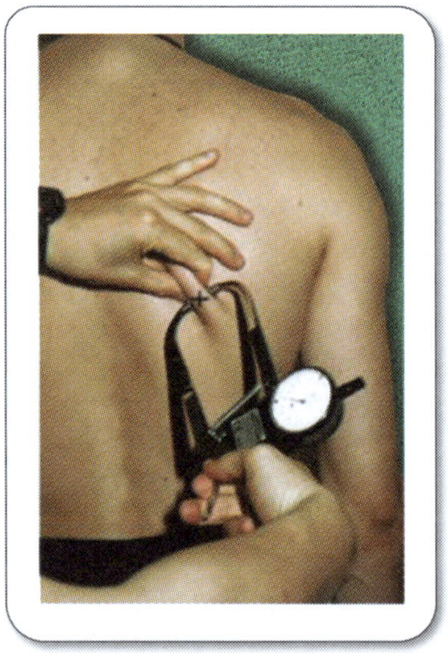

Harpenden Caliper

- Normal value
- 1–6 years is >10 mm
- If it is <6 mm—malnutrition
- Microcephaly: Head circumference <**–3 SD (standard deviation)**
- Macrocephaly: HC >2 SD

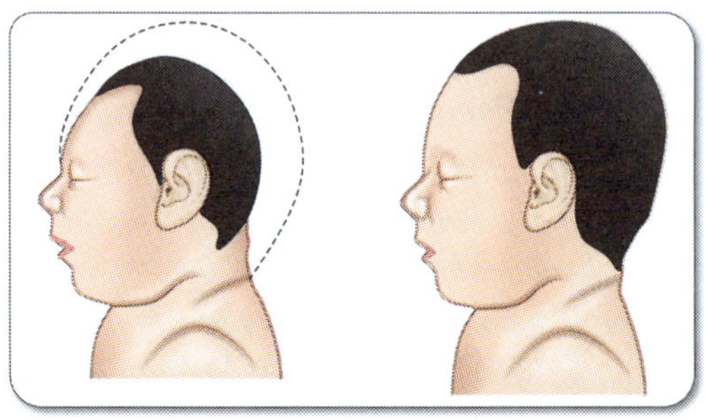

CAUSES OF MICROCEPHALY

Mnemonic

There were two babies—Rubin and Smith

- **Rubin:** Rubinstein—Taybi syndrome
- Smith: Smith-Lemli-Opitz syndrome

Their **Families** were **Crying** because they want to **Eat Corn** at **Pataya** beach

- **F:** Familial
- **C:** Cri du chat syndrome
- **E:** Edward syndrome
- **Corn:** Cornelia de Lange syndrome
- **Pataya:** Patau syndrome

Rubinstein-Taybi syndrome

- **GREAT**—Great toe deviated
- **MR**—Mental retardation
- **MICRO**—Microcephaly
- **THUMBS**—Thumbs are broad
- **ASD**—Atrial septal defect

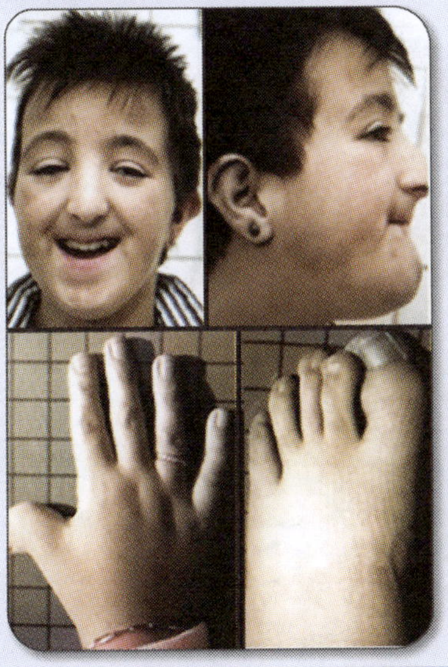

Cri du chat syndrome

- 5p deletion
- Microcephaly
- High pitch cry resembling a cat

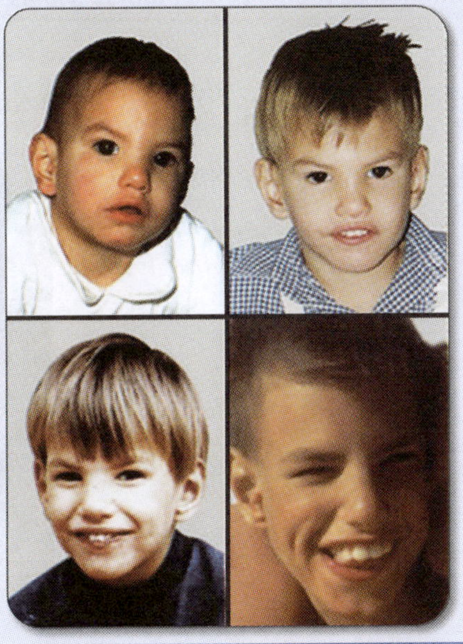

Edward syndrome

Trisomy 18

R: Rocker bottom feet
O: Overlapping digits
C: Cardiac defect
K: Kidney defect
Y: Microcephaly
M: Mental retardation

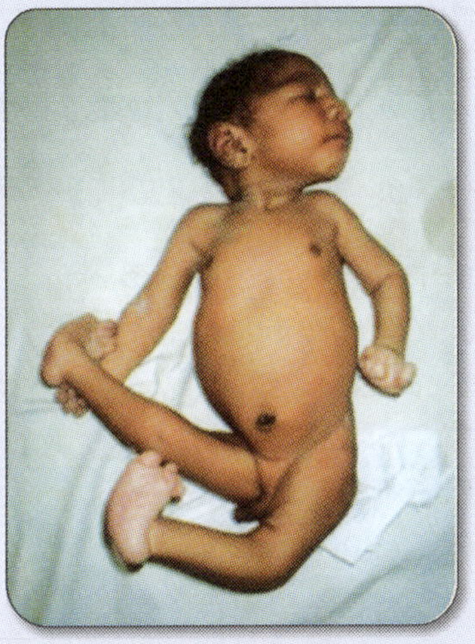

Upper Segment: Lower Segment Ratio

- Upper segment: Vertex to pubic symphysis
- Lower segment: Pubic symphysis to heel
- Normal ratio at birth: 1.7:1
- 3 years: 1.3:1
- 7–10 years: 1:1
- Adult: 0.9:1

Golden Points

- Growth of a child is cephal to caudal and distal to proximal
- That means during fetal life, head grows before the neck
- Distal parts of the body such as hands increase in size before the upper arms

DRUGS CONTRAINDICATED IN PREGNANCY

Maternal intake	Defect in the baby
Thalidomide	Phocomelia
Antimalarial	Deafness
Alcohol	Fetal alcohol syndrome/limb abnormalities
Carbamazepine	Spina bifida
Carbimazole	Scalp defects, choanal atresia, esophageal atresia

Contd...

Maternal intake	Defect in the baby
Cocaine	Microcephaly, LBW, IUGR
Danazol	Virilization
Lithium	Ebstein anomaly, macrosomia
Misoprostol	Mobius syndrome—cranial neuropathies
Phenytoin	Fetal hydantoin syndrome, neuroblastoma, bleeding (Vitamin K deficiency)
Quinine	Abortion, thrombocytopenia, deafness
Statins	Vacterl anomalies
Tetracyclines	Teeth pigmentation, cataract
Vitamin D	Supravalvular aortic stenosis, hypercalcemia
Warfarin	Fetal bleeding, hypoplastic nasal structures
Erythromycin	Congenital hypertrophic pyloric stenosis

- If the mother is a case of polyhydramnios, we should rule out trachea esophageal fistula (TEF) in the baby
- If the mother is a case of oligohydramnios, we should rule out renal agenesis in the baby

Renal agenesis and oligohydramnios are associated with Potter syndrome (image)

- **P**: Pulmonary hypoplasia
- **O**: Oligohydramnios
- **T**: Twisted skin (wrinkled skin)
- **T**: Twisted face (potter face)
- **E**: Extremities defect
- **R**: Renal agenesis

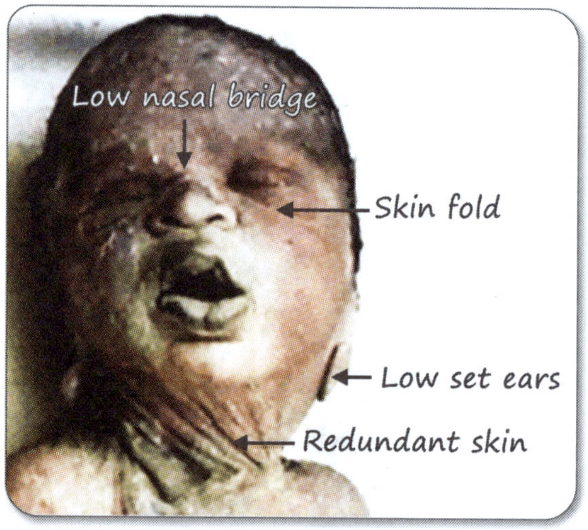

Potter syndrome

Turner syndrome	Noonan syndrome
Karyotype 45 XO	Karyotype normal
Infertile due to streak ovaries	Fertile but delayed puberty
Only females	Males or females
Intelligence normal	Intellectual disability present
	Heart: Pulmonary stenosis

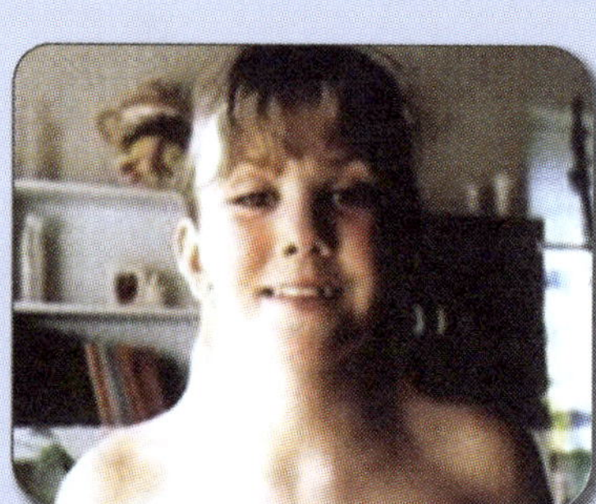

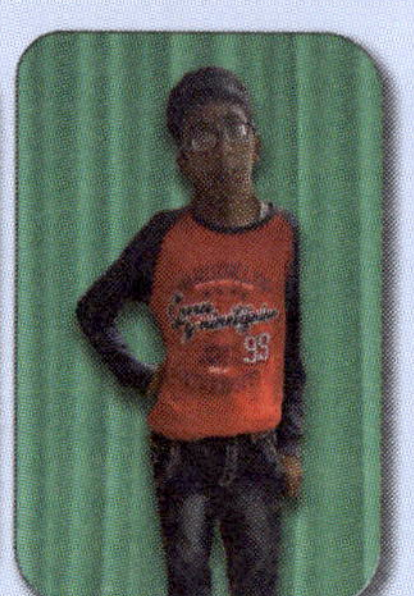

Fetal alcohol syndrome

- Microcephaly
- Short palpebral fissure
- Smooth philtrum
- Thin upper lip

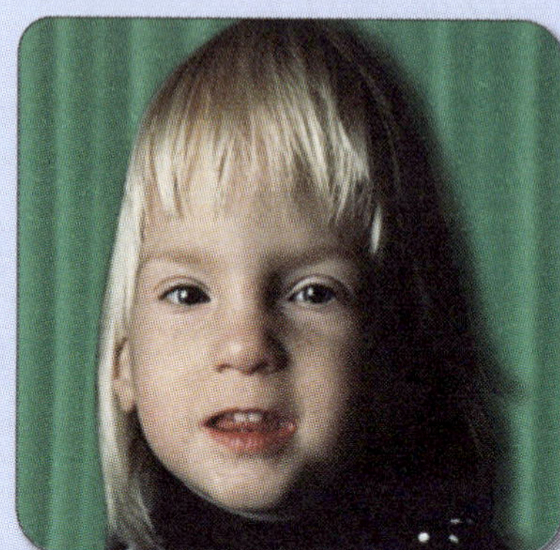

TURNER SYNDROME: MNEMONIC—LOW CABINS

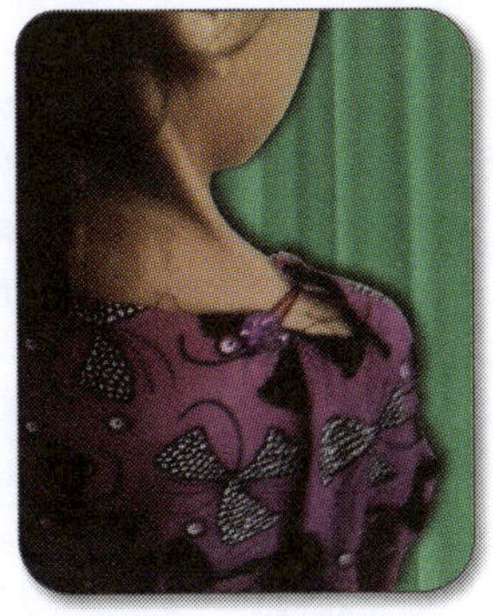

L : Low thyroid, lymphedema
O : Ovaries under developed, Streak ovaries
W : Webbed neck
C : Cystic hygroma
A : Primary amenorrhea, high arched palate
Bi : Bicuspid aortic valve (Most common heart disease in Turner) Absent Barr body**
N : Nipples widely spaced
S : Short stature, horseshoe shaped kidney** sensorineural hearing loss, short 4th metacarpal

Galactosemia

- Breastfeeding contraindicated
- Oil drop cataract
- Hypoglycemia

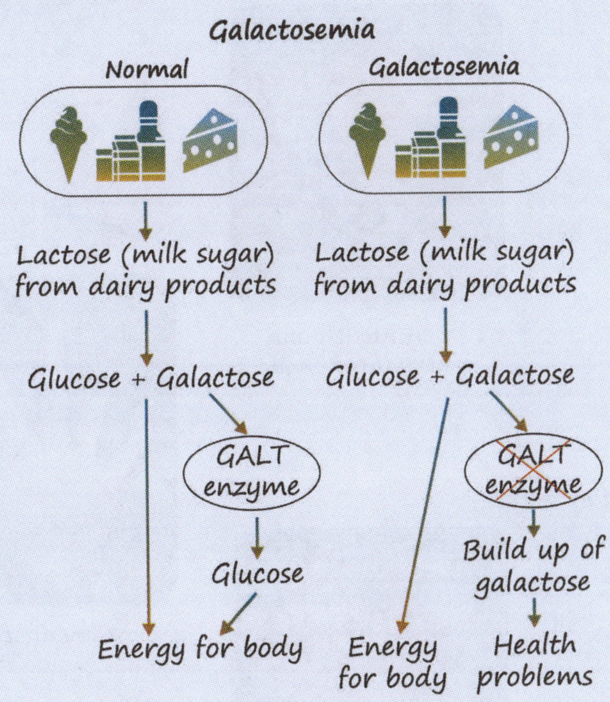

Rett syndrome

- Common in girls
- Acquired microcephaly
- Hand wringing movement
- Intellectual disability
- X-linked dominant

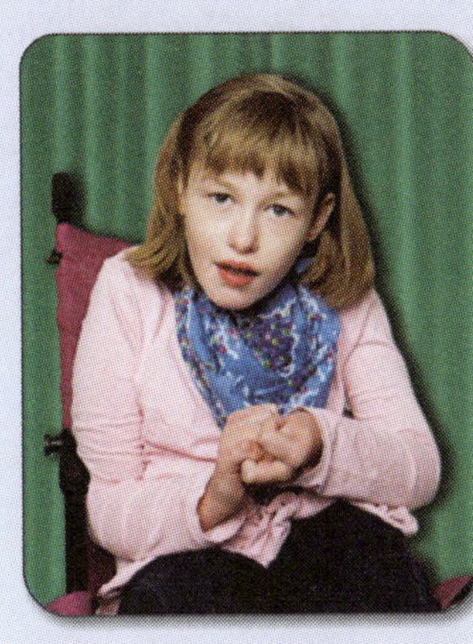

GENE MUTATION

- TCOF1: Treacher Collins
- FGFR1: Pfeiffer syndrome
- FGFR2: Crouzon syndrome
- FGFR3: Achondroplasia
- ATP7b: Wilson disease
- ATP7a: Menkes disease
- ABCC2: Dubin Johnson
- PTPN11: Noonan syndrome
- MECP2: Rett syndrome
- GABRA 1: Juvenile myoclonic epilepsy (JME)

MARFAN SYNDROME

- M — Mitral valve prolapse
- A — Arachnodactyly/camptodactyly (contracture of the fingers) + autosomal dominant**
- R — Retinal detachment
- F — Fibrillin deficiency FBN1 ch.15q21/flat feet, facial features (flattening of midface—malar hypoplasia), flexible joints (joint laxity)
- A — Aortic aneurysm, arm span > height, arch (high arch palate)
- N — -ve urinary cyanide-nitroprusside test/pneumothorax/nasal voice (high arch palate)/near sightedness
- S — Superolateral subluxation of lens/scoliosis/sternal-excavatum or carinatum, signs

Most common congenital heart disease is mitral valve prolapse.
Most common cause of death is aortic dissection.

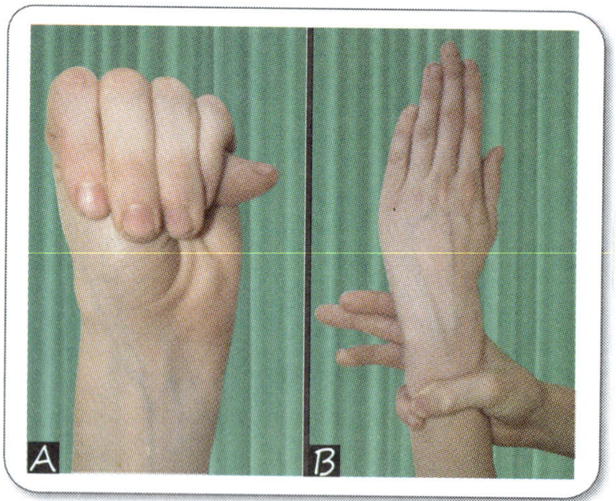

A. Steinberg sign/Thumb sign B. Walker Murdoch sign/Wrist sign

DOWN SYNDROME

Mnemonic: "Do Eyes Checkup Along Side"
- Depressed nasal bridge
- Decreased intellectual disability (IQ)
- Down ear (low set ears)

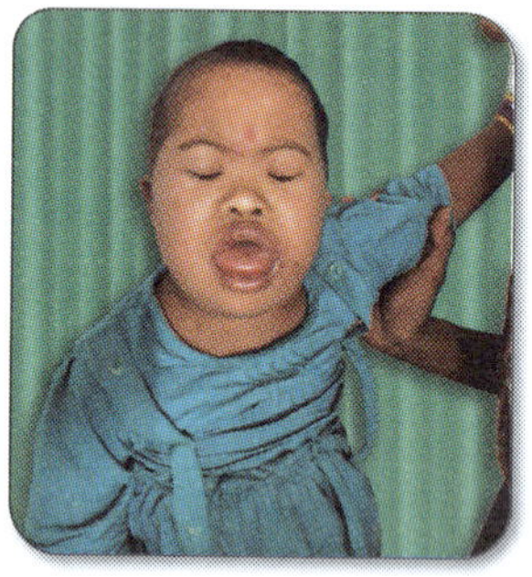

Open mouth and protruding tongue

Eyes

- Brushfield spots in iris
- Epicanthal folds
- Eyes mongoloid slant

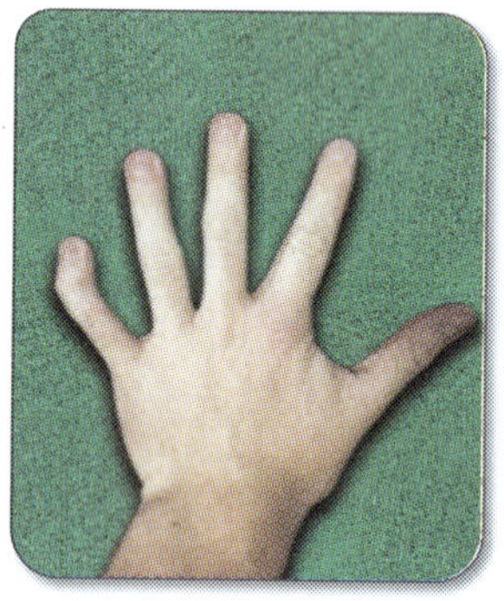

Clinodactyly

Checkup

- Congenital Heart—most specific endocardial cushion defect, most common ostium primum ASD, VSD*
- Congenital hypothyroidism (open posterior font**)
- Clinodactyly (incurvature of finger)

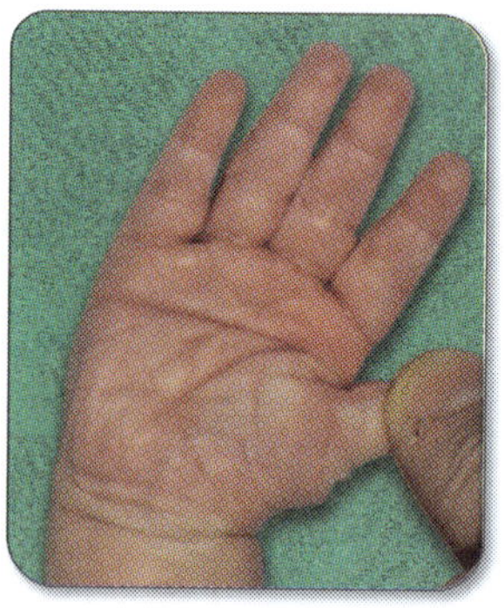

Single palmer crease

Along

- Atlanto axial instability
- AML acute promyeloblastic leukemia M_7**
- Alzheimer's

Along

- Occiput flat
- Open wide fontanel
- O face means round

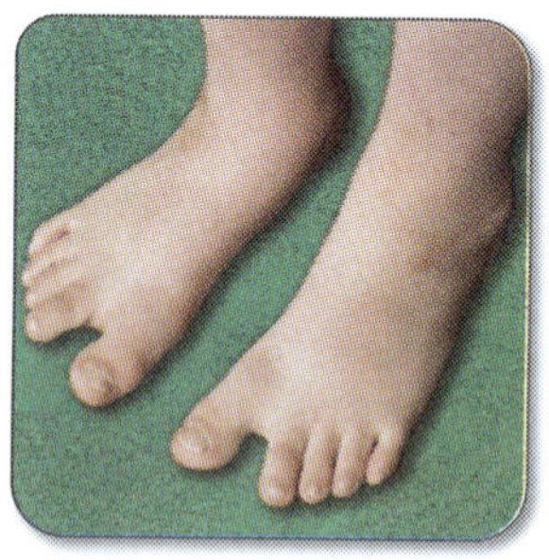

Sandal gap

Side

- Simian crease
- Sandal gap
- Short head: Brachycephaly (image)

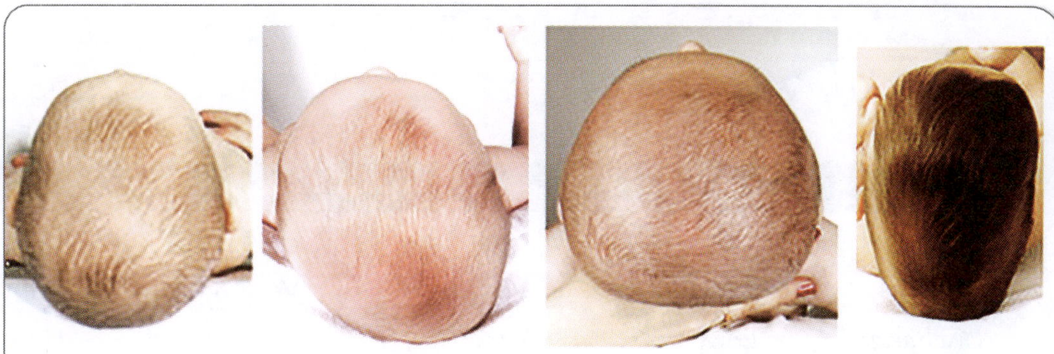

Normal Plagiocephaly Brachycephaly Dolichocephaly

Extra Points

- **Most common GIT abnormality in Down syndrome is:** Duodenal atresia (X-ray: Double bubble sign)

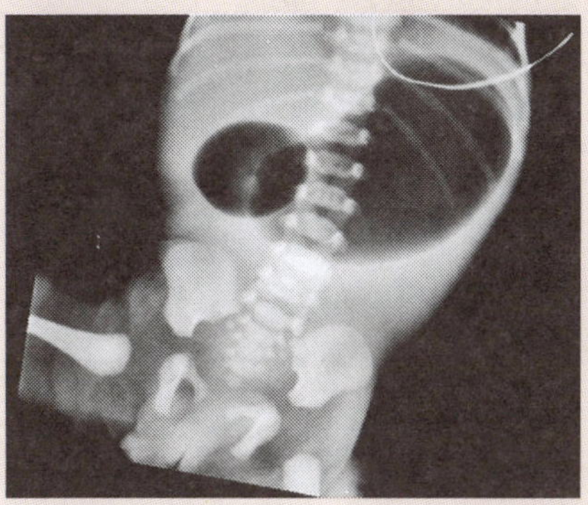

- **Single bubble sign is seen in:** Pyloric stenosis

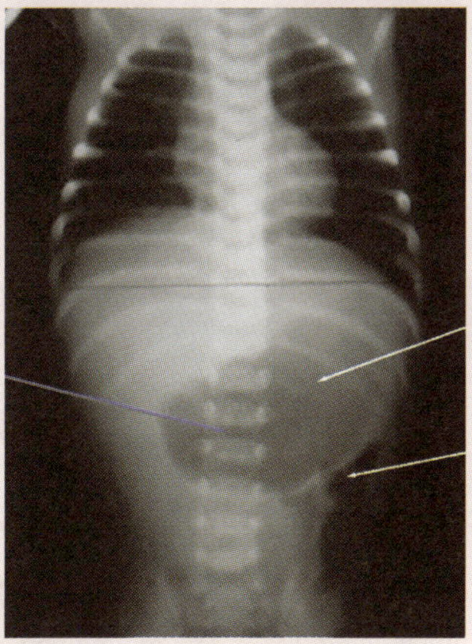

- **Triple bubble sign:** Jejunal atresia

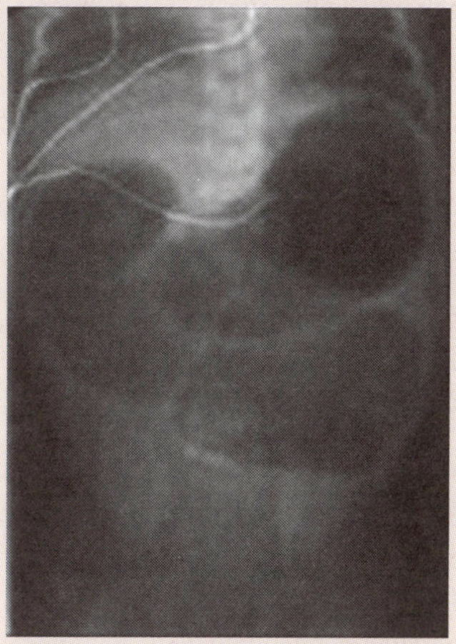

- Most common congenital
- Heart disease in Down's syndrome

For the antenatal screening of down syndrome in 1st trimester:

1. Nuchal thickness >3 mm
2. β-hCG and pregnancy-associated plasma protein A (PAPP-A)

2nd trimester:

Triple scan AFP, unconjugated estriol, β-hCG

Quadruple scan: All 3 + inhibin A

Imp PYQs

Q: Which is the syndrome where IQ will not be affected?

Ans: Turner syndrome

	AFP	Estriol	hCG	Inhibin A	Levels
Down	Low	Low	High	High	High
Turner	Low	Low	Very high	Very high	High
Edward	Unchanged	Low	Very low	Unchan ged	HE is low
Patau	Increased	Normal	Normal	Normal	AFPatau is high

FONTANELLE AND SUTURE

Fontanelle: 6

Total number of fontanelle in a newborn: 6

Anterior fontanel

- Present between frontal and parietal suture
- Closes by 8–18 months
- It is the last fontanel to close

Posterior

- Posterior fontanelle (1)
- Sphenoid: pair (means total 2)
- Mastoid: pair (means total 2)

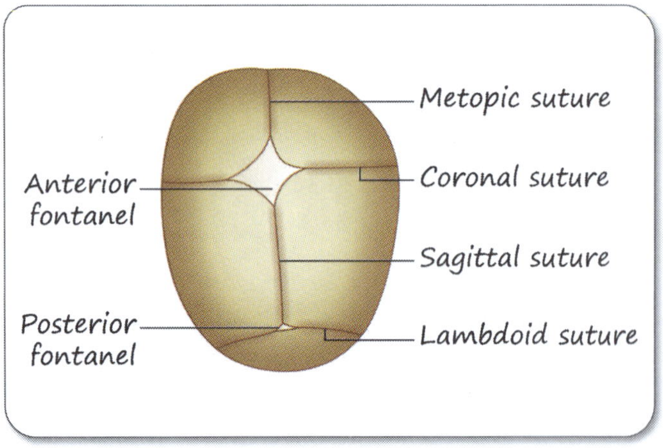

Suture: 4

Total number of sutures in a newborn: 4

- Metopic suture
- Coronal suture
- Sagital suture
- Lambdoid suture

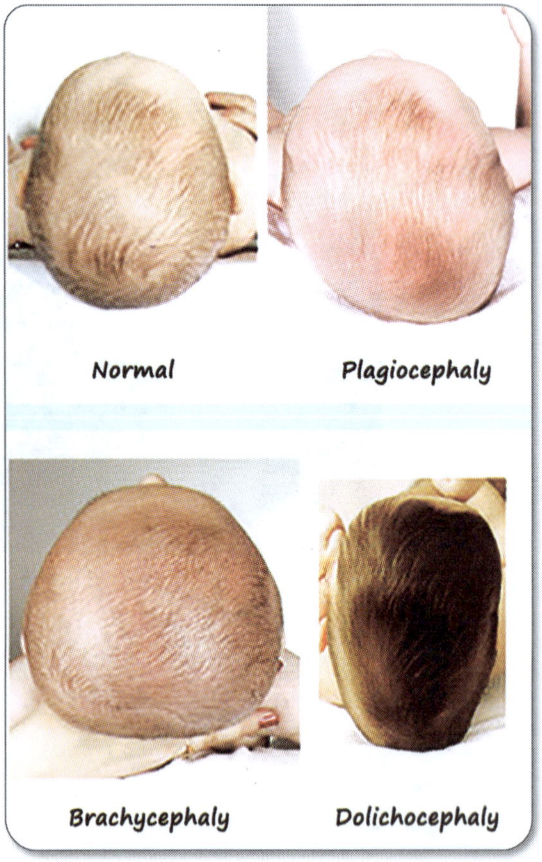

CRANIOSYNOSTOSIS

Premature fusion of suture is known as craniosynostosis.

- If it involves metopic suture, it will cause trigonocephaly
- Coronal suture—brachycephaly

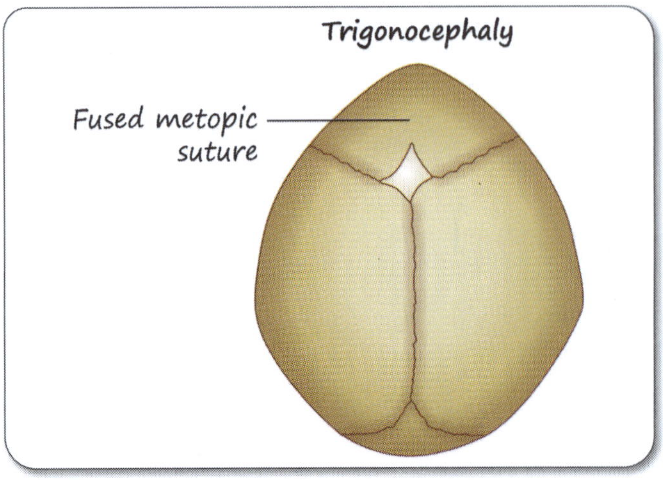

- Sagittal suture—dolicocephaly/scaphocephaly (most common among all)
- Lambdoid suture—plagiocephaly

CROUZON SYNDROME

- Autosomal dominant FGFR2 gene
- Craniosynostosis—coronal suture
- Beaked nose
- Maxillary hypoplasia
- Exophthalmos
- Hypertelorism
- Brachydactyly
- Protruding lower jaw—mandibular prognathism
- Dental problem, hearing loss and high risk of hydrocephalus
- Low set ears
- The most common craniosynostosis syndrome is Crouzon syndrome

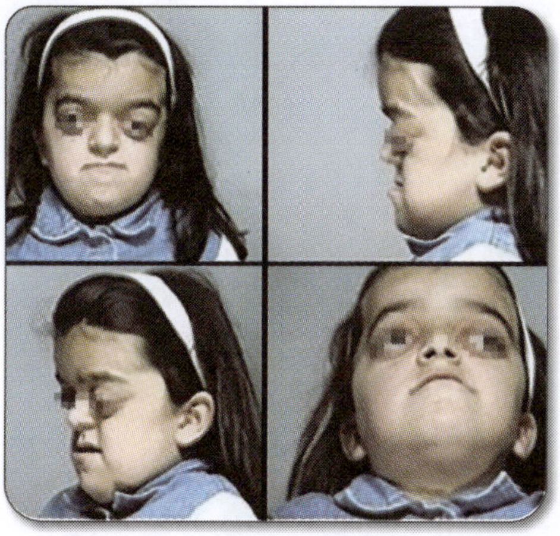

CLEIDOCRANIAL DYSOSTOSIS

- Absent clavicle
- Patient will have drooping shoulders + delayed ossification of the cranial bones with multiple ossification centers (wormian bones), and delayed ossification of pelvic bones.

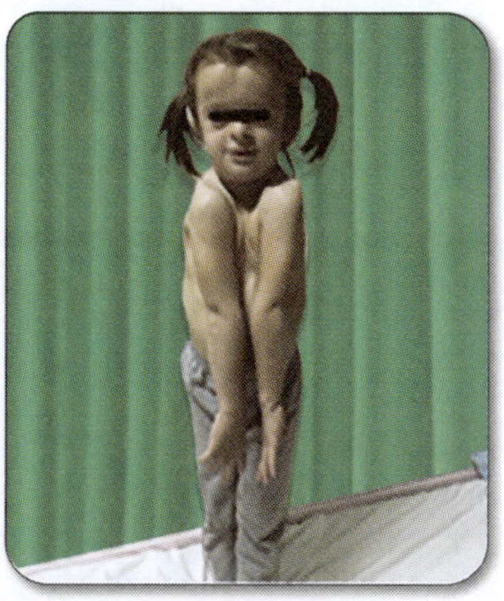

WAARDENBURG SYNDROME: "IMAGINE HOSTEL WARDEN"

- Who cannot see: Heterochromia iridis
- Who cannot hear: Hearing loss
- Who has white bunch of hair: Distinctive hair coloring

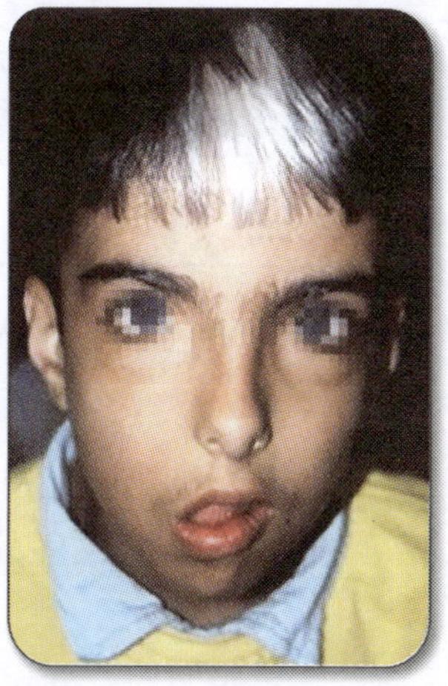

- Autosomal dominant*
- PAX3 mutation

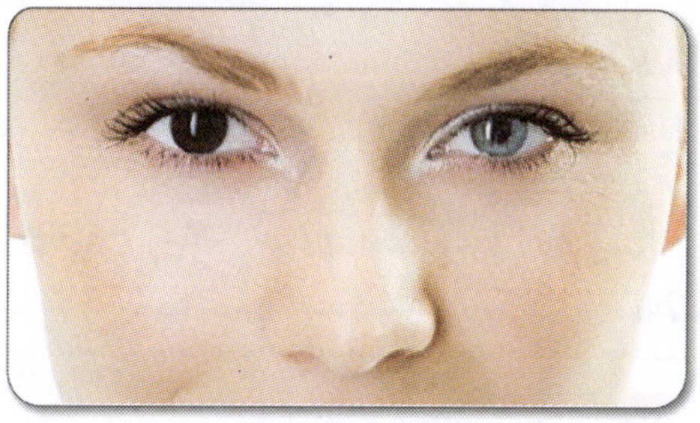

TREACHER COLLINS SYNDROME

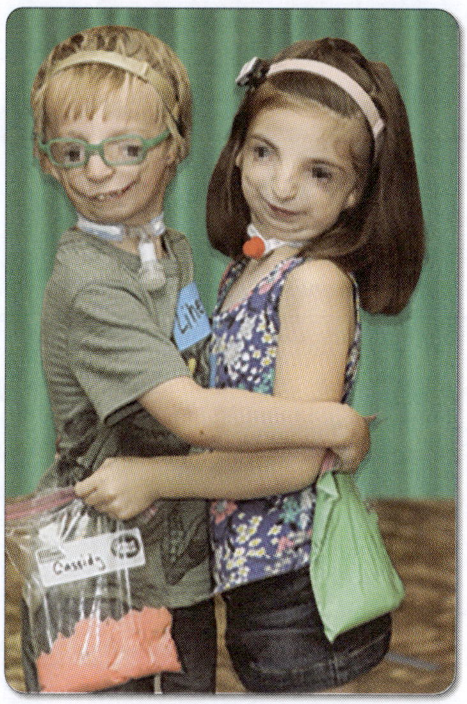

"You are unique and that is the best thing about you."

Mnemonic

Gandhi ji's three monkeys

- "Bura mat dekho/don't see bad"—coloboma of eyes
- "Bura mat suno/don't hear bad"—deafness
- "Bura mat bolo/don't speak bad"—hypoplasia of cheeks, micrognathia
- Autosomal dominant
- TCOF1 gene mutation
- Intelligence is not affected*

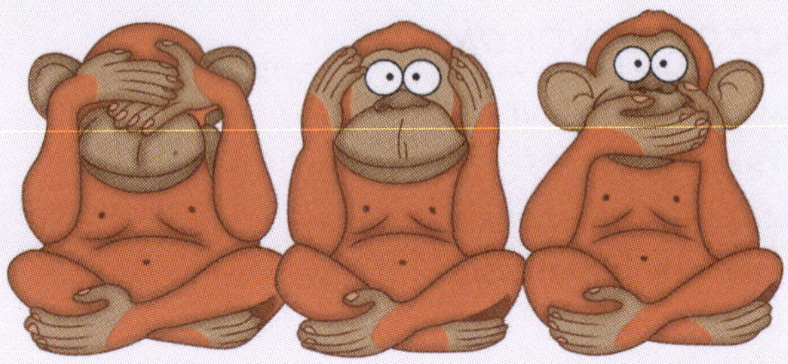

Causes: Macrocephaly: Mnemonic: "ARO Saves My Health"

- A : Anemia (chronic)
- R : Rickets
- O : Osteogenesis imperfecta
- S : Subdural hematoma, Syndromes like—Galactosemia, Weaver syndrome, Sotos syndrome, Morquio syndrome
- M : Megalencephaly
- H : Hydranencephaly
- H : Hydrocephalus

X-RAY WRIST

"Be humble, we all have a past."

	Hamate	Capitate	Trapezoid	Trapezium	
Medial					Lateral
	Pisiform	Triquetral	Lunate	Schaphoid	

1st carpal bone to appear: Capitate comes by 2 months
2nd carpal bone to appear: Hamate comes by 3 months
3rd—triquetral comes by 3 years
4th lunate comes by 4 years
5th scaphoid comes by 5 years
Last carpal bone to appear: Pisiform

Mnemonic

3—3 means 3-year-old will have 3 carpal bones
4—4 means 4-year-old will have 4 carpal bones
5—5 means 5-year-old will have 5 carpal bones

Age	X-ray for bone age estimation	X-ray is compared with
Newborn	Knee joint	Greulich and Pyle atlas and Tanner-Whitehouse methods
3-9 months	Shoulder joint	
1-13 years	Wrist joint	
12-14 years	Elbow/hip	

DENTITION

"Be stronger than your excuse!"

Dental formula: 2123/2123

First and last primary teeth: Lower central incisor and M_2

First and last permanent teeth: M_1 and M_3

Define delayed dentition: No teeth by 13 months

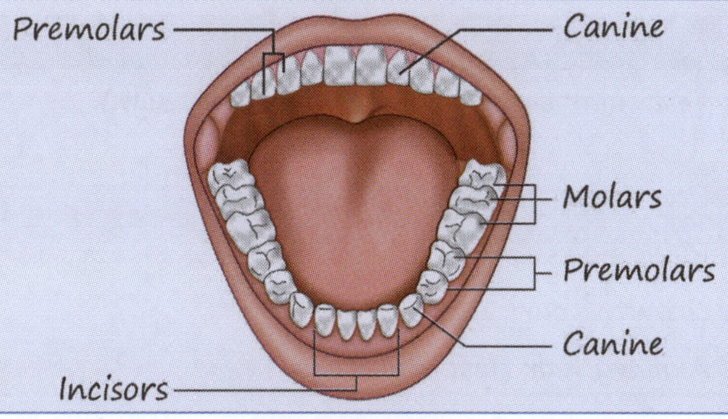

Causes of natal teeth: mnemonic: PEES	Causes of delayed dentition: (FRIED CAP)	Most common location of supernumerary teeth: incisor Causes:
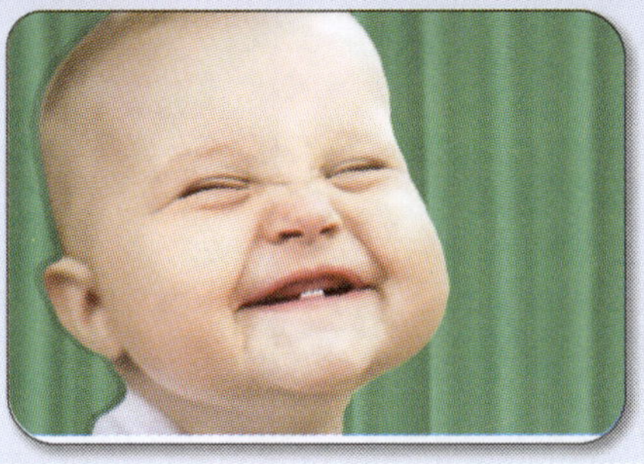	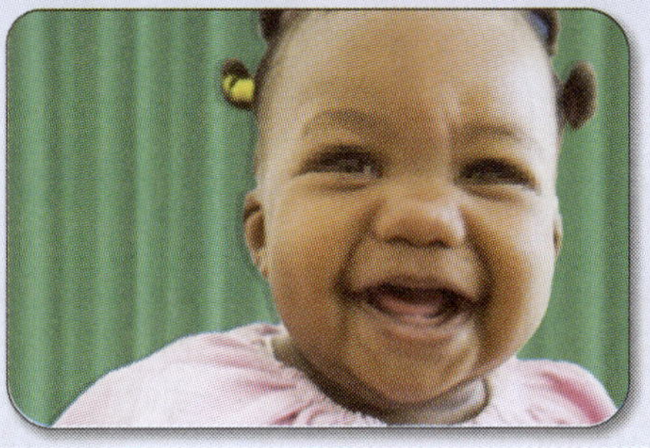	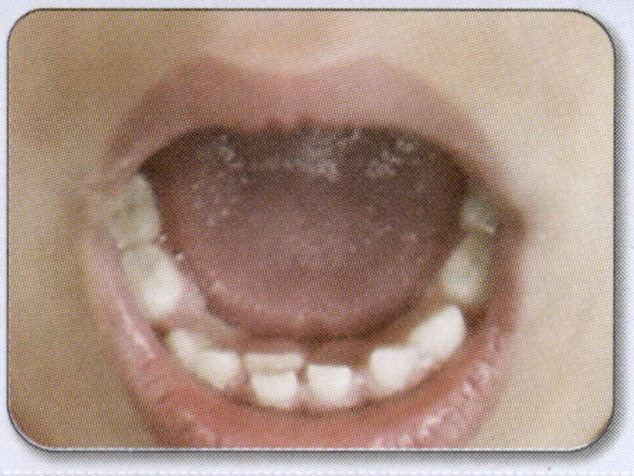
P: Pierre Robin syndrome E: Ellis-van Creveld syndrome E: Epidermolysis bullosa S: Sotos syndrome: points Macrocephaly Flushed cheeks Pointed chin	Familial Rickets Idiopathic Endocrine causes: Hypothyroidism, hypopituitarism, hypoparathyroidism D: Down syndrome Cap: Cleidocranial dysostosis (absent clavicle)	C: Cleft lip C: Cleft palate C: Cleidocranial dysostosis Gard: Gardner syndrome

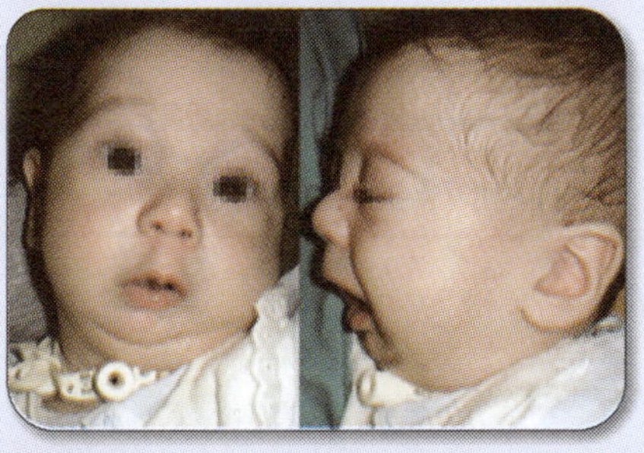

- Micrognathia
- Glossoptosis
- Difficult bag and mask ventilation
- Cleft palate
- Autosomal dominant

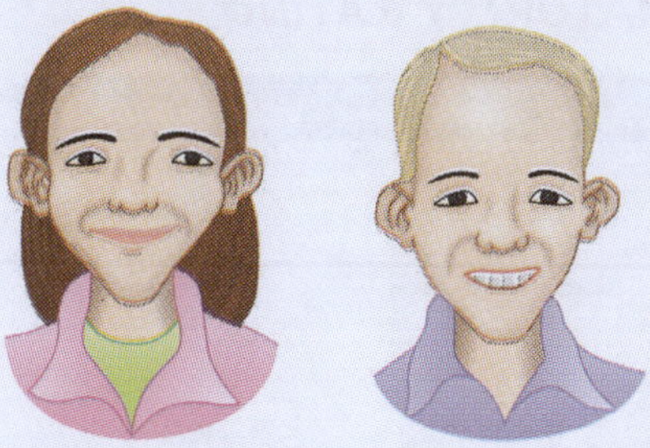

- Macrocephaly
- Flushed cheeks
- Pointed chin

SEQUENCE OF CHANGES OF PUBERTY

"If the plan doesn't work, change the plan, not the goal."

Boys	Girls
1. Testicular enlargement (first visible sign)	1. Thelarche (breast development) 8–12 years (first visible sign)
2. Penis enlargement	2. Pubarche
3. Pubic hairs	3. Growth spurt
4. Growth spurt	4. Menarche (last visible sign)
5. Axillary hair (last visible sign)	

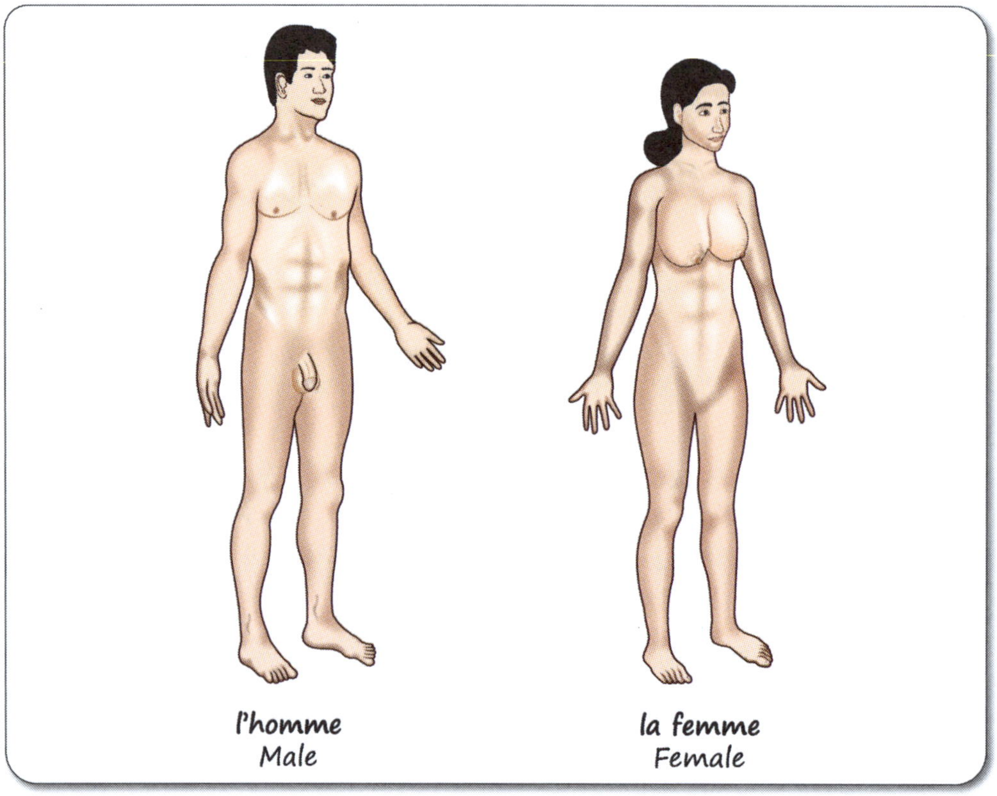

SEXUAL MATURITY RATING

Stage	Volume and size of testis	Characteristic feature
1. 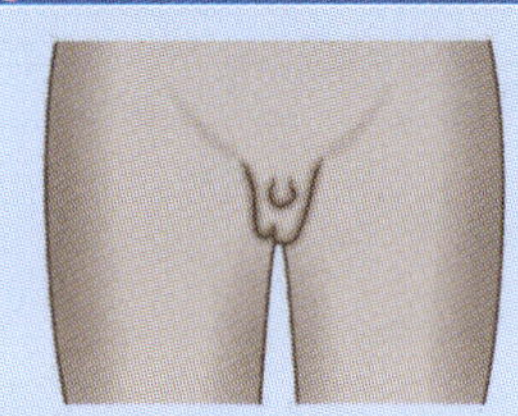	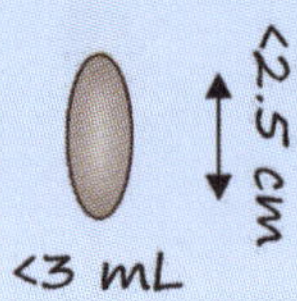	Prepubertal
2. 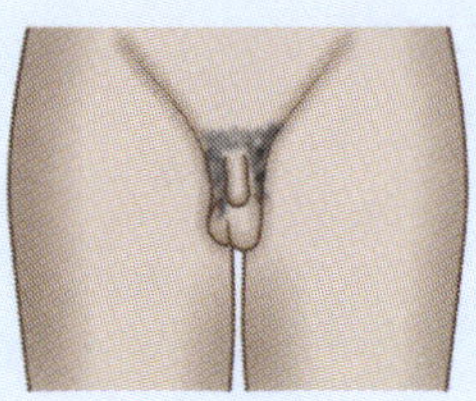	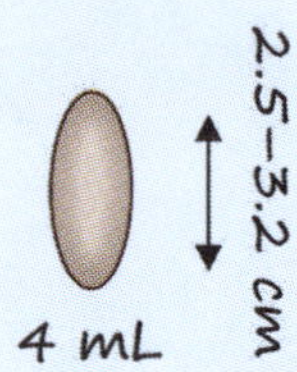	Reddening of scrotum Scanty hair at penile base

Contd...

Stage	Volume and size of testis	Characteristic feature
3. 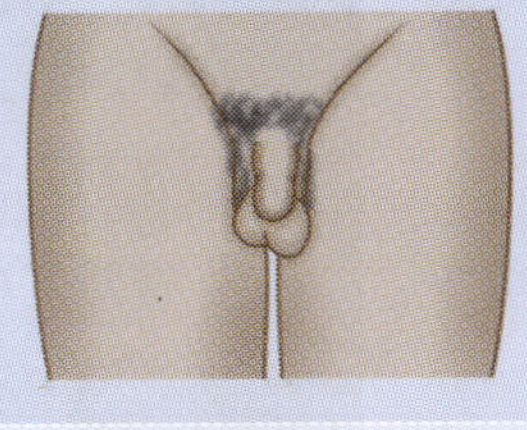	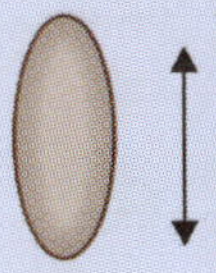 3.3–4.0 cm 10 mL	Increase in length of penile shaft, hair begins to curl and darken
4. 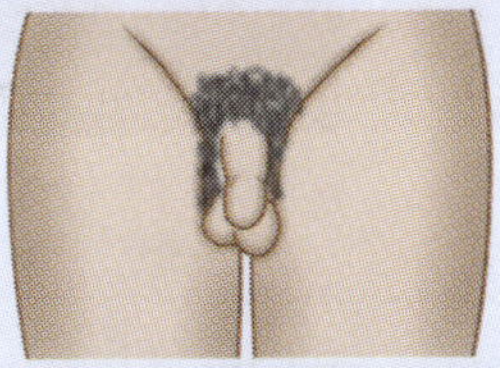	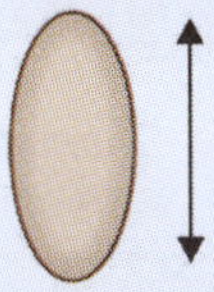 4.1–4.5 cm 16 mL	• Increase in girth of penis and glans • Darkening of scrotum • Coarse abundant and curly hair
5. 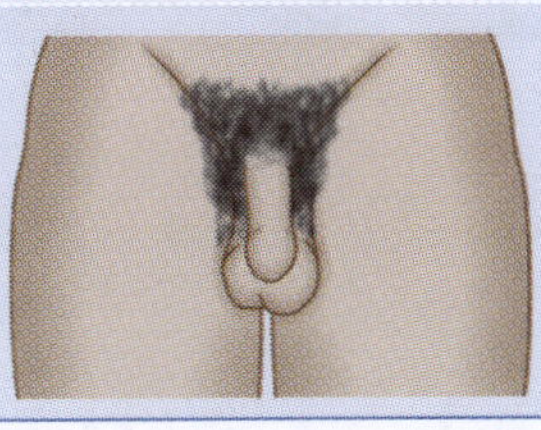	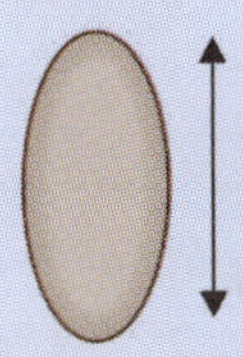 >4.5 cm	Adult type • Adult size scrotting • Adult type penis • Hair spreading to medial side of thigh

CMR stage	Features
Grade 1	Prepubertal, no terminal hair
2. 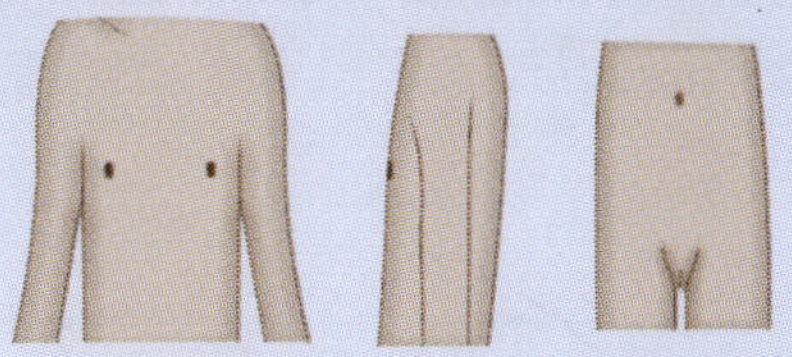	Breast bud, sparse straight hair along the labia
3. 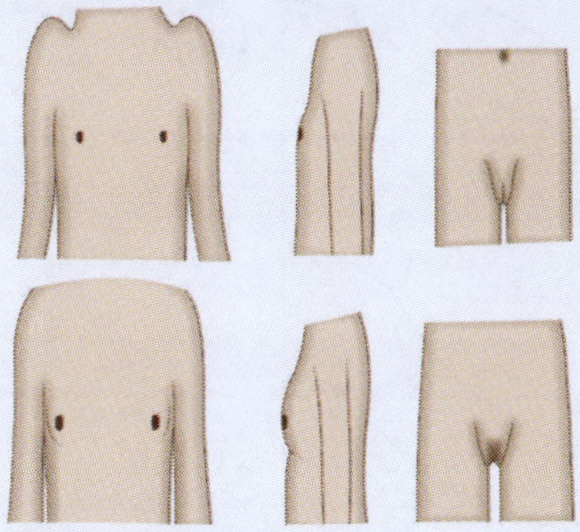	Generalized breast development (extending beyond the areola), hair begins to curl
4. 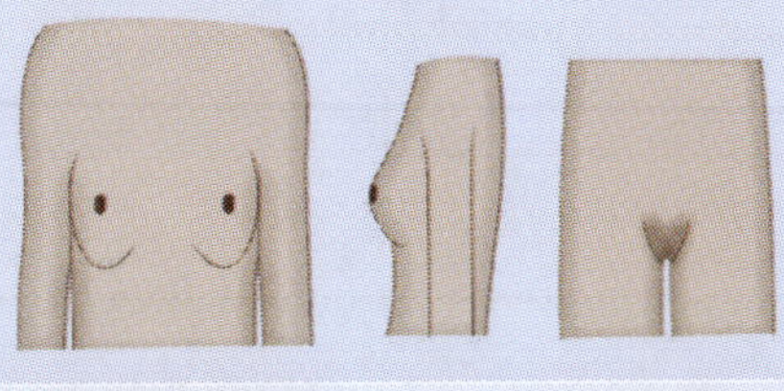	Nipple and areola form a second mound over the breast with increase in amount of hair over the entire mons.
5. 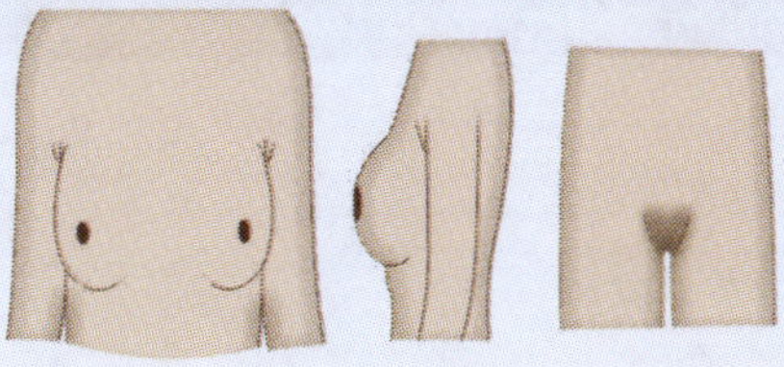	Mature adult type Nipple projects and areola receds with adult type pubic hair in triangle spreading over to medial part of thigh.

Imp PYQs

Q: What is the function?

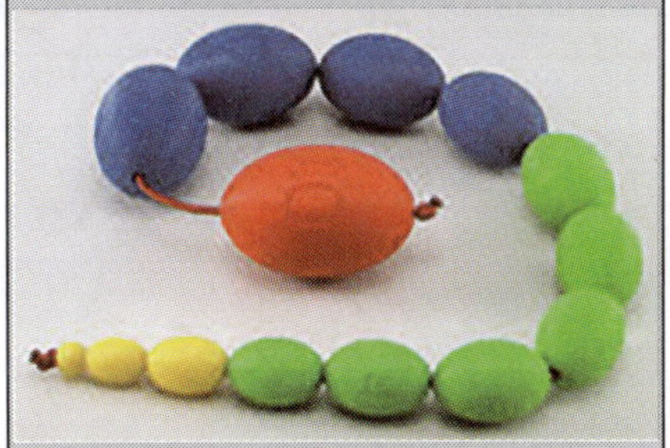

Ans: Orchidometer. The instrument used for testis volume/hypogonodisim.

SHORT STATURE

- Definition: Height <3rd percentile
- Types:
    - Physiological
    - Pathological (subtypes)
        1. Proportionate: US : LS ratio is normal
        2. Disproportionate: US : LS segment is abnormal (subtypes)
            1a. Short trunk dwarfism: US : LS ratio is decreased
            1b. Short limb dwarfism: US : LS ratio is increased
- MC cause of short stature: Constitutional delay in growth and puberty (CDGP)

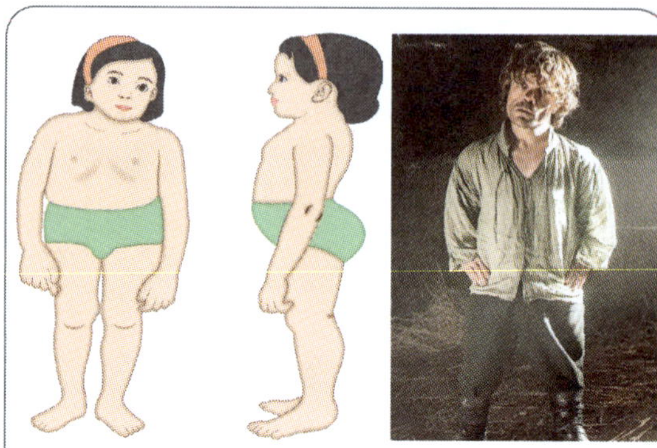

Short trunk dwarfism | Short limb dwarfism

Short trunk dwarfism decrease US : LS	Short limb dwarfism increase US : LS
Mucopolysaccharidosis	Rickets
TB spine Marfan syndrome*	Achondroplasia
Hemivertebrae kyphoscoliosis	Pseudoachondroplasia
Spondylo epiphyseal dysplasia	Hypochondroplasia
Alagille syndrome	Hypothyroidism

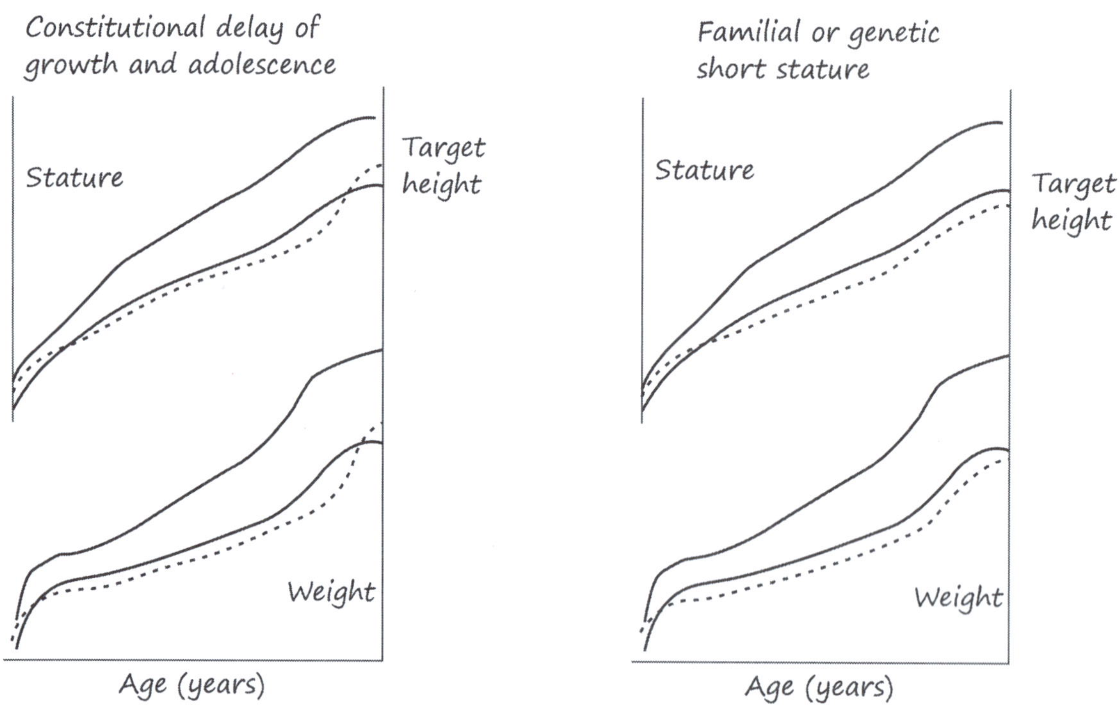

Features	Constitutional growth delay	Familial short structure
Height	Short	Short
Height velocity	Normal	Normal
Family history	Delayed puberty	Short stature
Bone age	Less than chronolgical age	Normal

Contd...

Features	Constitutional growth delay	Familial short structure
Puberty	Delayed	Normal
Final height	Normal	Low but normal for target height

ACHONDROPLASIA

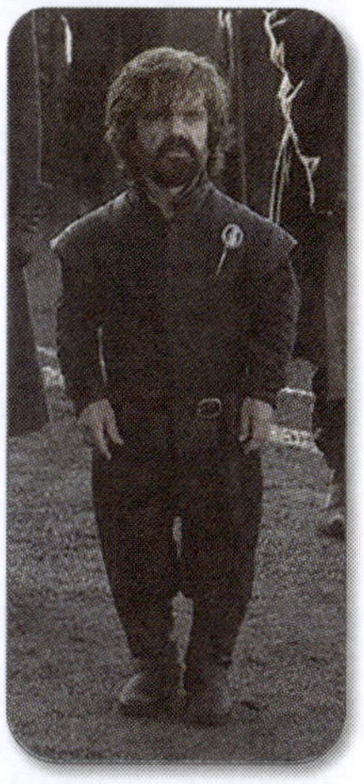

Achondroplasia

A – Autosomal dominant FGFR3 gene mutation
C – Champagne glass pelvis
H – Hand (trident)
O – Obesity
N – Neurological problems
D – Delayed motor milestones
R – Recognized at birth
O – Bowing of legs
P – Proximal limb shortening
La – Large head
S – Short stature
Ia – Decrease interpedicular distance

JOURNEY OF MILESTONES

- Neck holding: 3 months
- Roll over: 6 months
    - Sitting with support: 6 months
    - Sitting without support: 8 months
- Standing with support: 9 months
- Cruising: 9–12 months
- Pivoting: 9–12 months
- Standing without support: 12 months
- Walk with 1 hand held: 12–13 months
- Independently walk: 15 months
- Running: 18 months
- Open the doors of almirah: 18 months
- Turn 2–3 pages a time: 18 months
- Turn 1 page at a time: 24 months
- 15 months: p: pointing p: indicating wet pants
- 18 months: d: dry by day d: dry by day
- Dry by night: 36 months

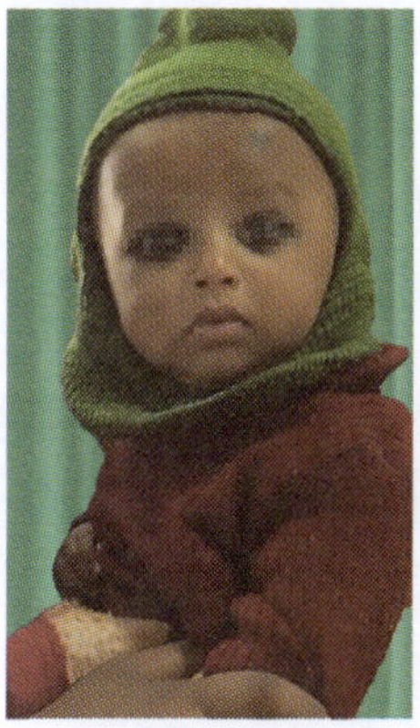

Neck holding (3 months)

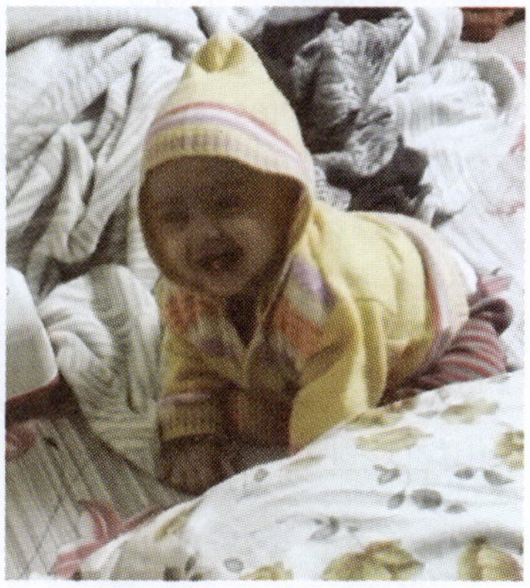

Sitting with support (6 months)

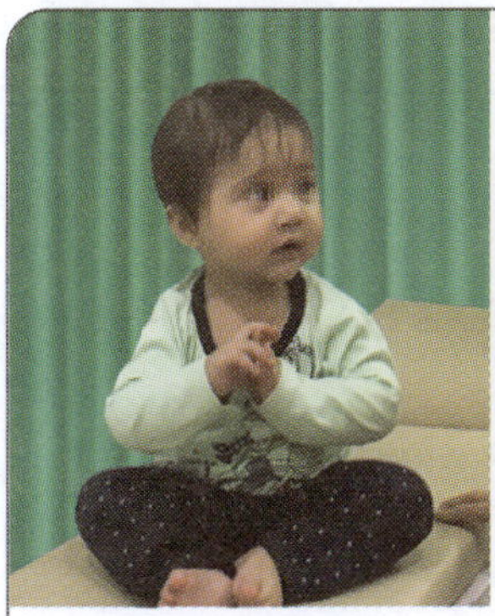

Sitting without support (8 months)

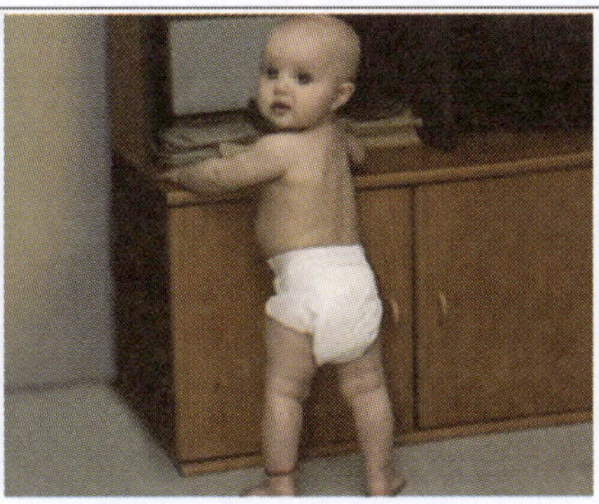

Standing with support (9 months)

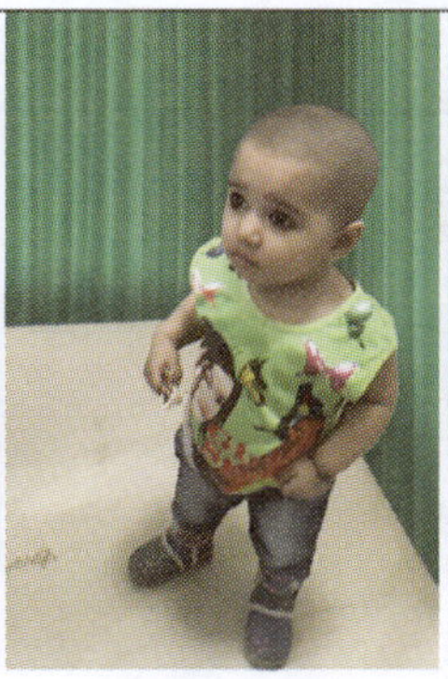

Standing without support (12 months)

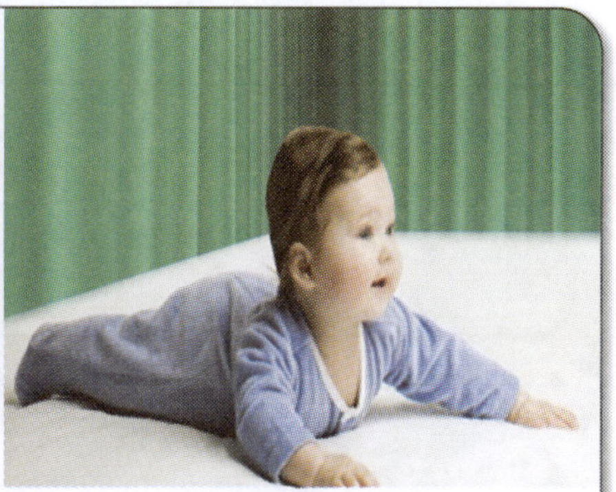

Crawling (8 months)

Nocturnal Enuresis

- Passing urine in the bed after 5 years
- Treatment of choice: Alarm/motivational therapy
- DOC: Desmopressin

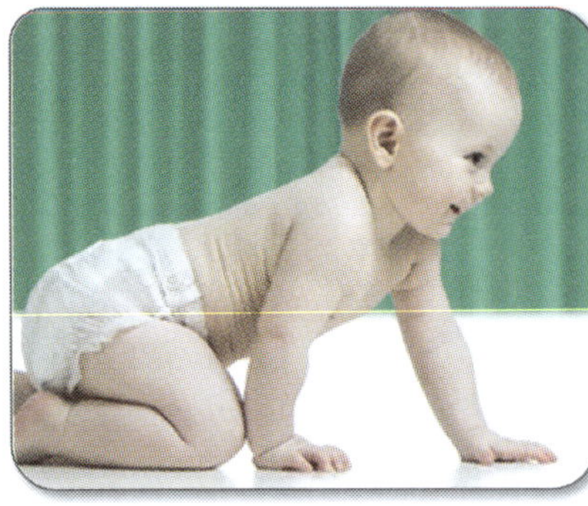

Creep

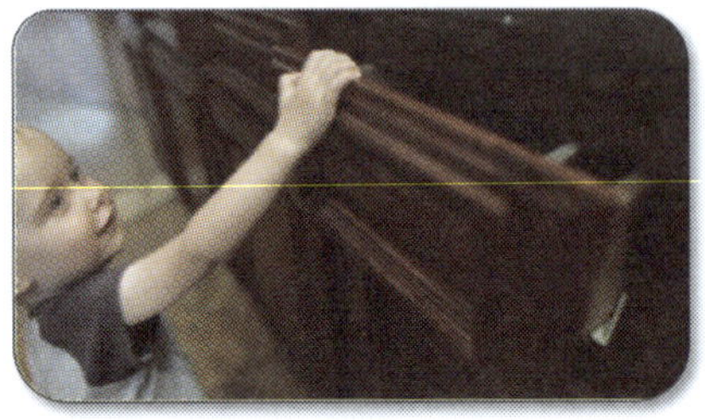

Opening drawer of almirah

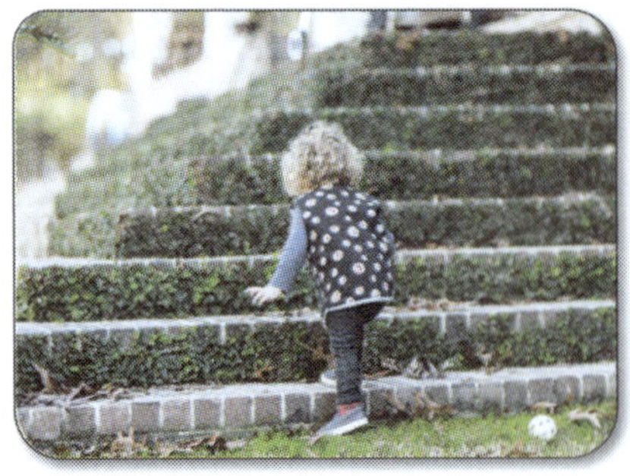

Climbing alternate steps (3 years)

- Baby knows his full name, age, sex: 3 years
- He can go to toilet alone: 4 years
- Tricycle: 3 years
- Hopping: 4 years
- Skipping: 5 years
- Hand regard: 3 months
- Hand comes in midline: 4 months
- Mouthing: 5 months
- Bidextrous approach: 4 months
- Unidextrous: 6 months
- Immature pincer grasp: 9 months
- Mature pincer grasp: 12 months
- Dressing/undressing: 3 years
- Buttoning: 4 years
- Tie shoelaces: 5 years
- Monosyllables: 6 months
- Bisyllables and bye bye: 9 months
- Drawing skills: Straight line 2 years, plus 4 years, diamond 7 years, cube 11 years
- Tower of cubes: Age* 3 : tower of 6 cubes by 2 years and 9 cubes by 3 years
- Developmental quotient (DQ): Developmental age/actual age 100
- Intelligence quotient (IQ): Mental age/chronological age 100

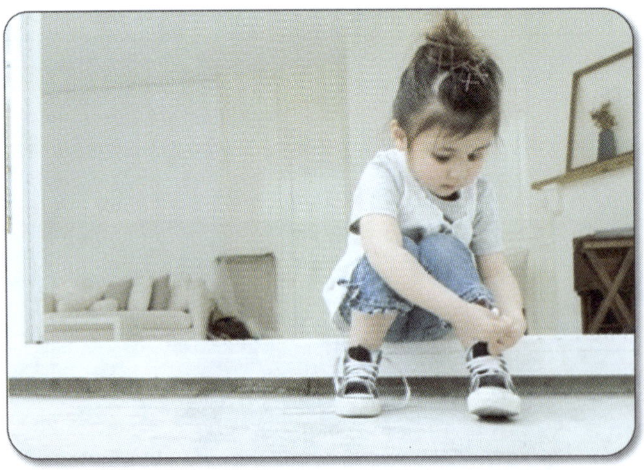

Tie shoelaces—5 years

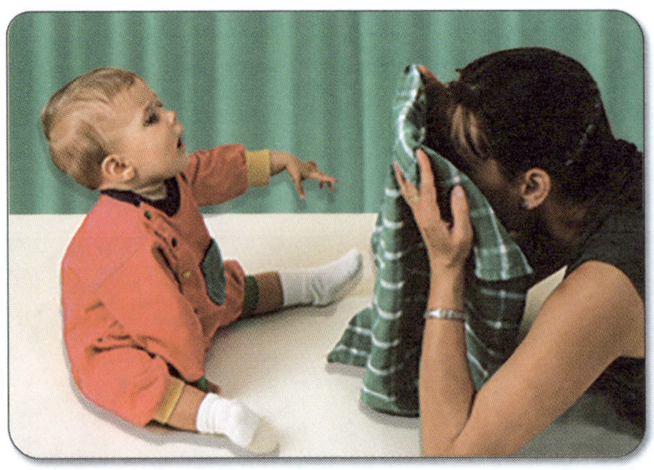

Peek-a-boo—10 months

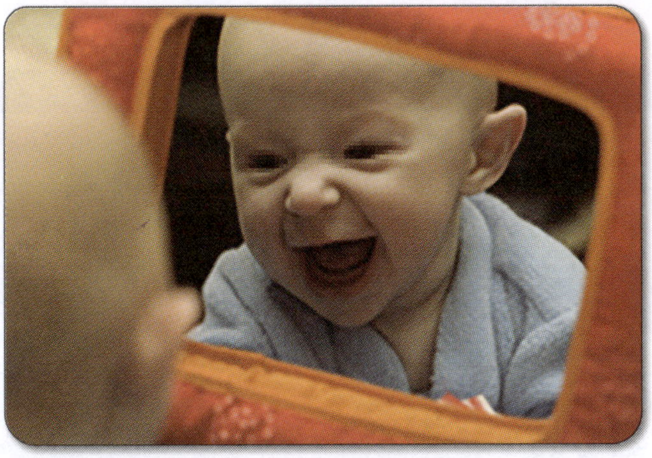

Mirror play—6 months

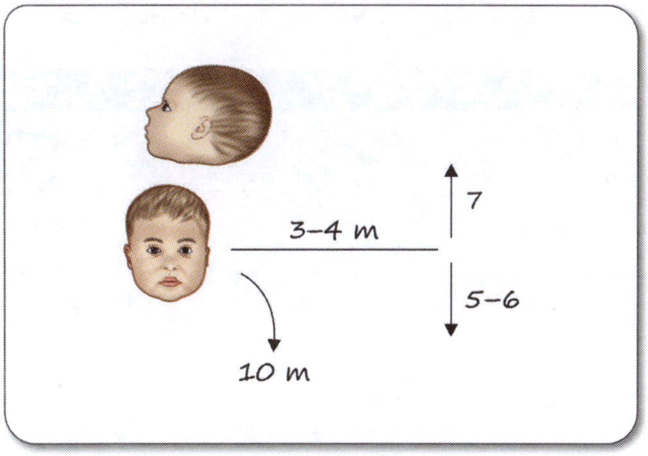

Vision and hearing

VISION AND HEARING

- A baby can turn toward the source of sound by 3–4 months.
- He can turn toward the source of sound and look downward by 5–6 months.
- Turn and look upward by 7 months.
- Look diagonally by 10 months.

Golden Points

- Doctor is aware that preschool children often display a developmental characteristic that makes them treat dolls and animals as if they have feelings or thoughts, this is an example of—animism.
- Toilet training needs to be initiated by 18 months
- Developmental quotient = $\frac{\text{Developmental age}}{\text{Actual age}} \times 100$
- Normal DQ is 100
- Intelligence quotient (IQ) = $\frac{\text{Mental age}}{\text{Chronological age}} \times 100$

Gross motor	Fine motor
3 months: Neck holding	1 month: Hands kept closed
Sitting with support: 6 months	2 months: Hands intermittently open
Sitting without support: 8 months	3 months: Hands regard appear
Standing with support: 9 months	4 months: Tries to reach out an object
Standing without support: 12 months	5 months: Bidextrous grasp, mouthing
Baby can walk with one hand held: 12–13 months	6 months: Unidextrous/palmar grasp*, takes biscuit to mouth
Independently walking: 15 months	7 months: Transfers objects
Running: 18 months	9 months: Immature/pincer grasp*
Baby can kick a ball and walk backward by 24 months	12 months: Mature pincer grasp/casting*

VISION AND HEARING

Age	Milestone
1 month	Alerts to sound
3 months	Coos (musical vowel sounds)
4 months	Laugh loud
6 months	Monosyllables (ba, da, pa), ahgoo sounds
9 months	Bisyllables (mama, baba, dada)
12 months	1–2 words with meaning
18 months	8–10 words vocabulary
2 years	2–3 words sentence, uses pronouns "I" , "Me", "You"
3 years	Asks questions; knows full name and gender
4 years	Says song or poem, tells stories
5 years	Asks meaning of words

2. NEONATOLOGY

"Mistakes are proof, that you are trying."

Vitals
HR: 120–160 bpm
RR: 40–60 per minute
Cyanosis: Acrocyanosis
Urine: Within 24 hours
Stool: Within 48 hours
Normal weight: 2.5–4 kg (image)
LBW <2.5 kg
VLBW <1.5 kg
ELBW <1.0 kg (image)
CFT: Capillary filling time <3 seconds
Length of umbilical cord: 50 cm
Normal BP: Half of normal—65/45 mm Hg
Blood volume in term: 60–80 mL/kg
Preterm: 90–110 mL/kg

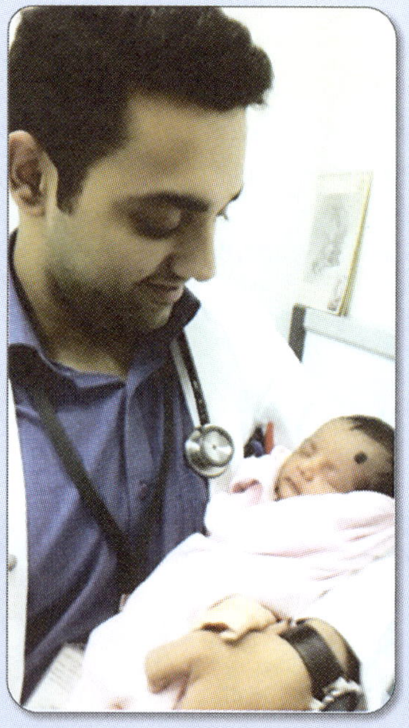

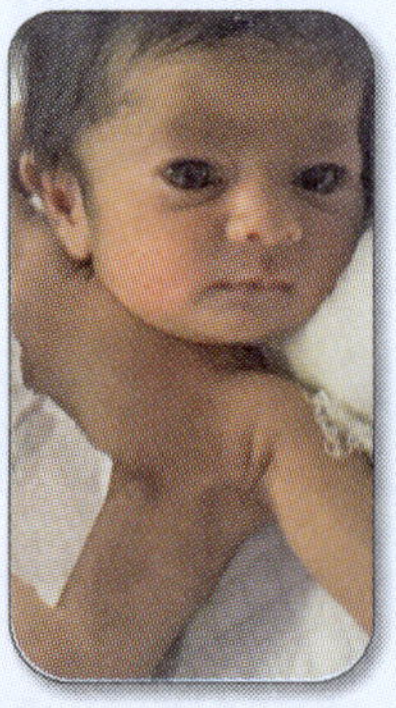

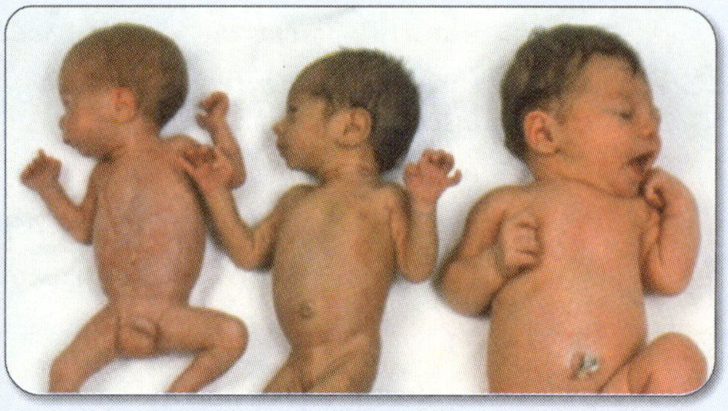

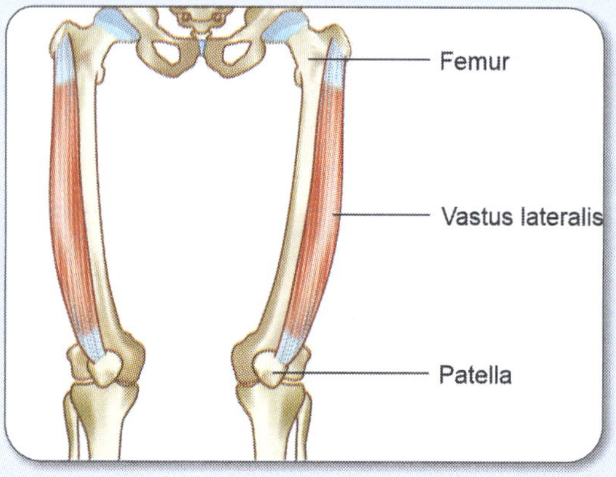

Contd...

Every newborn is given vitamin K injection, route: Intramuscular **Dose:** <1 kg: 0.5 mg 1 kg: 1 mg Site: Anterolateral aspect of thigh Muscle pierced: Vastus lateralis (image)	Every newborn is also given vitamin D drops Dose: For preterm—800 IU Term—400 IU Duration: Till 1 year

INTRODUCTION

- Extremely preterm: <28 weeks
- Very preterm: 28–31 weeks + 6 days
- Moderate preterm: 32–33 weeks + 6 days
- Late preterm: 34–36 weeks + 6 days
- Preterm: <37 weeks
- Post-term: >42 weeks
- Term: 37–41 completed weeks

PERLMAN SYNDROME

Features

- Fetal overgrowth disorder present @ birth
- Fetal gigantism
- Renal hamartomas
- It does not cause IUGR

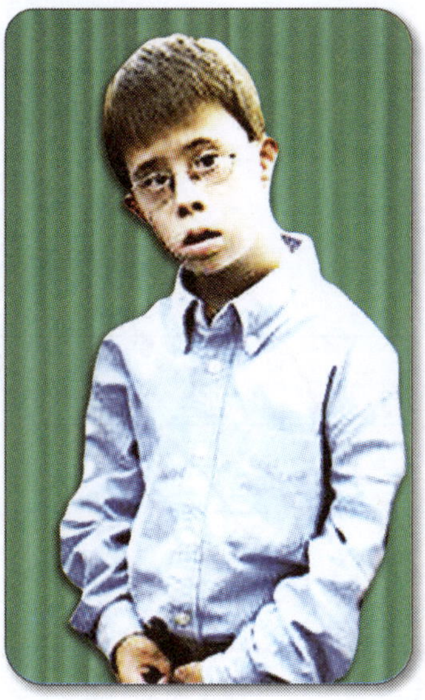

Perlman syndrome

Identify the finding in the image.

- Acrocyanosis: ACRO = periphery and cyanosis = bluish discoloration
- One of the conditions in a newborn which looks abnormal, but is normal

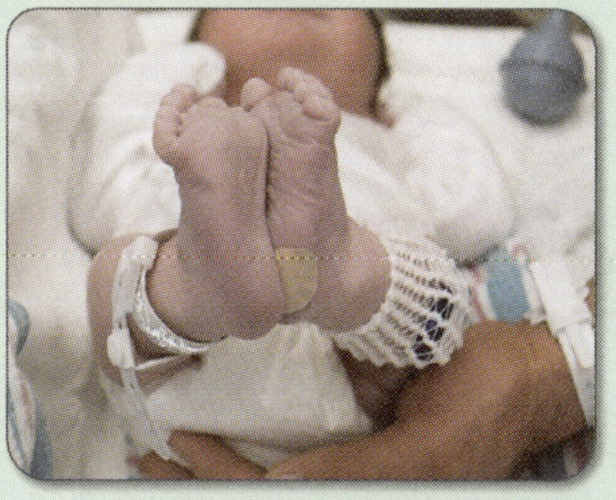

Acrocyanosis

APPROACH TO HEPATITIS B POSITIVE MOTHER

Hepatitis B immunoglobulin (within 48–72 hours) + hepatitis B vaccine on alternate thigh to the baby.

APPROACH TO HIV + MOTHER

- ART sufficient (>4 weeks): Nevirapine 10 mg once daily for 6 weeks.
- ART insufficient: (<4 weeks)
  - High risk of transmission then nevirapine + zidovudine for 12 weeks.
  - Low risk of transmission: Only nevirapine for 12 weeks.

APPROACH TO TB + MOTHER

Isoniazid to the baby 10 mg/kg/day for 6 months.

TYPES OF IUGR

Symmetrical IUGR	Asymmetrical IUGR
• Insult to the mother in 1st or early 2nd trimester • **Causes:** Chromosomal defect, genetic defects and torch infections • HC/WT/length equally affected • Ponderal index: Weight in height/length in cm (CUBE) Then multiply by 100 • Ponderal index (PI) >2 • PI >2.5 is seen in term babies • Poor prognosis	• Insult in late 2nd or 3rd trimester • Cause: Maternal anemia, not gaining weight, hypertension, uteroplacental insufficiency • Head circumference is normal; rest of body appears small (due to "Brain sparing" effect) • Ponderal index <2 • Good prognosis **Formula:** $\text{Pouderal Index} = \frac{\text{Weight in grams}}{(\text{Length in cm})^3} \times 100$

Color of stool—Day wise

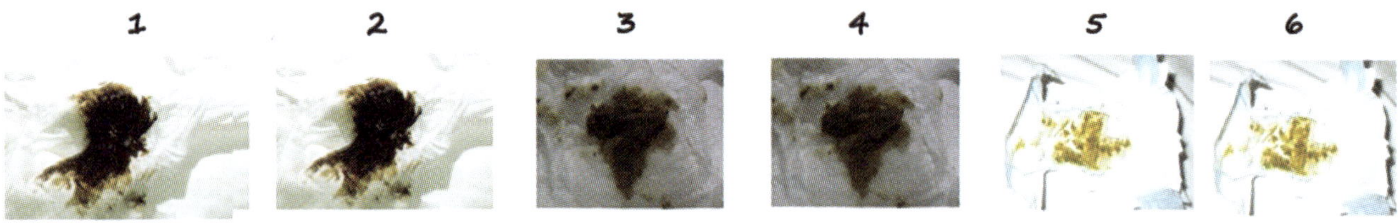

Birth Weight Related Terminology

- SGA: Weight for age <10th centile or <-2 SD
- AGA: B/W 10th and 90th centile or >2 SD
- LGA: >90th centile

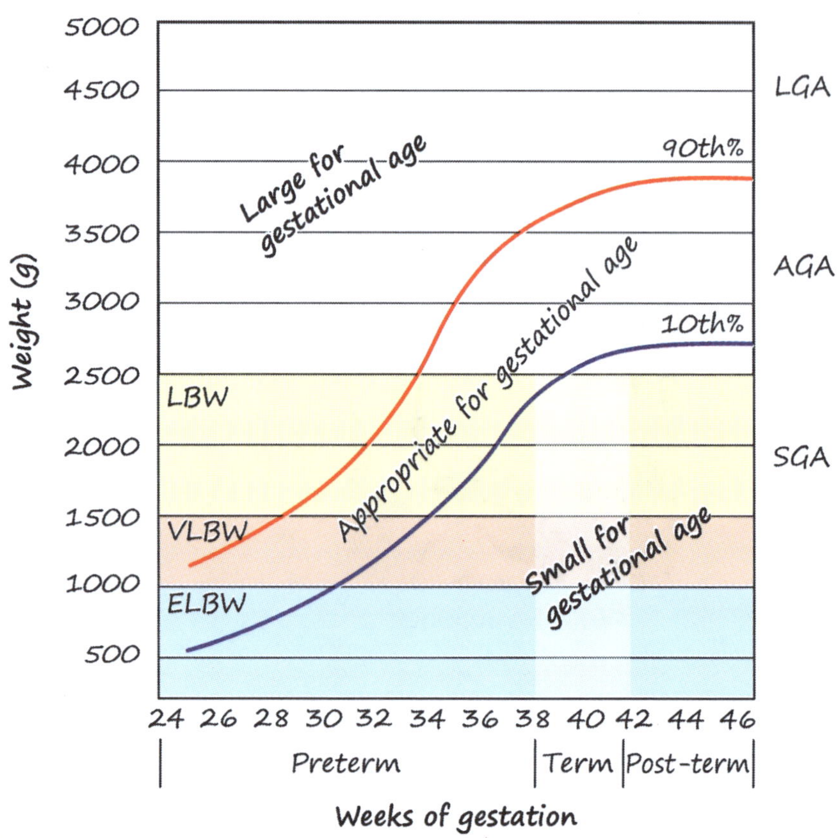

- Causes of LGA
  - S: Sotos syndrome
  - B: Beckwith-Wiedemann syndrome
  - I: Infant of diabetic mother
  - E: Erythroblastosis fetalis
  - Account: Constitutional causes

BECKWITH-WIEDEMANN SYNDROME

- Macroglossia
- Microcephaly
- Hemihypertrophy of limbs
- Omphalocele/umbilical hernia
- Increased incidence of Wilms tumor.
- Hypoglycemia due to IgF1 polymorphism
- Lateral earlobe fissure
- Mutations in the chromosome 11 p15.5

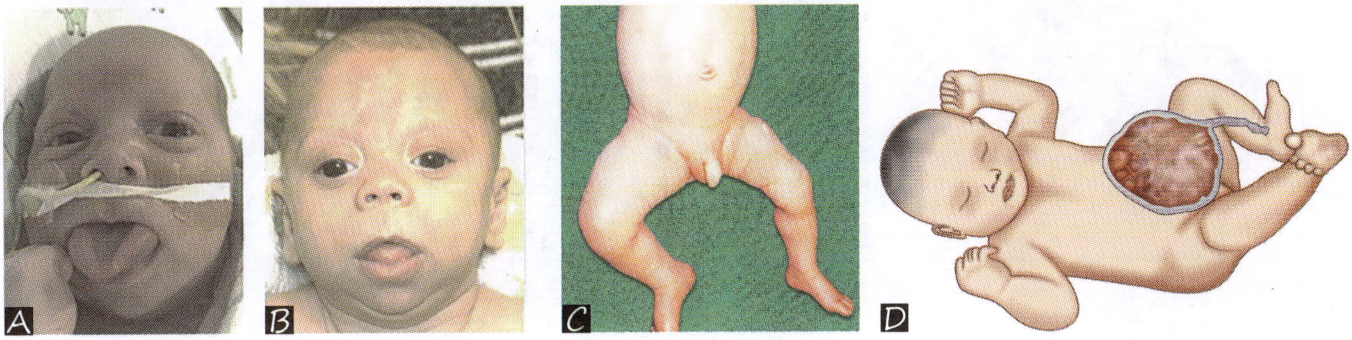

A: Macroglossia; B: Microcephaly Beckwith-Wiedemann syndrome; C: Hemihypertrophy of limbs; D: Omphalocele

Beckwith Wiedemann syndrome

Golden Points

Which three syndromes are associated with Wilms tumor?

1. Denys-Drash syndrome
2. WAGR syndrome
3. Beckwith-Wiedemann syndrome

Microdeletion syndromes	Gene deletion
Sotos syndrome	5 q
Langer-Giedion syndrome	8 q
Prader-Willi syndrome	15 q
Rubinstein-Taybi syndrome	16 p
Smith-Magenis syndrome	17 p
Digeorge syndrome	22 q

	Preterm	Term	Post-term
Scalp hair	Curly/fizzy	Smooth silky shiny	Smooth silky shiny
Lanugo	Present	Absent	Absent
Breast nodule	<5 mm	>5 mm	5–10 mm
Plantar creases	Faint red marks	Creases present	Creases present
Genitals female	Clitoris exposed out	Labia majora covering the minora and clitoris	Labia majora covering the minora and clitoris
Genitals male	Scrotal bag empty no darkening of scrotum rugosities absent	Scrotal bag full darkening of scrotum present rugosities present	Scrotal bag full darkening of scrotum present rugosities present

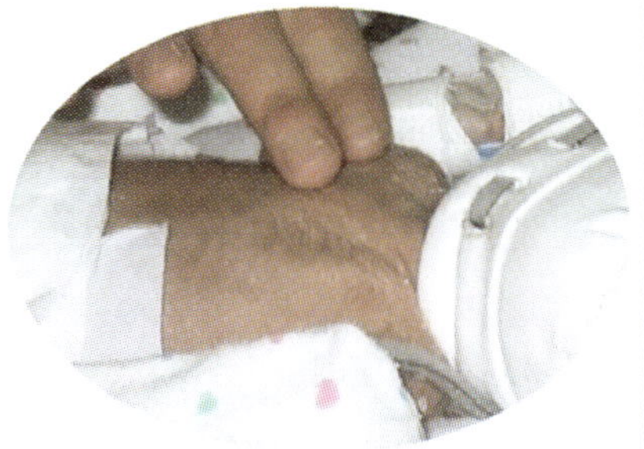

Lanugo: Hair at the back, seen in preterm

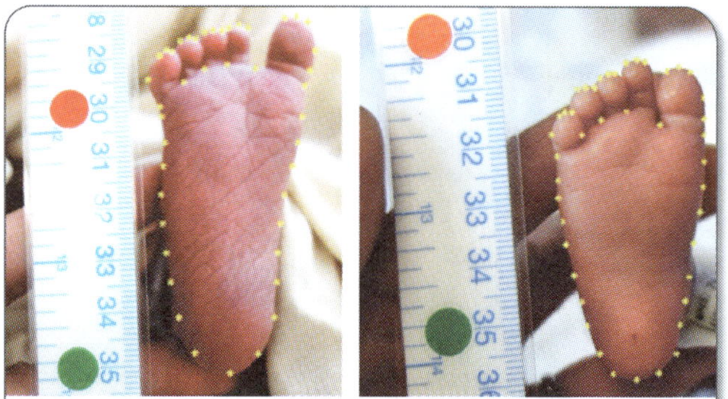

Term infant–multiple creases on foot

Preterm infant–very simple creases

Image of the umbilical cord demonstrates the difference between term and post-term: Green colored umbilical cord is present in post-term neonate.

Golden Points on Post-term Neonates

- Peeling of skin
- Green umbilical cord
- Green nails

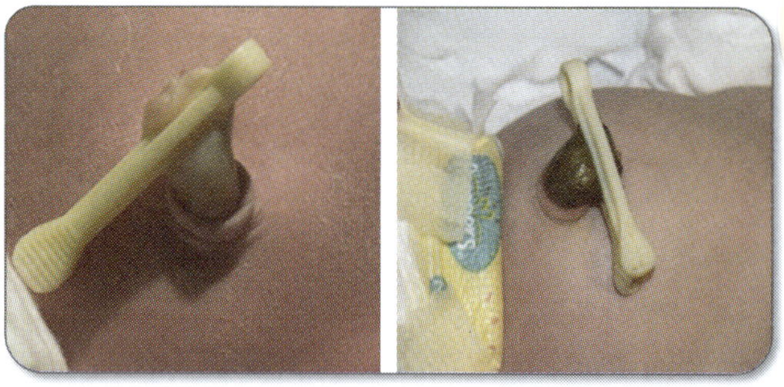

Normal umbilical cord

Green color umbilical cord

EXPANDED NEW BALLARD SCORE: 20–44 WEEKS (SCORE –10 TO 50)

"Your future needs you, your past doesn't."

- Used for the gestational age calculation
- Minimum score is –10 which corresponds to 20 weeks.
- Maximum score is 50 which corresponds to 44 weeks.
- Component with lowest score (–2) is plantar surface and eye/ear.
- Component with maximum score (+5) is popliteal angle and skin.

Score	–1	0	1	2	3	4	5
Posture	—						—
Square window (wrist)*	>90°	90°	60°	45°	30°	0°	—
Arm recoil	—	180°	140°–180°	110°–140°	90°–110°	<90°	—
Popliteal angle	180°	160°	140°	120°	100°	90°	<90°
Scarf sign*							—
Heel to ear							—

Skin	Sticky, iriable, transparent	Gelatinous, red, translucent	Smooth, pink visible veins	Superficial peeling and/ or rash few veins	Cracking; pale areas; rare veins	Parchment, deep cracking no vessels	Leathery cracked, wrinkled
Lanugo	None	Sparse	Abundant	Thinning	Bald areas	Mostly bald	
Plantar surface	Heel-toe 40–50 mm: -1 <40 mm: -2	>50 mm, no crease	Faint, red marks	Anterior transverse crease only	Creases anterior 2/3	Creases over entire sole	
Breast	Imperceptible	Barely perceptible	Flat areola, no bud	Stippled areola 1–2 mm bud	Raised areola 3–4 mm but	Full arola 5–10 mm bud	
Eye/ear	Lids fused, loosely: 1 tightly: -2	Lids open; pinna flat, stays folded	Slightly curved pinna; soft, slow recoil	Well curved pinna; soft but ready recoil	Formed and firm, instant recoil	Thick cartilage ear stiff	
Genitals (male)	Scrotum flat, smooth	Scrotum empty faint rugae	Testes in upper canal, rare rugae	Testes descending, few rugae	Testes down, good rugae	Testes pendulous, deep rugae	
Genitals (female)	Clitoris prominent, labia flat	Clitoris Prominent, small minora	Clitoris Prominent, enlarging minora	Majora and minora equally prominent	Majora large, mionora small	Majora cover clitoris and minora	

Score	Weeks
-10	20
-5	22
0	24
5	26
10	28
15	30
20	32
25	34
30	36
35	38
40	40
45	42
50	44

*Square Window Sign

If the fingers are touching the forearm: baby is term neonate.

*Scarf Sign

If elbow is crossing the midline—baby is preterm.

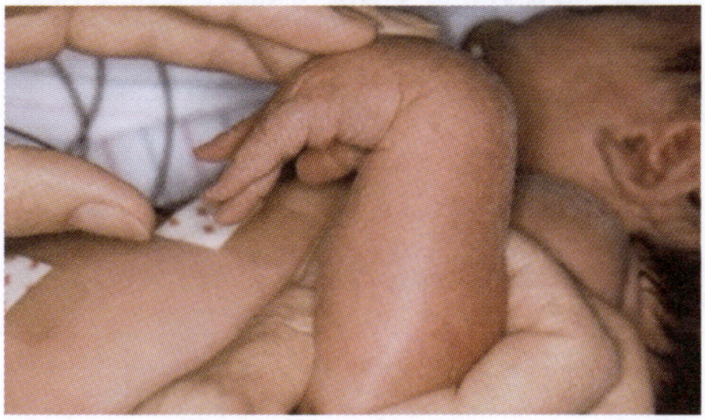

Square window sign

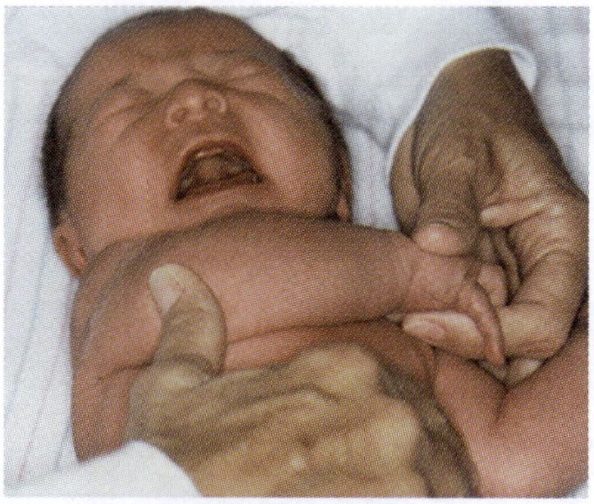

Scarf sign

GESTATION WISE FEEDING IN A NEWBORN

Feeding
<28 weeks: IV fluids
28–32 weeks: Nasogastric feed
32–34 weeks: Paladai feed (image)
>34 weeks: Breastfeeding

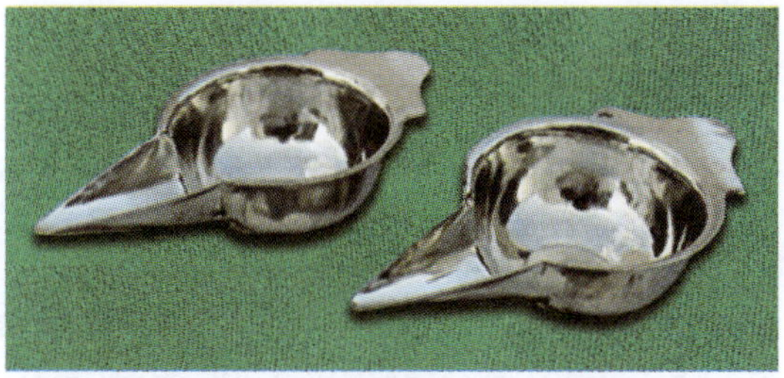

Paladai

Golden Points

- A baby can breathe while sucking due to higher position of larynx

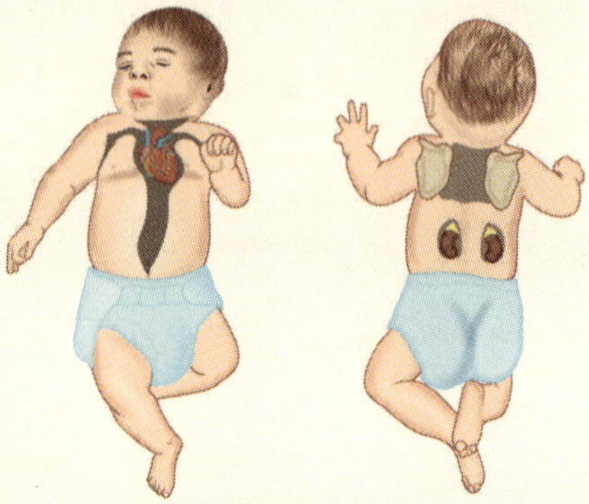

Location of brown fat

- Can newborn shiver? No
- They have nonshivering thermogenesis by the breakdown of brown fat (image showing brown fat location)
- Brown fat is absent in mesentery
- Do newborn have tears? No
- Are newborns color blind? Yes
- Newborn's pupils are constricted
  - ROP (retinopathy of prematurity) screening: @32 weeks of gestation or 4 weeks postnatal age (which ever is later)
  - Risk factor: Prematurity and oxygen toxicity
  - Keep the target SpO_2 in newborn 91–94%
  - Treatment: Bevacizumab (intravitreal)

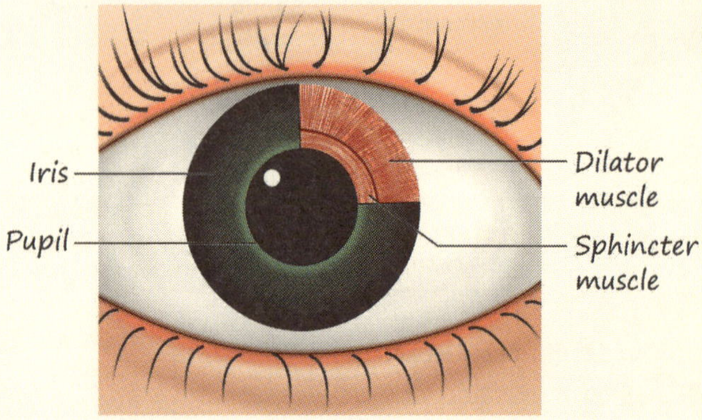

Immature dilator muscle in a newborn

Extra Points

Is babinski response (extensor plantar response) normal in newborn?

Yes it is normal (image attached)

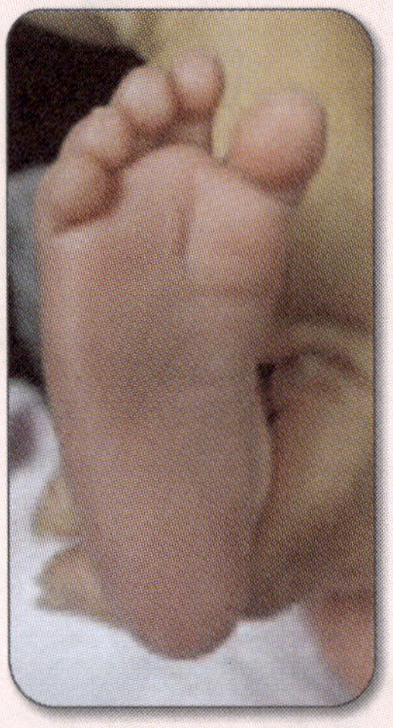

Normal temp of newborn	36.5°–37.5°C
Mild hypothermia/cold stress	36–36.5
Moderate	32–36
Severe	<32
Hyperthermia	>37.5

- Nursery temp should be kept: 22°–26°C (72°–78°F)
- Noise decibels allowed in NICU is 45 DB

Imp PYQs

Recent Question

Q: The range of environmental temp at which the BMR is at minimum, oxygen consumption is least and baby maintains its normal body temp is called:

A. Thermoneutral environment
B. Thermal comfort zone
C. Ambient environmental temp
D. Ideal thermal environment

Test for:
- B for barlow B for bad
- In barlow we are dislocating the hip (image)
- In Ortolani test we are relocating the hip (image)

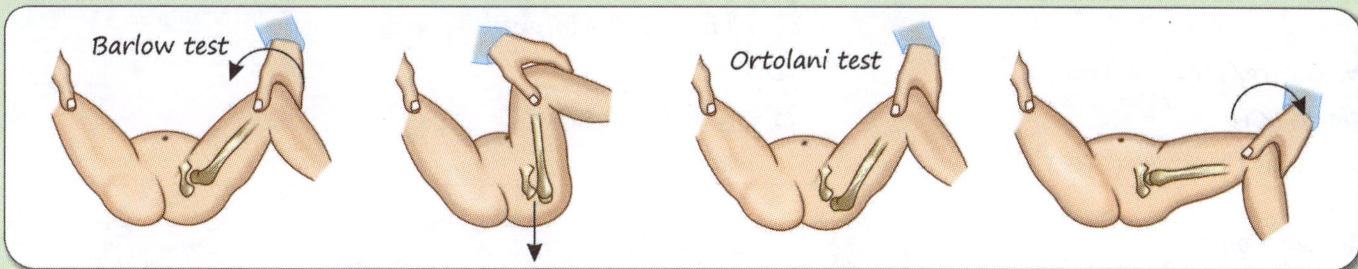

Method of Heat Loss in Newborn

A. **Conduction:** Directly in contact with cold surface
B. **Convection:** Fan/open window
C. **Radiation:** Inevitable: Have to happen, through skin*
D. **Evaporation:** Near a cold surface or near a cold wall of nursery

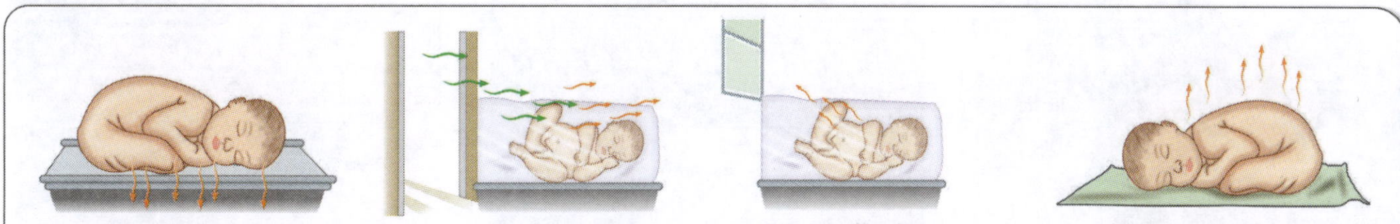

APGAR SCORE

	Indicator	0 point	1 point	2 points
A	Appearance (skin color)	Blue; pale	Pink body; blue extremities	Pink
P	Pulse	Absent	Below 100 bpm	Over 100 bpm
G	Grimace (reflex irritability)	Floppy	Minimal response to stimulation	Prompt response to stimulation
A	Activity (muscle tone)	Absent	Flexed arms and legs	Active
R	Respiration	Absent	Slow and irregular	Vigorous cry

- Normal APGAR >7
- Moderate birth asphyxia: 4–7
- Severe birth asphyxia: 0–3
- Respiratory rate is not a part of APGAR score

NEONATAL SEPSIS

"There is no shortcut to success, we all have taken the stairs."

Types
- Early-onset sepsis (EOS) <72 hours
- Late-onset sepsis (LOS) >72 hours
- MCC in India: Acinetobacter f/b klebsiella
- MCC throughout in the world: *E. coli*
- MCC overall in the world: Group B streptococci
- MCC of early onset sepsis: Group B streptococci
- Poor feeding (earliest clinical feature)
- Hypothermia (more common)/hyperthermia
- The most common manifestation of LOS neonatal sepsis: Meningitis
- Gold standard IOC: Blood culture
- Treatment: Antibiotics

SEPTIC SCREEN IN NEONATAL SEPSIS

Components	Abnormal value
Total leukocyte count	$<5000/mm^3$
Absolute neutrophil count	Low counts as per Manroe chart for term and Mouzinho's chart for VLBW infants
Immature/total neutrophil	>0.2
Micro-ESR	>15 mm in 1st hour
C-reactive protein (CRP)	>1 mg/dL

Golden Point

Which is the risk factor in EOS which warrants immediate antibiotic treatment?

Foul-smelling liquor

CONDITIONS IN A NEWBORN WHICH LOOKS ABNORMAL BUT ARE NORMAL & THEY ARE SELF RESOLVING WITH NO TREATMENT REQUIRED

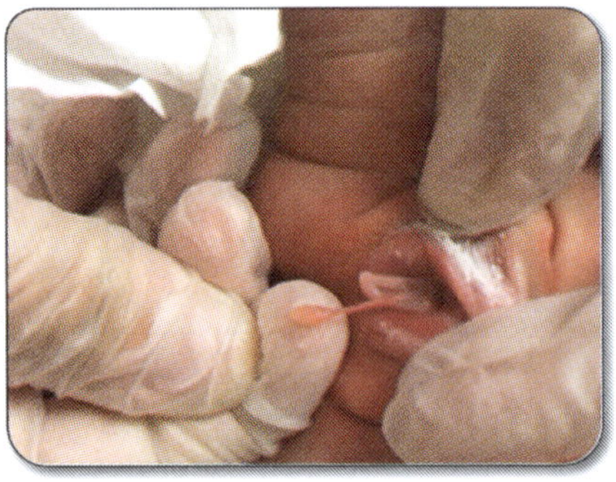

Hymental tag

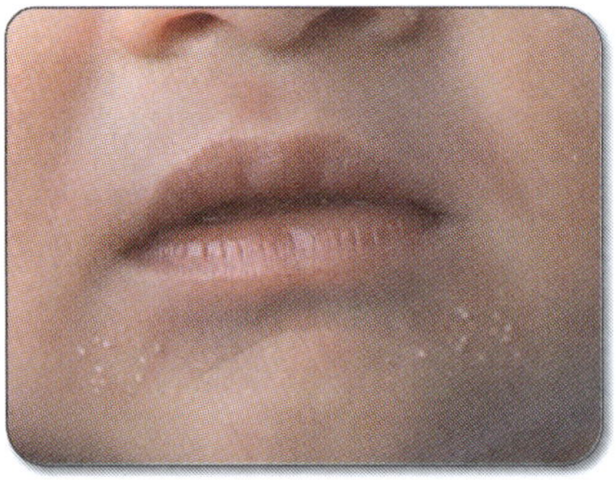

Milia: keratin deposition beneath the skin

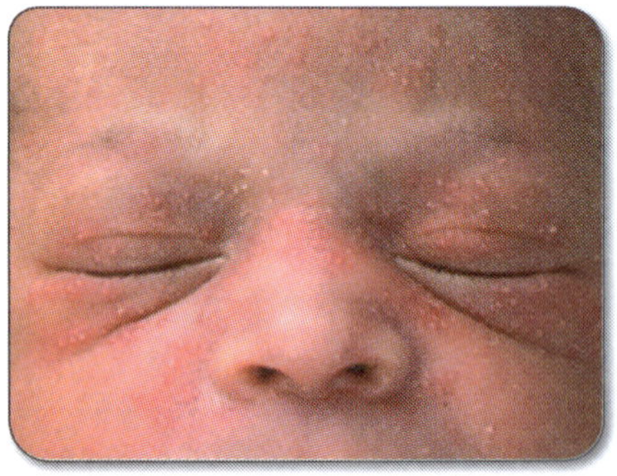

Erythema toxicum: maculopapular pustular rash with an erythematous base—it contains accumulation of eosinophils (remember e for erythema e for eosinophils)

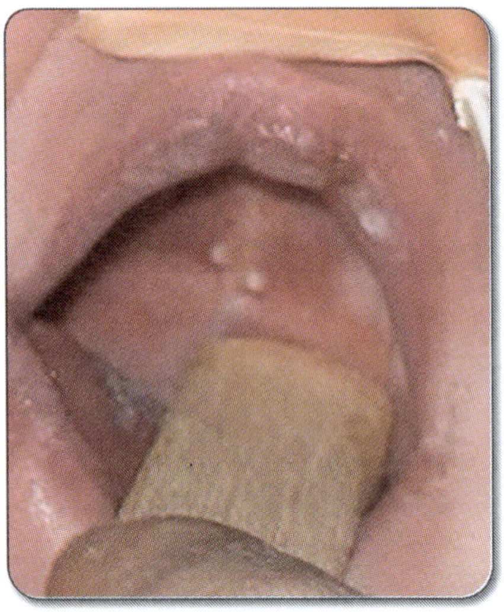

Epstein pears: inclusion cyst over the hard palate

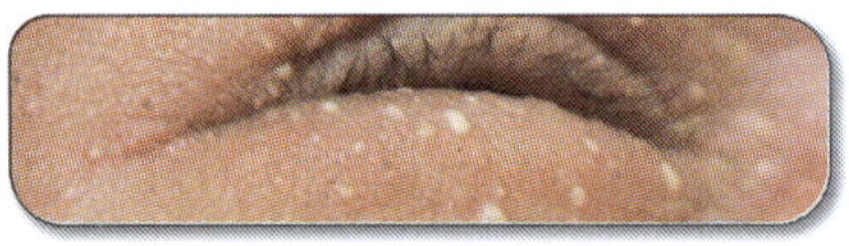

Neonatal pustular melanosis: maculopapular pustular rash without an erythematous base—contains accumulation of neutrophils (remember n for neonatal n for neutrophils)

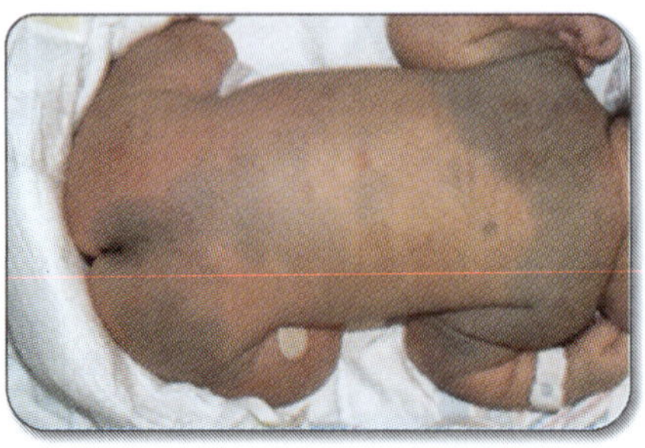

Mongolion spot—most common location is lumbosacral region

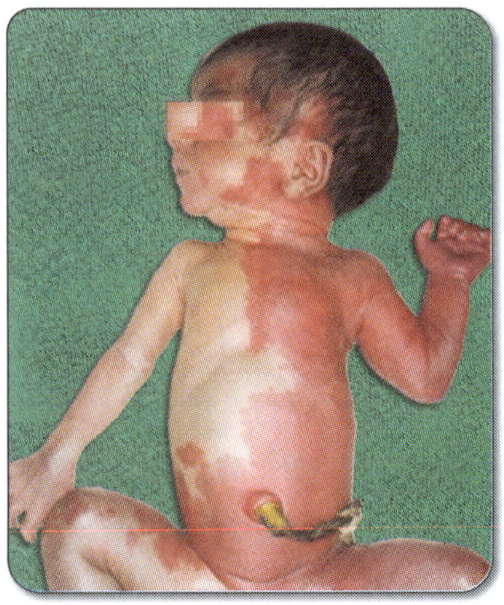

Harlequin color change

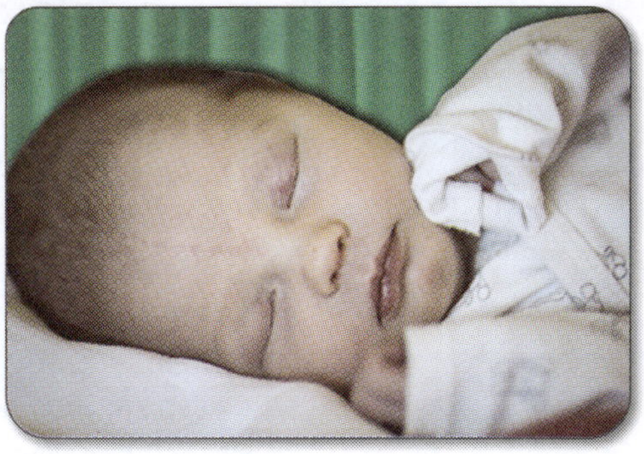

Stork bite/salmon patch/nevus simplex—these are small capillary hemangiomas

HEAD SWELLINGS IN A NEWBORN

Caput succedaneum	Cephalohematoma
• **Cause:** Prolonged labor • Not confined to suture line • Doesn't cause jaundice • Resolves in 3 days • Content: Fluid • Onset: Appears within few hours after birth • Location (plane of swellings): Subcutaneous plane 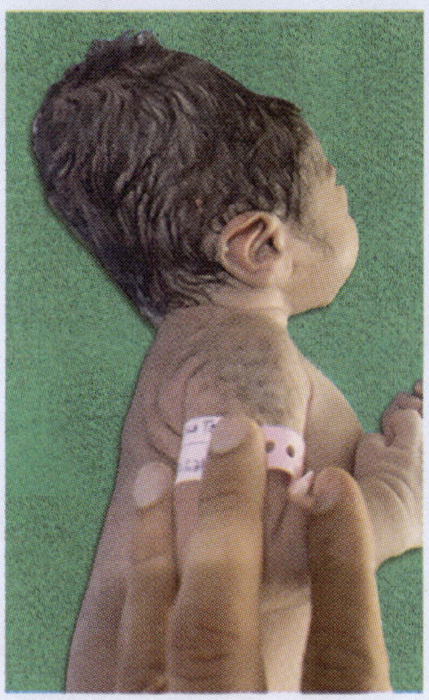	• **Cause:** Traumatic or forceps delivery • Confined to suture line • Causes jaundice • Resolves in 3–6 weeks • Content: Blood • Onset: Appears 3–5 days after birth • Location: Between skull and periosfeum (usually over parietal bone) 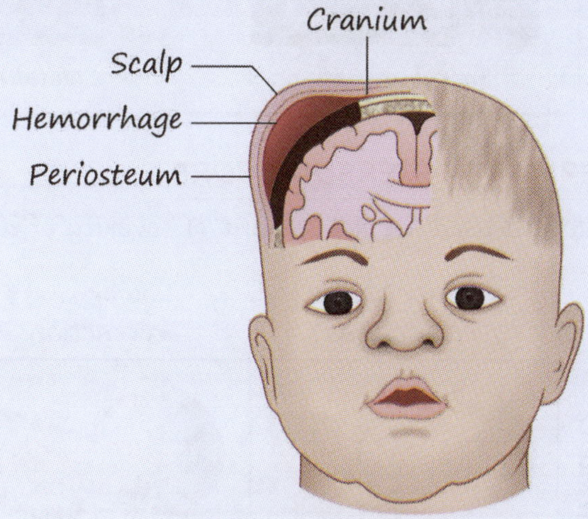

Layers of Scalp

- S – Skin
- C – Connective tissue
- A – Epicranial aponeurosis/galea aponeurotica
- CAPUT succedaneum swelling is b/w S and A
- L – Loose areolar tissue
- P – Pericranium/periosteum
- Cephalhematoma is b/w A and P

Ichthyosis Vulgaris

- Defective lipid transport
- Defective dev. of normal skin barrier

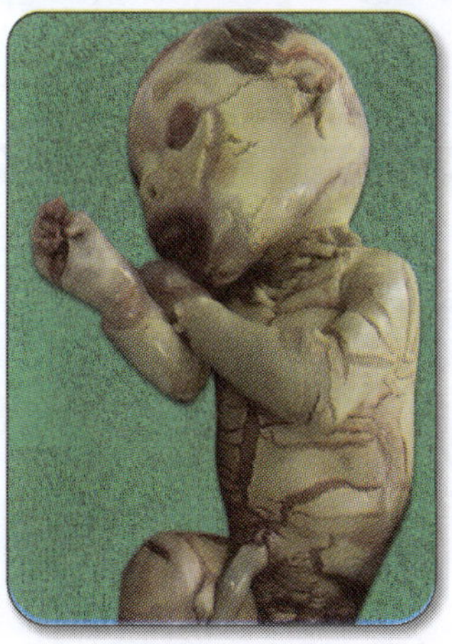

Icthyosis vulgaris

- Autosomal recessive
- Thickened, ridged, and cracked skin forms horny plates over the entire body, disfiguring and constricting the digits.
- Rx: Fluids—to avoid dehydration from transepidermal water loss
- Emulsifying agents
- Oral retinoids
- Hygiene
- MCC of distress in:
  - Preterm: HMD/RDS
  - Term: Transient tachypnea of newborn (TTN)
  - Post-term: Meconium aspiration syndrome (MAS)
- MCC of neonatal mortality is: Prematurity

INFANT OF DIABETIC MOTHER (IDM)

- Mother will be hyperglycemic and baby will be hypoglycemic
- Infant of diabetic mother will always be a macrosomic baby (>4 kg)
- IDM baby's will never be IUGR or low birth weight baby
- Most common congenital heart disease: Ventricular septal defect
- Most specific: TGA
- Most common neurological abnormality: Neural tube defect
- Most specific: Caudal regression syndrome/sacral agenesis
- All organs increase in size except brain

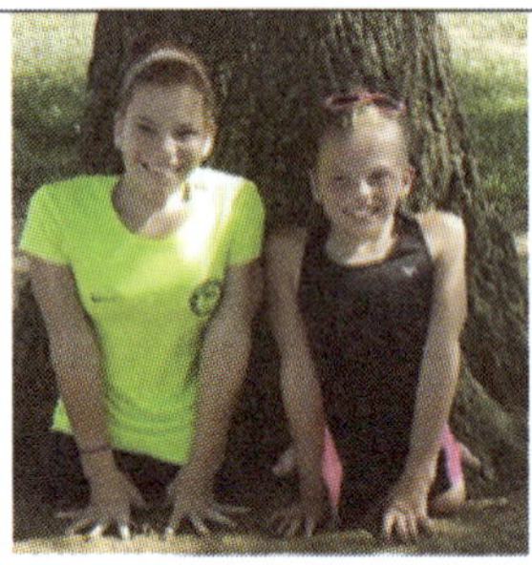

Sacral agenesis

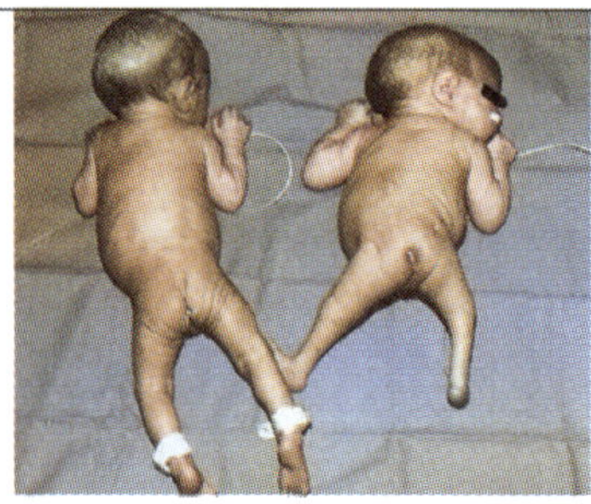

Caudal regression syndrome

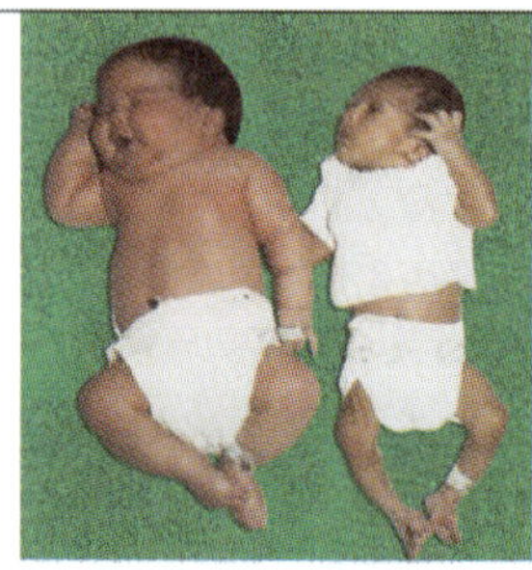

Macrosomic baby

SILVERMAN ANDERSON SCORE

This score is used for assessment of severity of distress in preterm

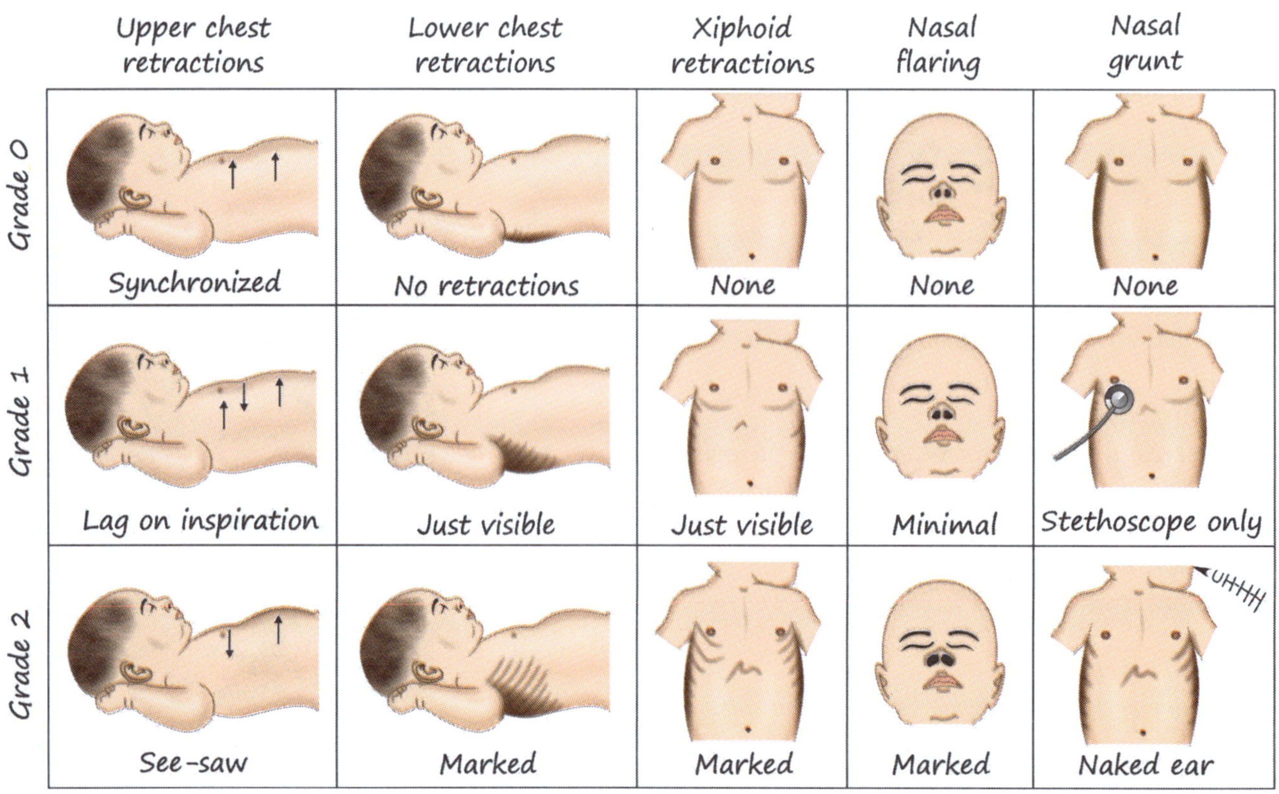

DOWNE SCORE

Used in term neonates for assessment of severity of distress.

Score	0	1	2
Respiratory rate (rate/min)	<60	60–80	>80
Cyanosis	None in room air	No cyanosis with oxygen support	Cyanosis in spite of oxygen support
Retractions	None	Mild	Moderate to severe
Grunting	None	Audible with stethoscope	Audible without stethoscope
Air entry	Good	Decreased	Barely audible

NEONATAL RESUSCITATION (LATEST UPDATE)

"Do smart work."

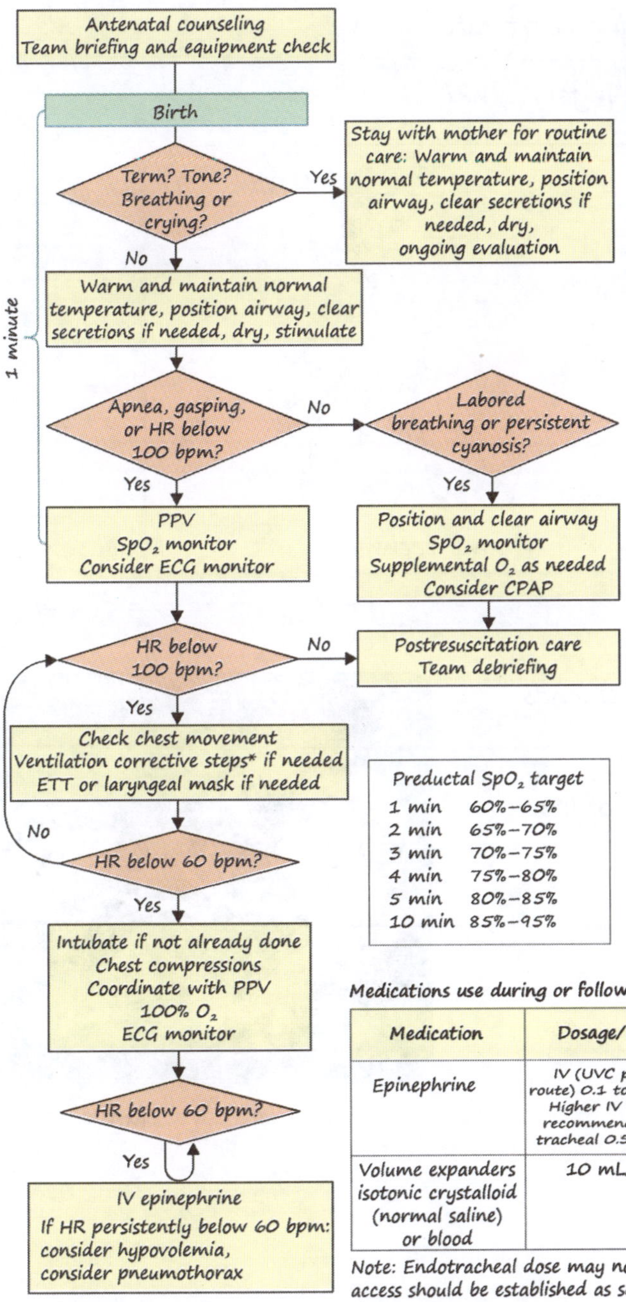

Preductal SpO_2 target	
1 min	60%–65%
2 min	65%–70%
3 min	70%–75%
4 min	75%–80%
5 min	80%–85%
10 min	85%–95%

A Airway
- Put baby's head in "sniffing" position
- Suction mouth, then nose
- Suction trachea if meconium-stained and NOT vigorous

B Breathing
- PPV for apnea, gasping, or pulse <100 bpm
- Ventilate at rates of 40–60 breaths/min
- Listen for rising heart rate, audible breath sounds
- Look for slight chest movement with each breath
- Use CO_2 detector after intubation
- Attach a pulse oximeter

C Circulation
- Start compressions if HR is <60 after 30 seconds of effective PPV
- Give (3 compressions: 1 breath) every 2 seconds
- Compress one-third of the anterior-posterior diameter of the chest

D Drugs
- Give epinephrine if HR is <60 after 45–60 seconds of compressions and ventilation
- Caution: epinephrine dosage is different for ET and IV routes

Corrective steps*(Ventilation corrective steps)

M	Mask adjustment
R	Reposition airway
S	Suction mouth and nose
O	Open mouth
P	Pressure increase
A	Airway alternative

If the baby's heart rate is <100 we do bag and mask ventilation for 30 seconds.

If the heart rate still persist to be <100 bpm then we do "MRSOPA" which are the ventilation corrective steps.

Endotracheal intubation

Gestational age (weeks)	Weight (kg)	ET tube size (ID, mm)	Depth of insertion* (on from upper lip)
<28	<1.0	2.5	6–7
28–34	1.0–2.0	3.0	7–8
34–38	2.0–3.0	3.5	8–9
>38	>3.0	3.5–4.0	9–10

*Depth of insertion (cm) = 6 + weight (in kg)

Medications use during or following resuscitation of the newborn

Medication	Dosage/Route*	Con-centration	Wt (kg)	Total IV volume (mL)	Precautions
Epinephrine	IV (UVC preferred route) 0.1 to 0.3 mL/kg Higher IV doses not recommended endo-tracheal 0.5–1 mL/kg	1:10,000	1 2 3 4	0.1–0.3 0.2–0.6 0.3–0.9 0.4–1.2	Give rapidly. Repeat every 3–5 minutes if HR <60 with chest compressions.
Volume expanders isotonic crystalloid (normal saline) or blood	10 mL/kg IV		1 2 3 4	10 20 30 40	Indicated for shock. Give over 5–10 minutes. Reassess after each bolus.

Note: Endotracheal dose may not result in effective plasma concentration of drug, so vascular access should be established as soon as possible. Drugs given endotracheally require higher dosing than when given IV.

• Baby crying—routine care	• HR <100: Bag and mask • HR <60: CC + BMV adrenaline
• Baby not crying-initial steps Warmth, position, suction, stimulation	• Most imp. Indicator: heart rate • Adrenaline: 0.2 mL/kg in 1:10,000 dilution
• TABCDE: Temp, airway, breathing, circulation, disability, exposure	• Ideal temp of labor room: 25° • Normal temp of newborn: 36.5-37.5

Indications of Giving Adrenaline

- After 60 seconds of CC (chest compressions) + BMV (Bag and mask ventilation), baby's heart rate is still <60 bpm then give adrenaline.

Ratio of CC + bmv: 3:1

Ratio of CC + bmv in infant or children: 15:2

Best IV access in neonates: Umbilical vein

Most important indicator for successful resuscitation: Ventilation

Most important indicator for successful ventilation: Rising heart rate

For CC: BMC—Thumb Technique is Better than the Finger Technique

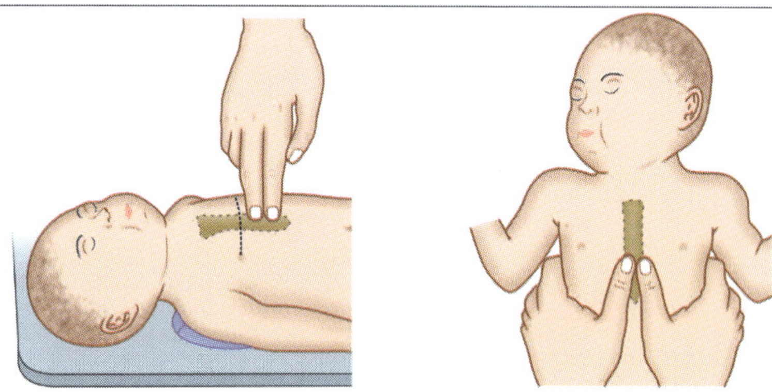

Two finger technique   Thumb technique

DELAYED CORD CLAMPING

Definition: Delay in clamping the umbilical cord by 60 seconds

Benefits:

- In term:
  - Prevents from iron def. anemia by 3–6 months of life
- In preterm:
  - Dec IVH
  - Higher BP and blood volume
  - Lesser anemia
  - Lesser blood transfusion

Side effects:

- Polycythemia (asymptomatic) and jaundice.

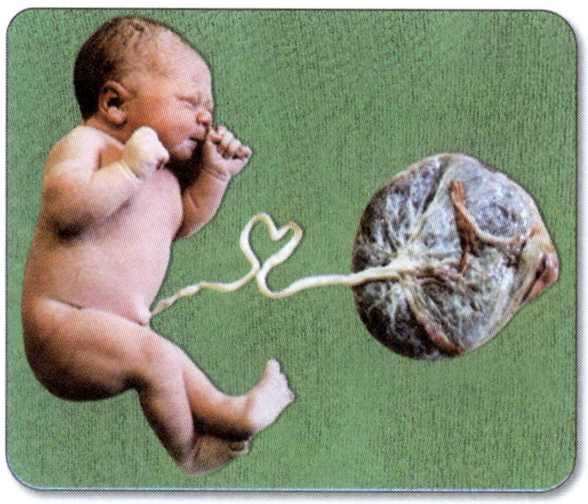

Delayed cord clamping

KANGAROO MOTHER CARE

What is KMC?

- Method of care of preterm or LBW
- Skin to skin (STS) contact
- Exclusive breastfeeding

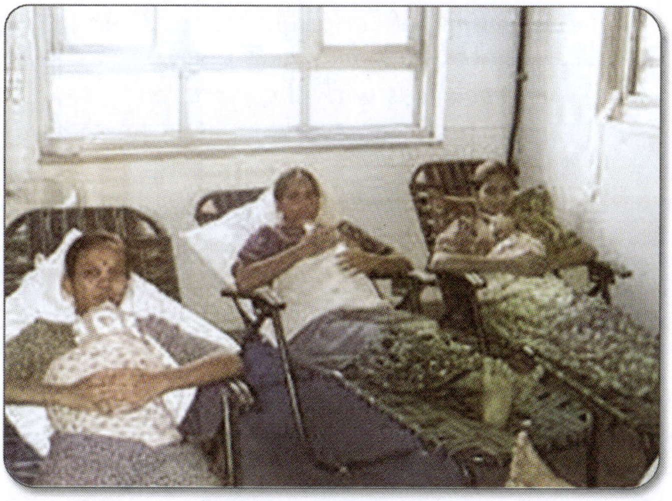

Kangaroo mother care

Benefits of KMC

- Improves breastfeeding at discharge
- Reduces risk of mortality
- Reduces sepsis
- Reduces length of hospital stay/hypothermia/ early discharge

Imp PYQs

Q: Which is the best weight to start KMC?

A: 1800 g

Q: When can I stop KMC?

A: 2.5 kg/when baby reaches term gestation.

INTRAVENTRICULAR HEMORRHAGE IN NEWBORN

Which is the most common site?

- Germinal matrix as vessels are immature with poor tissue support.
- There are 4 grades of IVH.
- Imaging of choice for screening and diagnosis: Ultrasonography cranium.
- Most common presentation of IVH in newborn is unexplained fall in hemoglobin.

Whom to screen for IVH?

- High risk babies <32 w/<1.5 kg or neonates with 32–34 weeks: who has a bad postnatal course.
- **Complications of IVH:**
  - PVHI—Periventricular hemorrhagic infarction.
  - PHH—Post hemorrhagic hydrocephalus.
  - Serial lumbar puncture.
  - Ventriculoperitoneal shunt (in 34% cases we do this).

TRANSIENT TACHYPNEA OF NEWBORN

- MCC of distress in term neonates
- Seen in LSCS delivery
- Delay in the clearance of secretions from the lung in LSCS
- X-ray: Fluid in the interlobar fissure
- Investigations: X-ray—fluid in the interlobar fissure
- Treatment: Self resolve in 48–72 hours

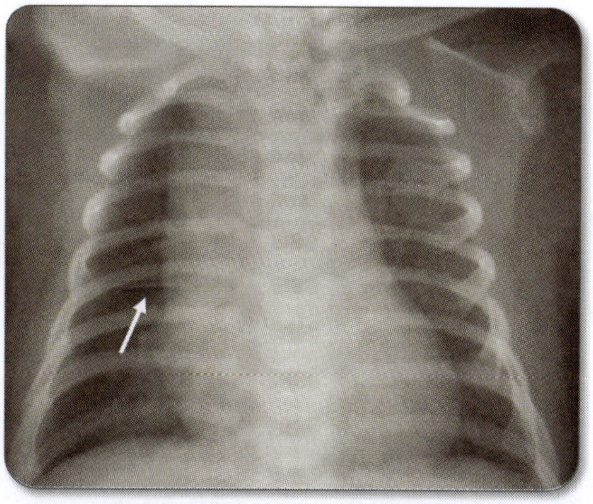

Fluid in interlobar fissure-TTN

APNEA OF PREMATURITY

- Definition: Temporary cessation of breathing for = >20 seconds with or without bradycardia <100 bpm
- Cause: Immature respiratory drive center due to prematurity
- Drug of choice: Caffeine citrate (it stimulates the respiratory center)

Golden Points

- Remember 45 and 54
  - <45 mg/dL random blood sugar is neonatal hypoglycemia
  - Most common clinical feature of hypoglycemia: Jitteriness or tremors
  - <54 mg/dL is hypoglycemia in SAM (severe acute malnutrition)
- Treatment in neonatal hypoglycemia
  - If asymptomatic hypoglycemia: Encourage breastfeeding
  - If symptomatic hypoglycemia like lethargy, seizure: 2 mL/kg 10% dextrose
- Treatment of hypoglycemia in SAM:
  - Asymptomatic: 50 mL of 10% glucose
  - Symptomatic: 5 mL/kg of 10% dextrose

NEONATAL HYPERBILIRUBINEMIA/JAUNDICE

Imp PYQs

Q: Why a newborn will have jaundice?

A: Whenever there will be hemolysis event—hemoglobin will breakdown into bilirubin and that will cause jaundice.

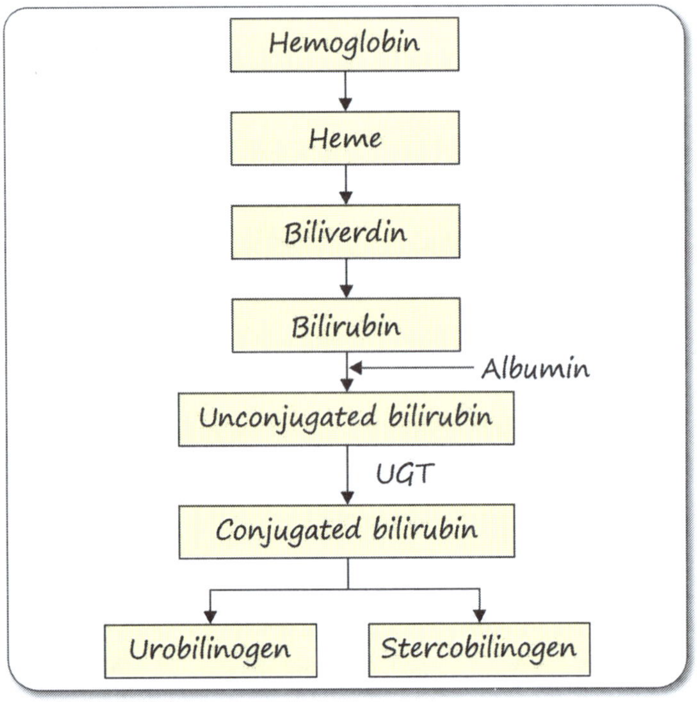

Causes of unconjugated hyperbilirubinemia:

- Rh incompatibility (means mother is negative blood group and baby is positive blood group)
- ABO incompatibility (means mother is O blood group and baby is A, B, AB blood group)
- Cephalohematoma (due to instrumental delivery)
- Breastfeeding jaundice (early onset 0–7 days of life, due to decrease breastfeeding)
- Breast milk jaundice (late onset—7–14 days of life, due to increase breastfeeding)
- Enzymopathies—G6PD enzyme deficiency
- Membranopathies: Hereditary spherocytosis, elliptocytosis
- Gilbert syndrome (unconjugated hyperbilirubinemia)
- Crigler-Najjar syndrome (unconjugated hyperbilirubinemia)

Causes of conjugated hyperbilirubinemia:

- Dubin-Johnson syndrome
  - Autosomal recessive
  - Prognosis: excellent
  - UGT enzyme is normal
  - Conversion of unconjugated bilirubin into conjugated bilirubin takes place
  - The problem is with the excretion
  - Therefore it causes conjugated hyperbilirubinemia
- Rotor syndrome (milder form of Dubin-Johnson syndrome)
  - Causes conjugated hyperbilirubinemia

Golden Points

- A newborn produces 6–10 mg of bilirubin/kg/day.
- 1 g of hemoglobin produces 34 mg of bilirubin.
- Physiological jaundice is also known as icterus neonatorum.
- In any case of jaundice, we will never stop breastfeeding.

Why does physiological jaundice appears?

- Shorter life span of RBC
- Poor hepatic uptake of bilirubin
- Less conjugation due to immature Glucronyl transferase (UDP), uridyl glucuronyl transferase (UGT) enzyme
- More ineffective erythropoiesis

Physiological jaundice	Pathological jaundice
Never appear in 1st 24 hours	May appear
Does not stain palm and soles	May stain
Urine does not stain diaper	High colored urine and clay colored stool
Does not persist beyond 3 weeks	May persist beyond 3 weeks

Extra Points

- Unconjugated bilirubin is more dangerous as it cannot get excreted by the kidneys and can cross the blood brain barrier causing kernicterus.
- Most common site of brain affected in kernicterus is: Basal ganglia.
- Most common cause of jaundice on day 1 is: erythroblastosis fetalis.

Treatment

- First clinically evaluate jaundice in the baby from cephal to caudal (means from top to bottom)
- We check by "Kramer's Rule"
- It is divided into 5 ZONES

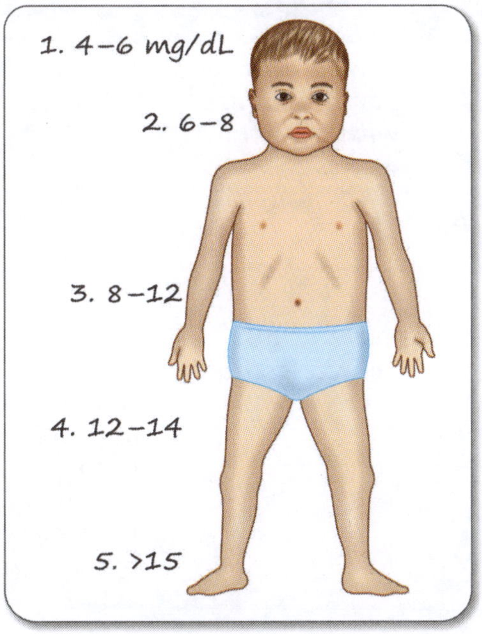

Krammer's rule

- **Zone 1:** Jaundice over head and neck – estimated Serum bil: 4–6 mg/dL
- **Zone 2:** Chest till umbilicus: 6–8 mg/dL
- **Zone 3:** Thigh: 8–10 mg/dL
- **Zone 4:** Lower legs: 10–15 mg/dL
- **Zone 5:** Palm and soles: >15 mg/dL

1st Line of Treatment: Phototherapy

- **Wavelength:** 460–490 nanometers.

Mechanism:

- Structural isomerization in which bilirubin gets converted into lumirubin which gets excreted.
- **Side effect:** Bronze baby syndrome.
- **Blue baby syndrome:** Amiodarone drug overuse.
- **Gray baby syndrome:** Chloramphenicol drug overuse.
- **Red man syndrome:** Vancomycin drug overuse.

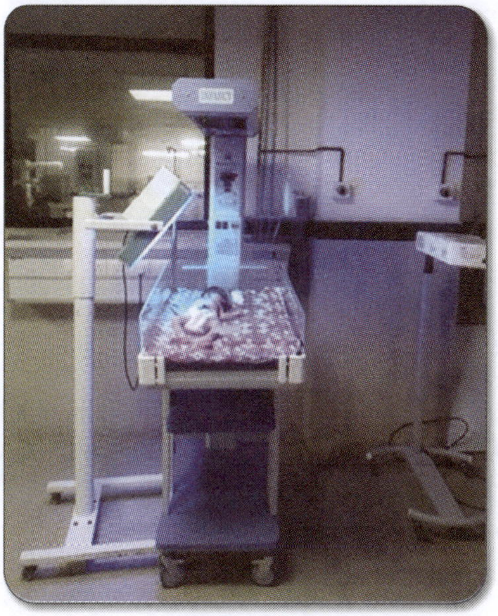

Phototherapy

2nd Line of Treatment

Exchange Transfusion

Indications:

- Cord hemoglobin <10 g/dL or cord bilirubin >5 mg/dL.
- DCT +ve.
- H/O kernicterus or Erythroblastosis in sibling.

NECROTIZING ENTEROCOLITIS (NEC)

"Why to follow when you can lead."

Stage	Systemic signs	Intestinal signs	Radiologic signs	Treatment
• **Suspected** ▪ A	Temperature instability, apnea, bradycardia	Elevated pregavage residuals, mild abdominal distension, occult blood in stool	Normal or mild ileus	NPO, antibiotics x 3 days
▪ B	Same as IA	Same as IA, plus gross blood in stool	Same as IA	Same as IA
• **Definite** ▪ Mildly ill	Same as IA	Same as I, plus absent bowel sounds, abdominal tenderness	Ileus, pneumatosis intestinalis	NPO, antibiotics x 7–10 days

Contd...

Stage	Systemic signs	Intestinal signs	Radiologic signs	Treatment
▪ Moderately ill	Same as I, plus mild metabolic acidosis, mild thrombocytopenia	Same as I, plus absent bowel sounds, definite abdominal tenderness abdominal cellulitis, right lower quadrant mass	Same as IIA, plus portal vein gas, with or without ascites	NPO, antibiotics x 14 days
• **Advanced** ▪ Severely ill, bowel intact	Same as IIB, plus hypotension, bradycardia, respiratory acidosis, metabolic acidosis, disseminated intravascular coagulation, neutropenia	Same as I and II, plus signs of generalized peritonitis, marked tenderness and distension of abdomen	Same as IIB, plus definite ascites	NPO, antibiotics x 14 days, fluid resuscitation, inotropic support, ventilator therapy, paracentesis
▪ Severely ill, bowel perforated	Same as IIIA	Same as IIIA	Same as IIB, plus pneumoperi-toneum	Same as IIA, plus surgery

Modified Bell's Staging

- Introduction: NEC is the most common life-threatening emergency of GIT in a neonate.
- Most important risk factor of NEC: Prematurity
- **Does Breast milk protect against NEC?**
  Yes
- Part of intestine involved is distal ileum and proximal colon
- Triad: Intestinal ischemia (injury), enteral nutrition and bacterial translocation
- Classification used: Modified Bell's Staging
  - Stage 1a: Occult blood in stool
  - Stage 1b: Gross blood in stool
  - Stage 2a: Pneumatosis intestinalis
  - Stage 2b: Portal venous gas
  - Stage 3a: Peritonitis
  - Stage 3b: Pneumoperitoneum (Football sign)

NEONATAL REFLEXES

Reflex	Onset	Fully developed	Disappears
Palmar grasp	28 weeks	32 weeks	4 months voluntary grasp comes (GHAI)
Rooting	32 weeks	36 weeks	Less prominent after 1 month
Moro	28	37	5–6 months
ATNR	35 weeks	1 month post natal	6–7 months

Reflex	Appears	Disappears
Parachute	7–8 m	Never disappears
Symmetric tonic neck reflex	4–6 m	8-12 months
Landau	3 m	24 m
Neck righting	4 m	24 m

MORO REFLEX

Components

- Opening of hands (28 weeks)
- Abduction and extension (32 weeks)
- Adduction and flexion (37 weeks)

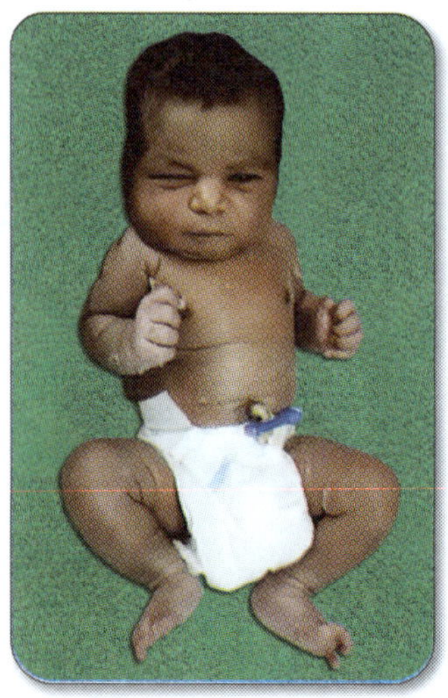

Moro reflex

- Disappear by 6 months
- Causes of asymmetric moro reflex:
  - Fracture clavicle
  - Erb's palsy—C5C6 (waiter's tip)
  - Klumpke's palsy
- Persistence of moro: Cerebral damage
- Exaggerated moro: Hypoglycemia, HIE stage 1
- Absent moro: Stage 3 HIE, Down syndrome, kernicterus
- Most common bone to fracture in a newborn: Clavicle

Golden Points

- Parachute reflex once appears, never disappears.
- When ATNR disappears, baby learn to roll over from prone to supine.
- Moro's reflex once disappears, never reappears.

NEONATAL SEIZURE

- **Most common cause:** Hypoxia
- **Most common type:** Subtle
- **Best prognosis:** Focal clonic seizure
- **Worst prognosis:** Myoclonic seizure

Jitteriness	Seizure
• Induced by a stimulus • If you hold the stimulus, jitteriness will stop • No change in autonomic system	• Not induced by a stimulus • Autonomic changes are present like tachycardia

- **Least common type:** Myoclonic
- **IOC:** Transcranial ultrasound
- **Drug of choice:** Phenobarbitone

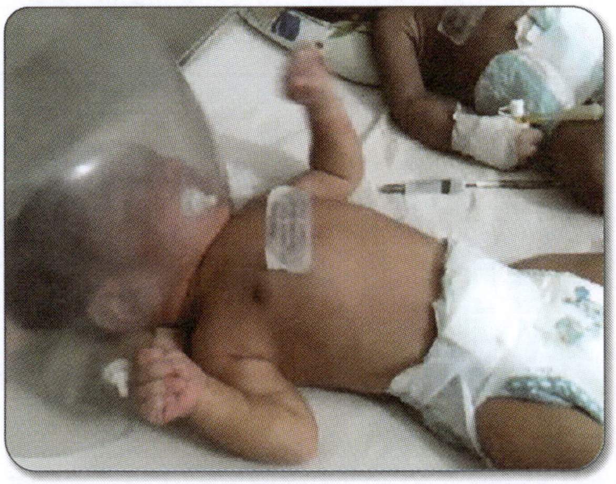

Jitteriness

Extra Points

- One condition in neonatology where Sildenafil is used is: PPHN (persistent pulmonary hypertension of newborn)

  What is pulse oximetry screening (POxS) and where do we use it?
  - It is done if we are suspecting a congenital heart disease in a newborn.
  - It is done after 24 hours of birth.
  - We check the saturation in right hand and foot.
  - If the saturation is <90% in either of the limbs that means the test is +ve and patient has likely (CHD) congenital heart disease.

MECONIUM ASPIRATION SYNDROME

- Meconium is a sterile, thick, blackish green, oderless material that results from the accumulation of debris in the fetal intestine during the 3rd month of gestation.
- Contains 72–80% water
- X-ray bilateral diffuse patchy opacities.
- **Clinical features:**
  - Peeling of skin
  - Green color umbilical cord
  - Green nails

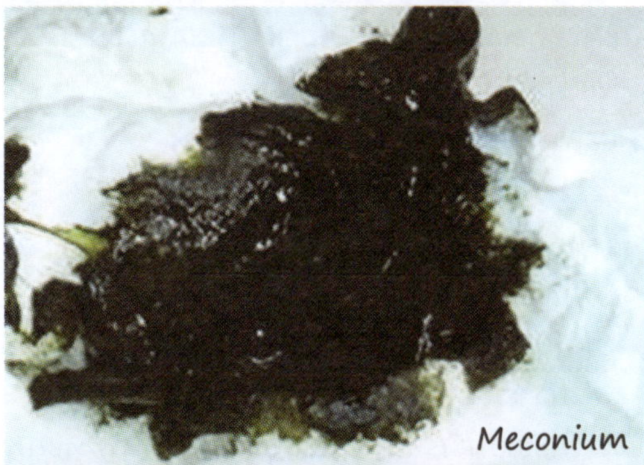

Meconium

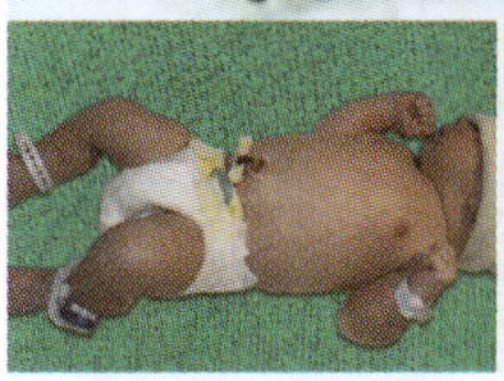

Peeling of skin

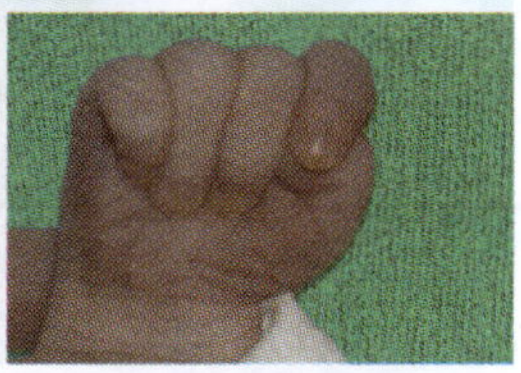

Green nails

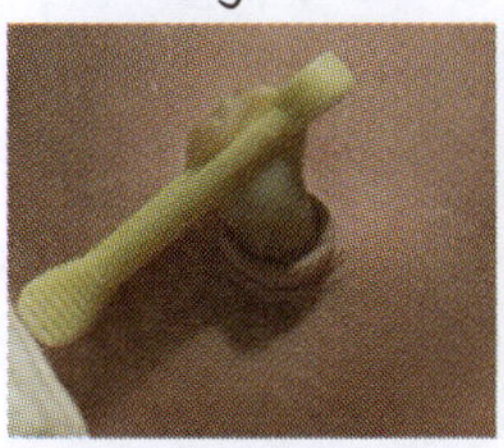

Normal umbilical cord

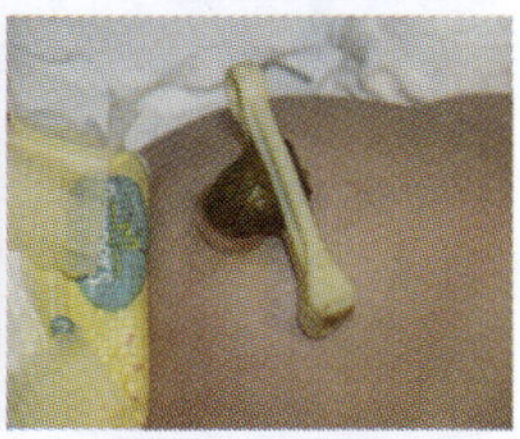

Green umbilical cord

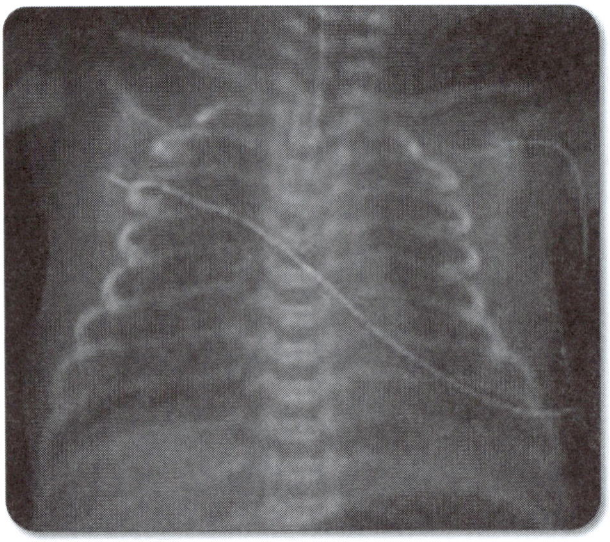

Patchy infiltrates with hyperinflated chest
Meconium aspiration syndrome

- Complication of MAS: PPHN (persistent pulmonary hypertension of newbron) and pneumothorax

What is vigorous and nonvigorous meconium stained?

- HR >100, good tone, good efforts
- Nonvigorous: HR <100, poor tone, poor efforts
- Tracheal suctioning is never done

HYALINE MEMBRANE DISEASE/ RESPIRATORY DISTRESS SYNDROME

- Incidence: Seen in preterm neonates
- Risk factors:
  - Prematurity
  - Maternal diabetes
- Etiology: Deficiency of surfactant
- Pathophysiology
- If the baby is premature, lungs will not mature due to deficiency of surfactant:
  - Surfactant is formed by type 2 pneumocytes of the lung
  - Surfactant appears in amniotic fluid by 28 weeks and lungs by 33–35 weeks
  - For the lung maturity of the baby, mother is given antenatal steroids
  - Betamethasone: 12 × 2 = 24 (12 mg 2 doses 24 hours apart)
  - Dexamethasone: 6 mg 4 doses 12 hours apart

Absolute Contraindication of Giving Steroids to the Mother?

Chorioamnionitis

X-ray: (image)

White out lung with air bronchogram

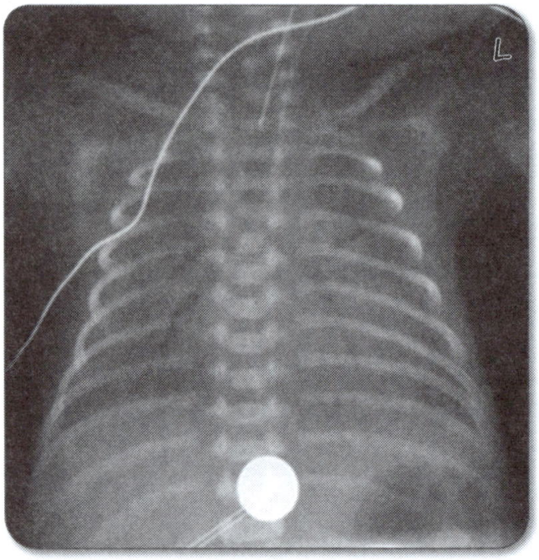

Air bronchogram—HMD/RD S

Investigations

- Lecithin/sphingomyelin ratio >2 means lung is mature
- Lamellar body counts: >50,000 lamellar bodies/ microliter predicts lung maturity.
- Treatment: Surfactant therapy
- Timing
- Prophylactic treatment: Within minutes of birth
- Selective/Rescue treatment: When symptoms are present
- Route: Intratracheal

> **Golden Points**
>
> **Differential diagnosis of white out lung:**
>
> - HMD
> - Obstructive/infracardiac total anomalous pulmonary venous connection (TAPVC)
> - Pulmonary alveolar proteinosis
> - Surfactant protein B deficiency Surfactant protein B
> - Massive pleural effusion

TRANSIENT TACHYPNEA OF NEWBORN (TTN)

It is the most common cause of distress in term babies.
Seen in babies born from LSCS.
Benign self limiting condition.

Clinical Features

Tachypnea within few hours after birth.

Mechanism

- In NVD: There is clearance of secretions from the lung.
- In LSCS: There is delay in the clearance of secretions from the lung (image).

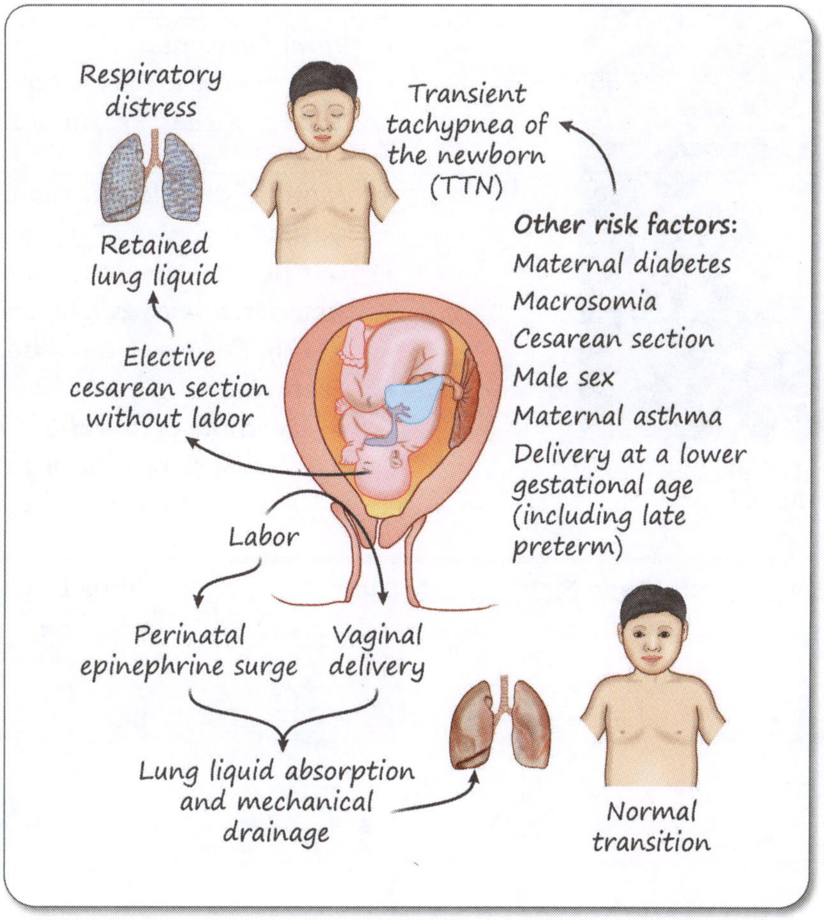

Management

Investigations

X-ray chest: fluid in the interloper fissure (image)

- Hyperinflated lung
- Increased perihilar
- Interstitial markings

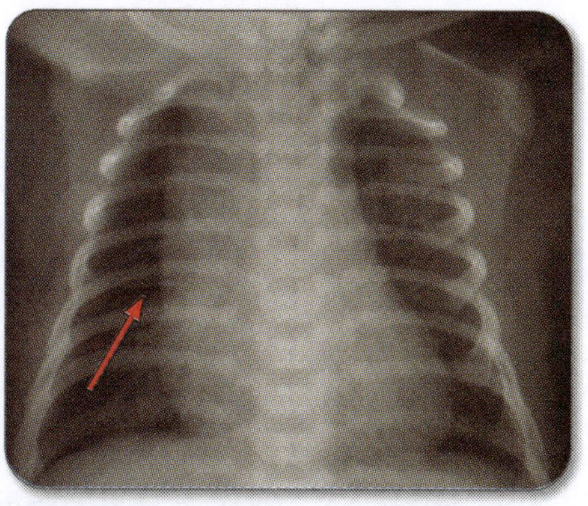

Treatment

Self-resolving condition, symptoms subside by 48–72 hours

3. RESPIRATORY SYSTEM

"He who doesn't hope to win, has already lost."

CONGENITAL DIAPHRAGMATIC HERNIA

- Bag and mask ventilation contraindicated.
- Bowel sounds in the chest.
- Most common variety: Posterolateral/bochdalek diaphragmatic hernia.
- Scaphoid-shaped abdomen.

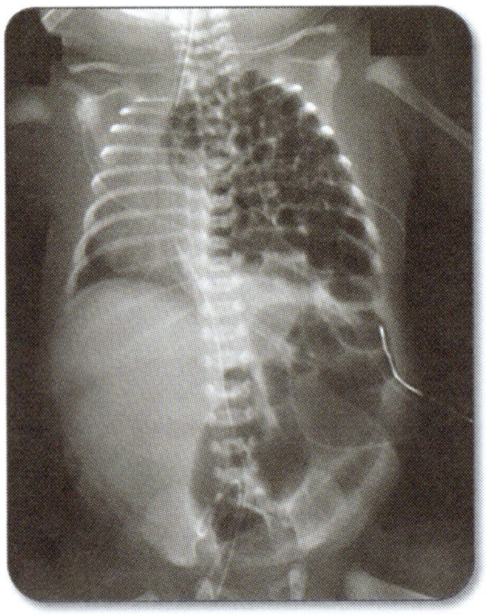

Congenital diaphragmatic hernia

- Neonatal distress.
- **Surgical repair:** Ideally done after 48 hours of life.
- If not done → indications → mentioned.
- **Management:** ECMO, iNO
- **Poor prognostic factor:** LHR <1
- **Recent advances:** Exit procedure or FETO

TRACHEOESOPHAGEAL FISTULA

- Total five types.
- Most common type is type C followed by type A.
- Type C means proximal esophageal atresia with distal TEF.
- Name of the classification: Gross classification.
- Gasless abdomen: Type A and B.
- Gas in the abdomen: Type C, D, E.
- Associated with polyhydramnios.
- X-ray: Coiling of the nasogastric tube.
- Features:
  - Frothing of secretions and dribbling of saliva
  - Cyanosis, respiratory distress
  - Maternal history of polyhydramnios

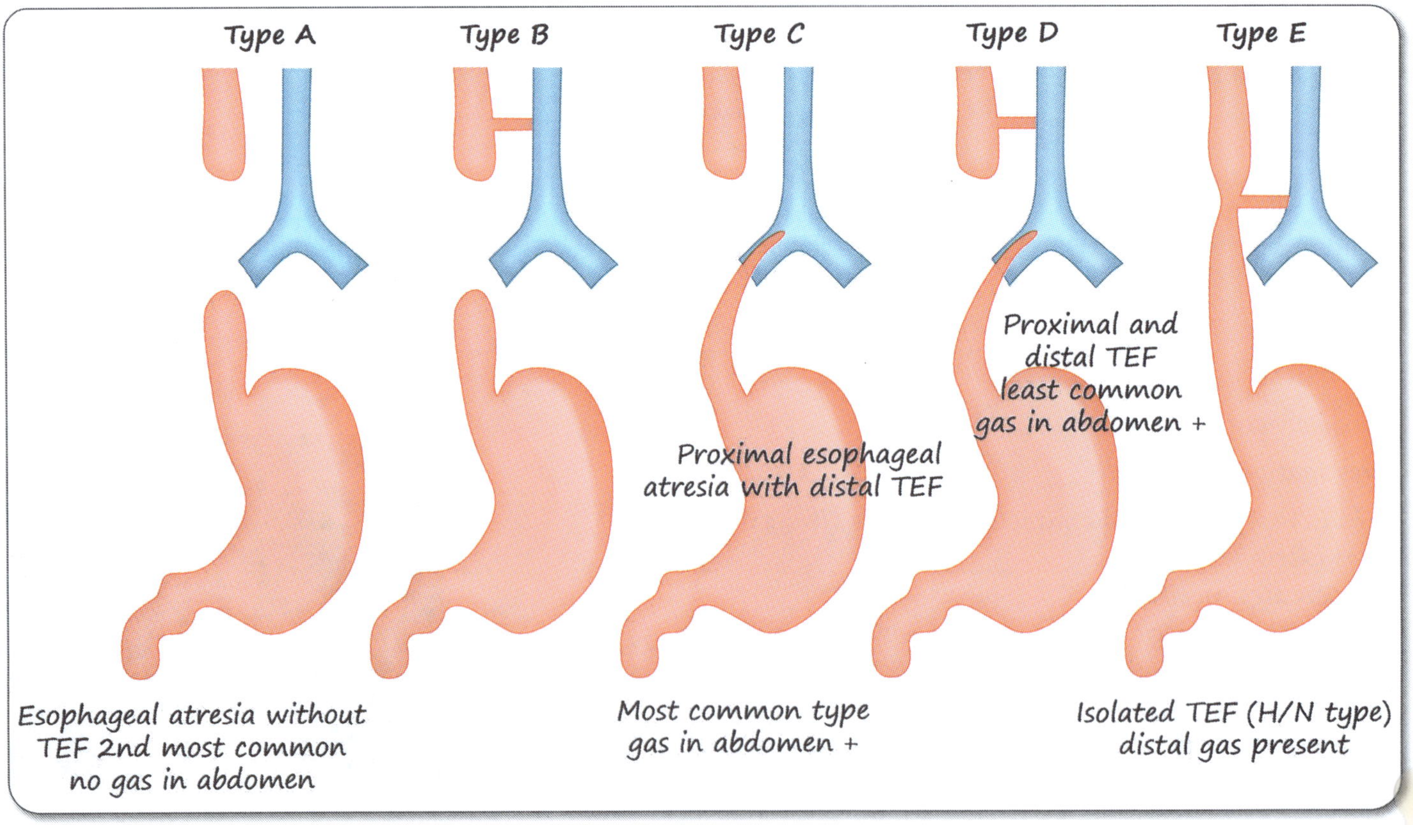

Gross classification—TEF

Tracheoesophageal Fistula is Associated with VACTERL Anomaly

- V - vertebral
- A - anorectal
- C - cardiac
- T - tracheal
- E - esophageal
- R - renal
- L - limb abnormalities

NAMES OF CLASSIFICATION

- West Haven classification: Acute hepatic encephalopathy.
- Silence classification: Osteogenesis imperfecta
- Gross classification: Tracheoesophageal fistula
- Becker score: Asthma
- Sarnat and sarnat: Hypoxic-ischemic encephalopathy
- Modified Bell's staging: Necrotizing enterocolitis
- Tanner chart/staging: Sexual maturity rating (SMR)
- Global initiative for asthma (GINA) guidelines: Asthma
- Modified Duke's criteria: Infective endocarditis
- Modified Jone's criteria: Acute rheumatic fever
- SLICC criteria: Systemic lupus erythematosus
- Rome criteria: Irritable bowel disease
- Kerosene oil poisoning: Gupta scoring
- Westley scoring: Croup
- Silverman-Anderson Score: For distress assessment in preterm
- Downe score: For distress assessment in term

CHOANAL ATRESIA

"Work hard in silence."

- Most common congenital anomaly of nose.
- Failure to pass the nasogastric tube.
- Distress and cyanosis improve on crying.
- On X-ray: Coiling of nasogastric tube.

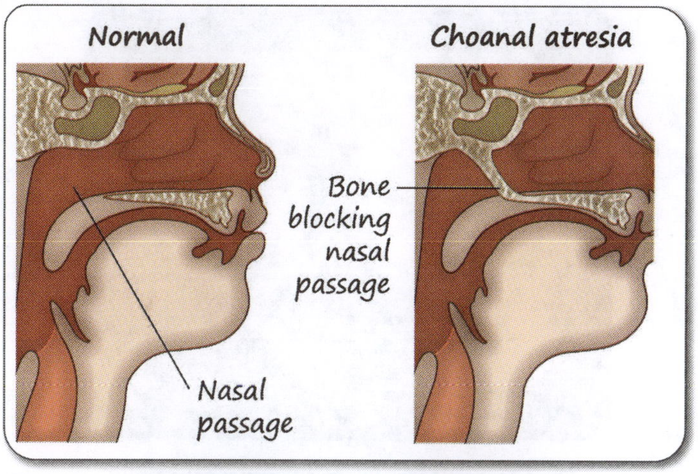

KARTAGENER'S SYNDROME/IMMOTILE-CILIA SYNDROME

- Impaired mucociliary clearance
- Triad
  1. Chronic sinusitis
  2. Bronchiectasis
  3. Dextrocardia

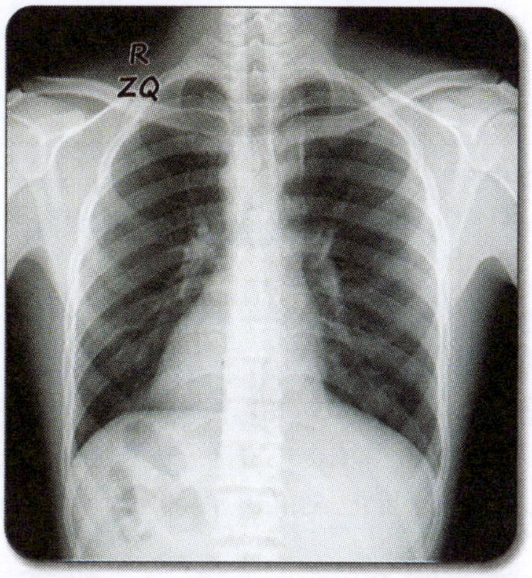

Kartagener syndrome (dextrocardia)

YOUNG SYNDROME

Triad

1. Chronic sinusistis
2. Bronchiectasis
3. Azoospermia

STRIDOR

- Definition: Forced expiratory sound against a partially closed glottis.
- Second most common cause is congenital subglottic stenosis.
- It is an upper respiratory tract problem.
- Most common case of stridor is laryngomalacia.
- Distress increases on lying and relieves on prone.
- Diagnosis: Omega shape epiglottis.
- Investigation: Flexible laryngoscopy.
- Treatment: Resolves spontaneously.

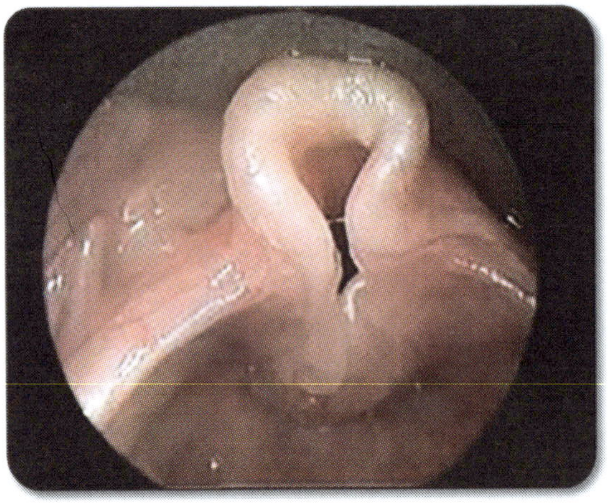

Omega snape epiglottis—laryngomalolia

ACUTE PHARYNGITIS

- Etiology: Rhinovirus.
- C/f: Fever, sore throat, cervical lymphadenopathy, malaise.
- Diagnosis: Throat swab rapid antigen detection test (RADT).
- Rx: Penicillin/amoxicillin for 10 days.
- Complications: Rheumatic fever, acute glomerulonephritis, peritonsillar abscess.

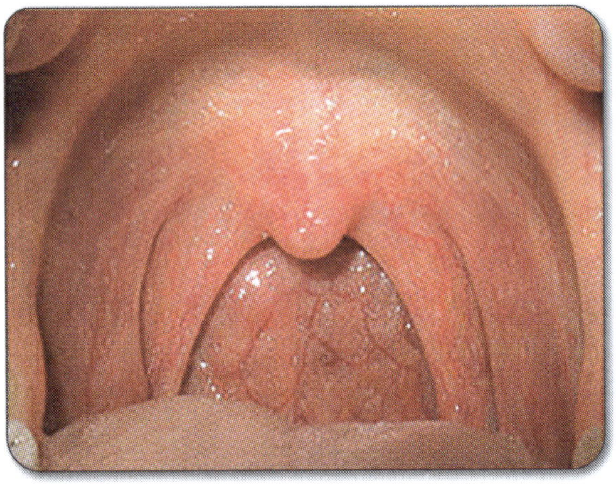

Acute pharyngitis

Most Common Cause

- Common cold: Rhinovirus
- Pharyngitis: Adenovirus
- Croup: Parainfluenza virus
- Whooping cough: Bordetella pertussis
- Bronchiolitis: Respiratory syncitial virus

ACTUE EPIGLOTTIS

- Cause: H. influenzae type b

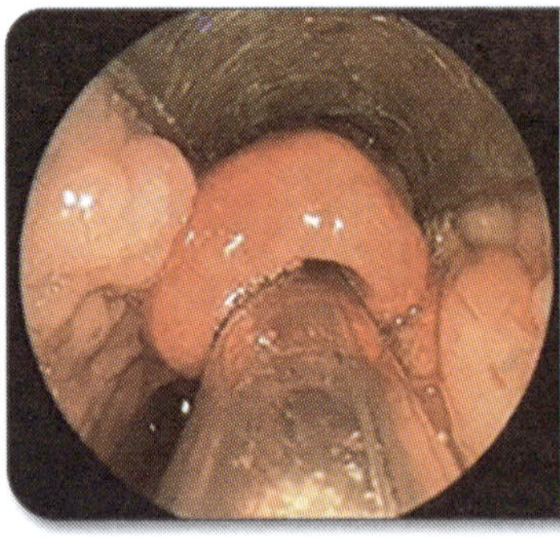

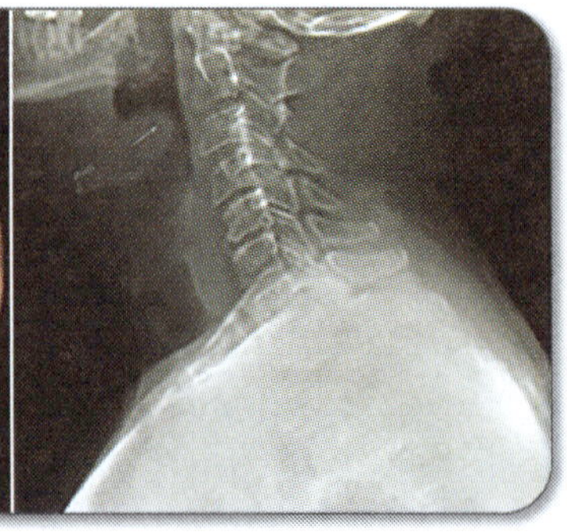

Cherry red epiglottis *Thumb sign*

- Sign: Thumb sign → X-ray neck shows
- 5 Ds of acute epiglottitis
  1. Dyspnea
  2. Dysphagia
  3. Dysphonia
  4. Drooling
  5. Distressed (rapid progression within hours)
- Child sits in tripod position, sitting upright, leaning forward with chin up
- Treatment: Antibiotics—cephalosporin 3rd generation → IV ceftriaxone

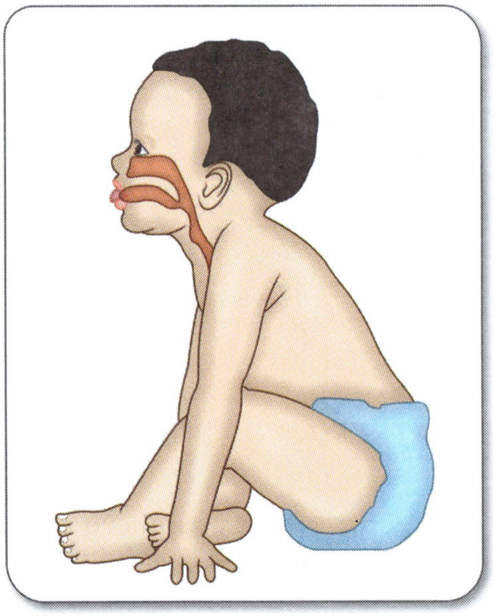

Tripod position seen in acute epiglottitis

CROUP

- Cause: Parainfluenza virus, less severe
- Symptoms: Hoarse voice, coryza, mild tachypnea
- Types: Mild, moderate, severe
- Investigations: Clinical diagnosis
- Sign: Steeple sign in X-ray
- Treatment: Dexamethasone + adrenaline nebulization, heliop mixture, hydration, antibiotic, morphine, salbutamol have no role.

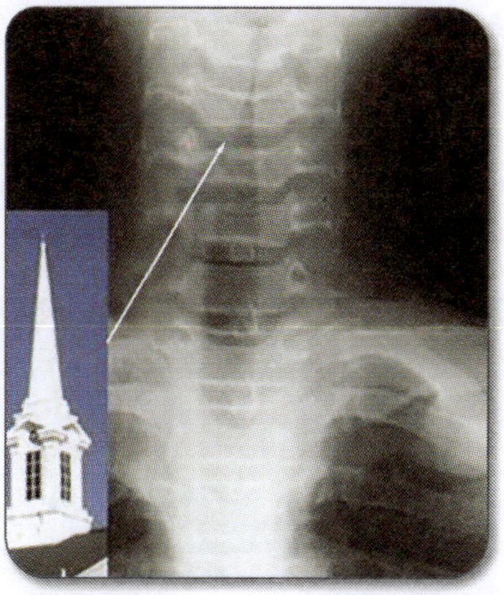

Steeple sign-Croup/Acute laryngotracheobronchitis

Classification of Croup

Mild	Moderate	Severe
Feed well	Irritated	Restless/agitated
Stridor on coughing	Rest	Rest + agitation
SpO_2 >92%	SpO_2 >92%	SpO_2 <92%
No distress	Tachypnea + chest retr.	Marked tachypnea

Diamond Points

- Croup decreases on lying down position.
- Laryngomalacia increases on lying down.

BRONCHIOLITIS

- Age group: 1-6 months but can affect up to 2-3 years*
- Most common cause: respiratory syncytial virus (RSV)
- Clinical features: distress, tachypnea (fast breathing)
- Inv: X-ray: hyperinflation and infiltrates (image)

Treatment

- Symptomatic management
- MOIST O_2 inhalation
- Antibiotic have no role
- Ribavirin- antiviral (it shortens the course of illness in HIV patient)
- RSV Ig and palivizumab*: should be considered for infants with chronic lung disease, prematurity.
- Ribavirin comes in powder form reconstitute with water 100 mL vial has 6 g of ribavirin 20 mg/mL given through SPAG nebulizer (small particle aerosol generator)

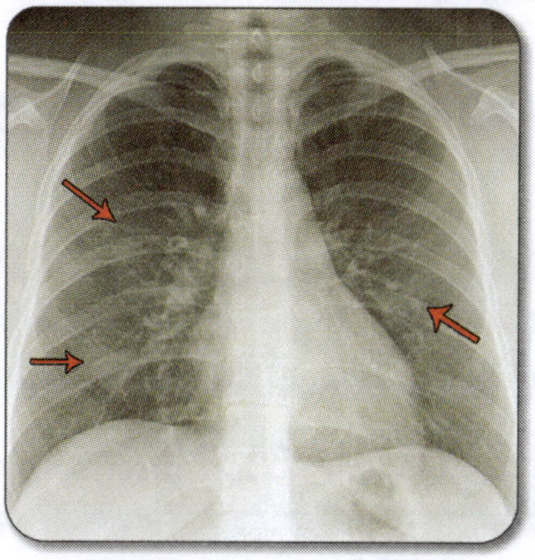

Chest X-ray of bronchiolitis

	Croup	Epiglottitis	Tracheitis
Incidence	Common	Rare	Rare
Age	6 months –3 years	2–7 years	6 months –14 years
Etiology	Viral	Bacterial	Bacterial
Speed of onset	Slow	Very rapid	Rapid
Fever	Rarely >39°	Normally >39°	Normally >39°
Cough	Barking	Suppressed	Present
Voice	Hoarse	Muffled	Hoarse
Position	Supine	Sitting forward, neck extended	Supine
Neck X-ray AP	Steeple sign*	Normal	Steeple sign*
Neck X-ray Lateral	Normal	Thumb print	Hazy
Response to adrenaline	Very good	No response	Partial or no response

WHOOPING COUGH

- Cause: Bordetella pertussis
- A well-appearing young child begins to choke, gasp and flail the extremities with face reddened.
- Stages: Catarrhal, paroxysmal, convalescent stage
- Hallmark: Apnea, bradycardia, cyanosis
- Treatment: Azithromycin

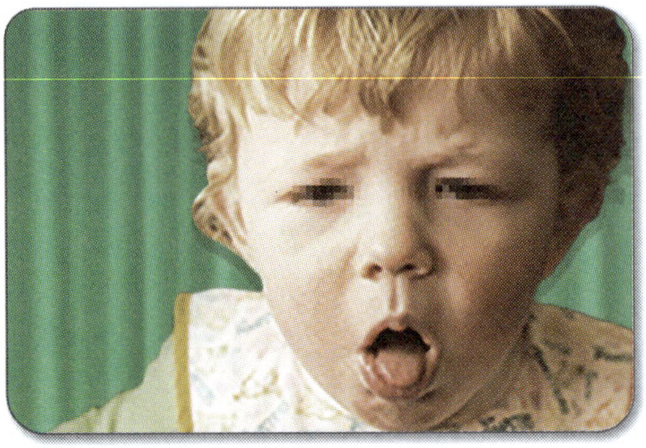

Whooping cough

Stages of Whooping Cough

Stage	Duration	Signs and symptoms
Catarrhal	1–2 weeks	Insidious onset with gradual progression No or mild fever, rhinorrhea, lacrimation, dry cough, malaise, Highly contagious
Paroxysmal	1–6 weeks (up to 10 weeks)	Paroxysms (i.e., periods of coughing occurring in rapid succession during one exhalation) Inspiratory whoop may follow coughing spell Post-tussive emesis, cyanosis, and exhaustion Leukocytosis, lymphocytosis, and weight loss.
Convalescent	2–3 weeks	Coughing lessens Susceptibility to respiratory tract infections

- Bacterial pneumonia in children—*Streptococcus pneumoniae*
- 2nd most common bacterial pneumonia in children—*H. influenzae* type B
- Viral pneumonia in children—RSV
- Pneumonia in neonates—group B Streptococci, *E. coli*
- Pneumonia in infants with HIV—*H. influenzae* type B
- Chest X-ray findings:
  - Pneumococcal pneumonia: Lobar consolidation > patchy

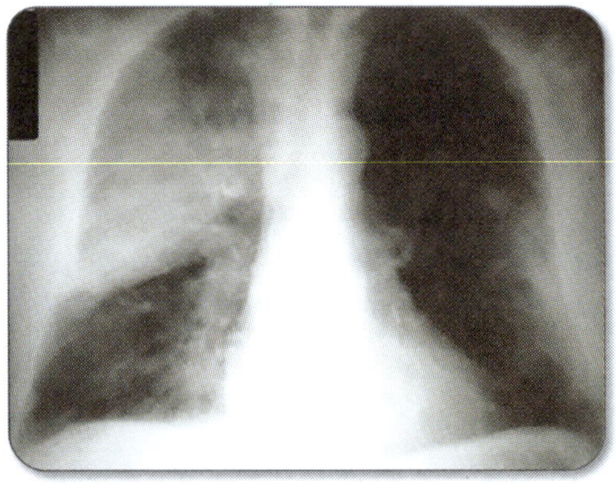

Consolidation

  - Staphylococcal pneumonia: Pneumatoceles, empyema

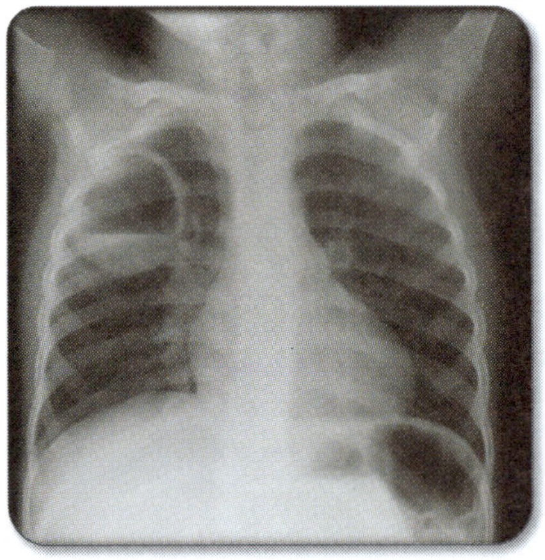

Pneumatocele

- Strep. pneumonia: Interstitial pneumonia, segmental involvement.

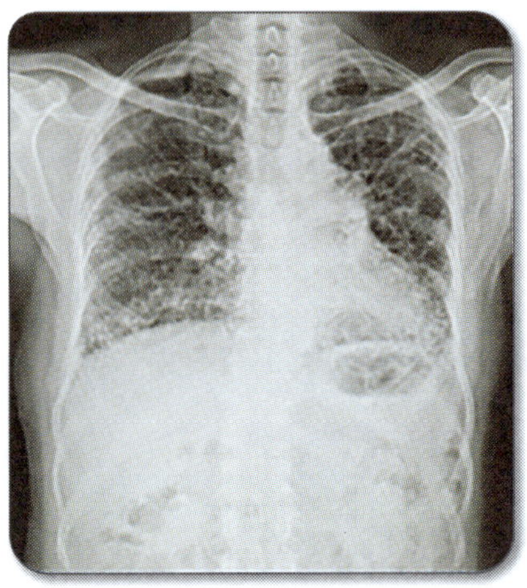

Interstitial pneumonia

ASTHMA

- Definition: Increased responsiveness of the airways to various stimuli.

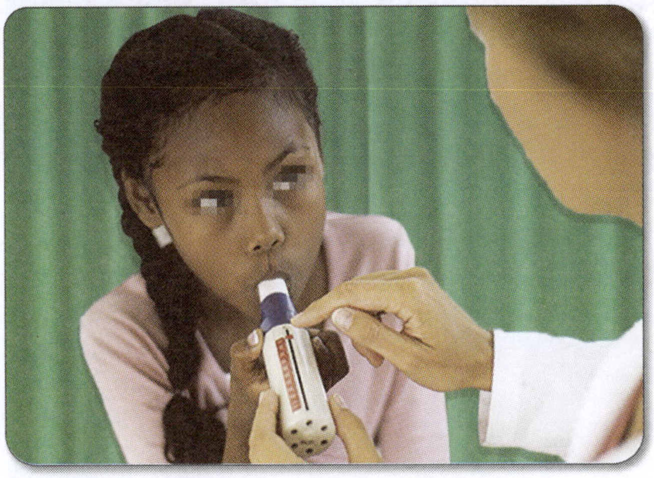

- Classification:
  - Extrinsic (atopic): IgE mediated, triggered by allergens
  - Intrinsic (nonatopic): Non-IgE mediated, triggered by infection
  - C/f: Dyspnea, wheezing or cough
- Peak expiratory flow rate (PEFR) is a person's maximum speed of expiration, as measured with a peak flow meter like the unit.
- Forced expiratory volume in first second (FEV_1): In one second how much we can expire out forcefully
- N-97% we can expire in 1 second
- Forced vital capacity (FVC): After each deep respiration how much we can forcefully expire
- ***Obstructive lung disease***
  - FEV_1 will decrease but FVC will remain same
  - Because lung capacity is not affected
  - COPD, emphysema, bronchial asthma, bronchiectasis
  - Spirometry we do use and we take a ratio:
  - FEV1/FVC ratio will decrease
  - So, in obstructive lung disease, this ratio will decrease
- ***Restrictive lung disease***
  - There is reduced expansion of lung parenchyma
  - Fibrosis, sarcoidosis, interstitial lung disease, chest wall neuromuscular disease
  - FEV_1 and FVC both will decrease
  - Ratio of FEV_1/FVC will not change, it will be normal.
  - Because both will decrease

Management of Asthma

- Bronchodilators
- Short-acting
  - Adrenaline alpha + beta (can be given S/C)
  - Salbutamol—specific β_2-agonist
  - Terbutaline—specific β_2-agonist (can be given S/C*)
  - Others—oral, inhalational, parenteral
- **Long-acting**
  - Salmeterol
  - Formoterol
  - Onset—action is delayed by 30–60 minutes but lasts for 24 hours

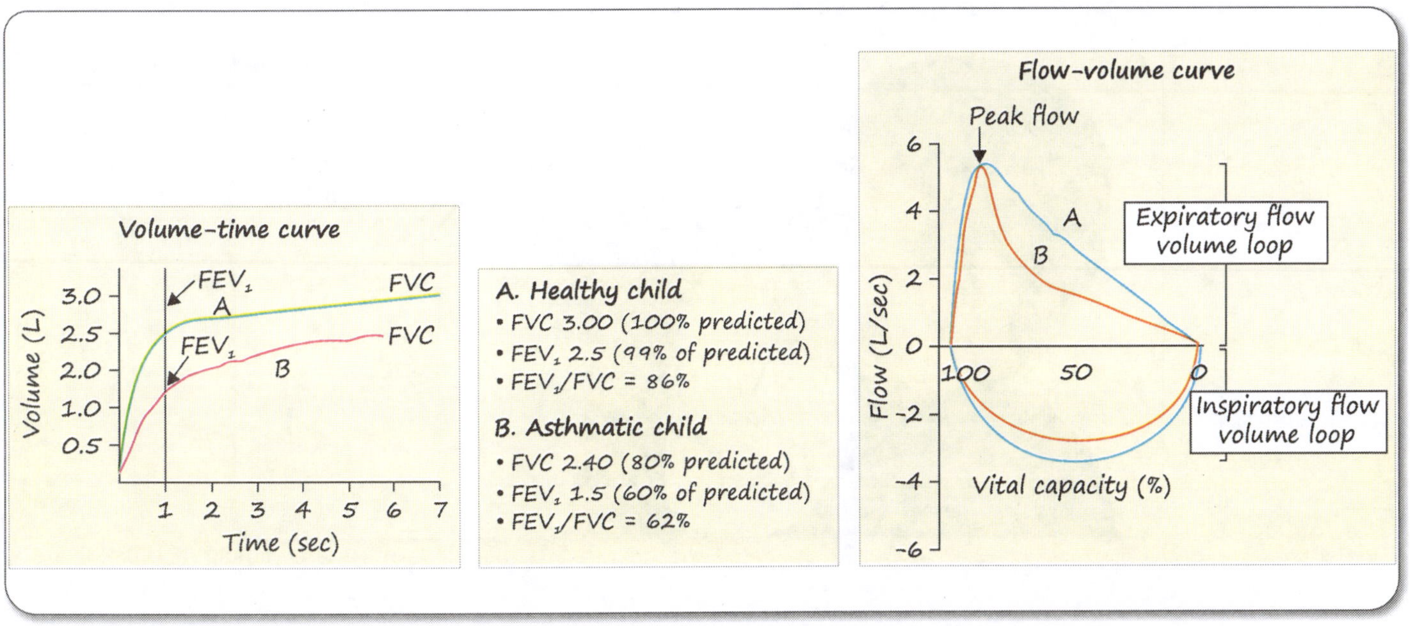

ASSESSMENT OF SYMPTOM CONTROL

Features	Controlled: All of the following	Partially Controlled: Any Measure present in any Week	Uncontrolled
Daytime symptoms	None (twice a week or less)	More than twice per week	Three or more features of partially controlled asthma present in any week
Limitation of activity	None	Any	
Nocturnal symptoms, awakening	None	Any	
Need for reliever of rescue drugs	None (less than twice a week)	More than twice per week	

SABA: *Short-acting β_2 agonists*
ICS: *Inhaled corticosteroids*
LABA: *Long-acting β_2 agonists*
LAMA: *Long-acting anticholinergics*
LTRA: *Leukotriene receptor antagonists*
OCS: *Oral corticosteroids*

	Step 1	Step 2	Step 3	Step 4	Step 5
Preferred controller treatment		Low dose ICS	Low dose ICS + LABA	Medium-high dose ICS + LABA ICS + LABA + LTRA	+ Anti IgE or + Anti-IL5 or + Macrolides (phenotype dependent)
Other controller options		Medium-high dose ICS initially or in periods	Low dose ICS + LTRA	+ LTRA + LAMA	+ OCS
Reliever	SABA		SABA or ICS + formoterol		

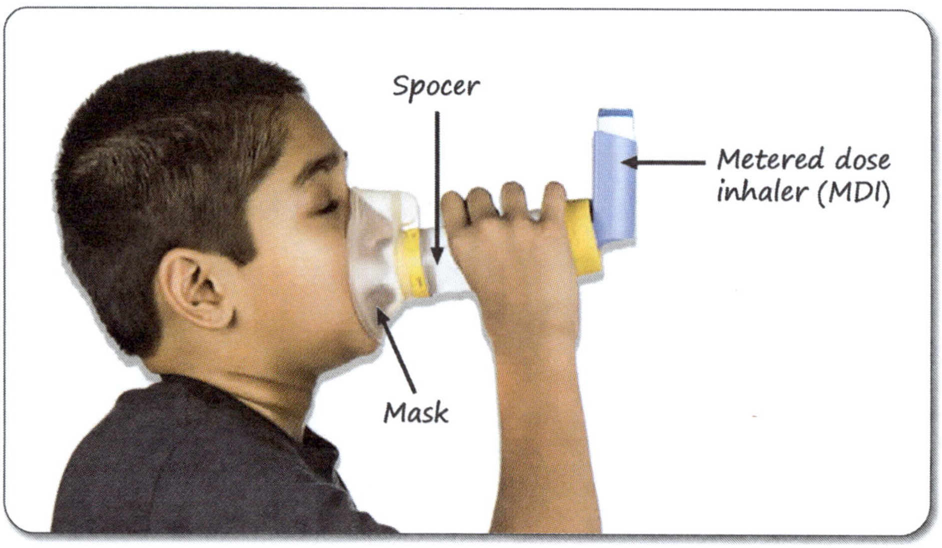

Types of Asthma

	Day time symptoms	Night time symptoms	PEFR	Long-term prevention
Step 1: Intermittent	**<1 time a week** Asymptomatic and normal PEFR between attack	<2 times a month	>80% predicted, variability <20%	**Inhaled short-acting β-agonist SOS** If they are needed more than 3 times a week, move to step 2.
Step 2: Mild persistent	**>1 times a week** But <1 time a day	>2 time a month	>80% variability 20–30%	Inhaled short-acting β-agonist SOS + **low dose inhaled steroid** + sustained release + leukotriene modifiers
Step 3: Moderate persistent	Daily use β_2 agonist, attacks affect activity	>1 times a week	**60–80%** predicted; variability >30%	Inhaled short-acting β-agonist sos + **medium dose infield steroids + long acing** β_2 agonist + sustained release theophylline
Step 4: Severe persistent	Continuous, limited physical activity	Frequent	**<60% predicted;** variability <30%	**Inhaled short-acting β-agonist SOS + inhaled corticosteroids (high dose) + long acting** bronchodilator + oral steroids low dose alternate day.

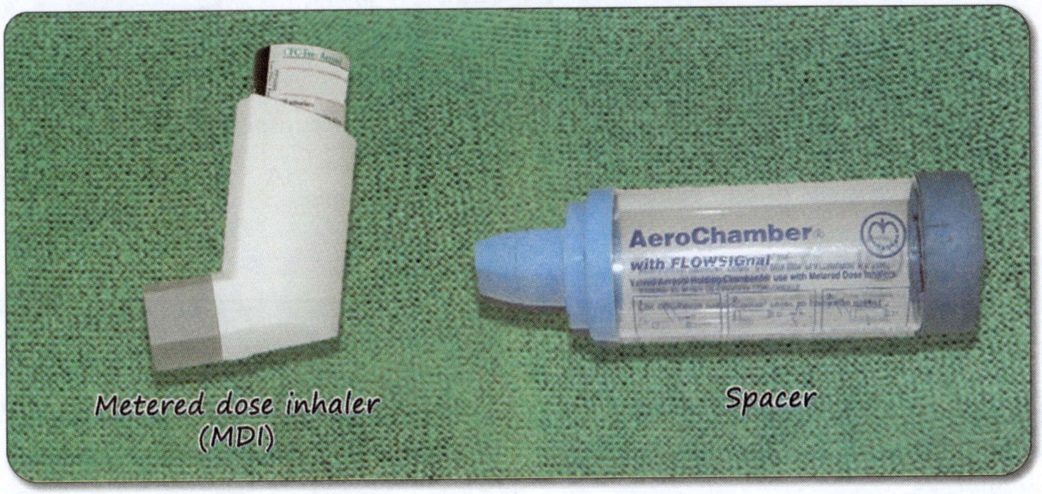

Diamond Points

- Newer drugs in asthma
- Omalizumab—anti IgE
- Mepolizumab—anti IL 5 AB
- Dupilumab—anti IL 4 receptor Ab

CYSTIC FIBROSIS

- Hallmark: Elevated sweat chloride levels >60 mEq/L in two occasions
- Channels affected: Sodium channels, chloride and potassium channels
- Important feature: Mother while kissing her child found her child skin salty tasting
- Patient should be screened for diabetes because there is stagnation of secretions that leads to scarring & damage to pancreas.
- Inheritance: Autosomal recessive condition
- Chromosome: 7 deletion
- Chromosome 5p deletion is seen in cri du chat syndrome
- Gene mutation: CFTR gene
- Hallmark: Sweat chloride levels >60 mEq/L
- Channels: Sodium channels
- Patients should be screened for: Diabetes
- Azoospermia: Yes it can happen
- Organism associated: *H. influenzae*
- If sweat chloride level is not correct, what is the next

  INV: NTPD—nasal transmembrane potential difference

  Clinical features: Respiratory—URTI, LRTI, atelectasis, cough, bronchiectasis, nasal polyp

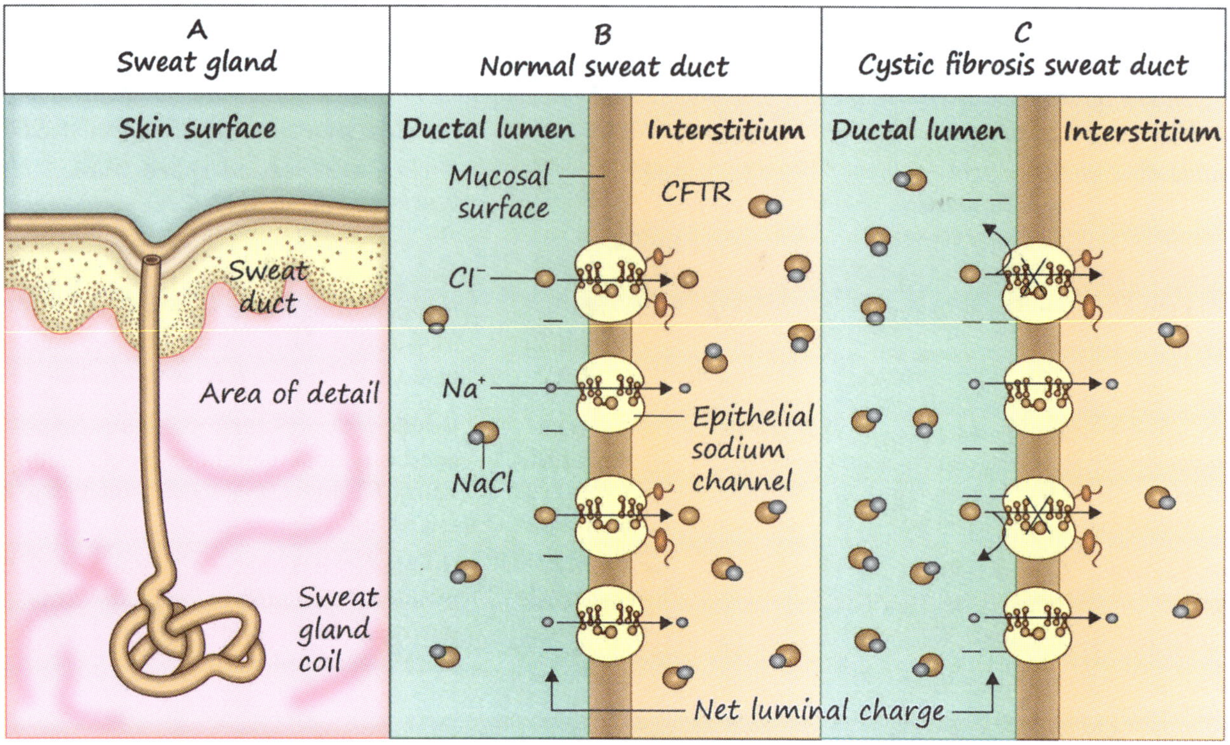

- H. influenzae, S. aureus are the first organisms recovered from lung secretions f/b P. aeruginosa*
- Mortality in cystic fibrosis is due to Burkholderia cepacia
- Genitourinary: Azoospermia, infertility
- Intestinal: Meconium ileus is the most common complication at birth
- Pancreatic: Foul smelling stool
- Medical management:
  - High protein diet
  - Bronchodilators
  - Hypertonic saline
  - Antibiotics
  - Ivacaftor

PNEUMONIA

- Normal RR of newborn: 40–60

Who cut off for fast breathing?

- 0–2 months RR >60 cpm
- 3 months–1 year RR >50 cpm
- 1–5 years RR >40 cpm
- Pneumonia: Fast breathing with or without chest indrawing
- Severe pneumonia: With danger signs like
- Refusal to feed
  - Lethargy
  - Seizures
  - Shock

	Typical pneumonia	Atypical pneumonia
Prodrome	Short (<2 days)	Atypical pneumonia
Fever	High (>102°F [38.9°C])	Long (>3 days)
Chest radiograph	One distinct lobe Involved	Diffuse or multilobe involvement
Etiology	Streptococcus pneumoniae	Mycoplasma, chlamydia spp
Antibiotic	Ceftriaxone, broad spectrum	Macrolides (e.g., azithromycin), doxycycline, or certain fluoroquinolones (e.g., levofloxacin, moxifloxacin)

"You are your only hope, do something magical."

4. PEDIATRIC CARDIOLOGY

"You will not always be motivated, so you must learn to be disciplined."

Important Points

- **Most common congenital heart disease:** Ventricular septal defect.
- **Most common cyanotic congenital heart disease:** ventricular septal defect.
- **Most common cyanotic congenital heart disease at day of life 1:** Transposition of great arteries (TGA).
- **Most common cyanotic congenital heart disease after day of life 1:** Tetralogy of Fallot (TOF).

TETRALOGY OF FALLOT COMPONENTS

- R: Right ventricular hypertrophy
- A: Atrial septal defect
- P: Pulmonary stenosis

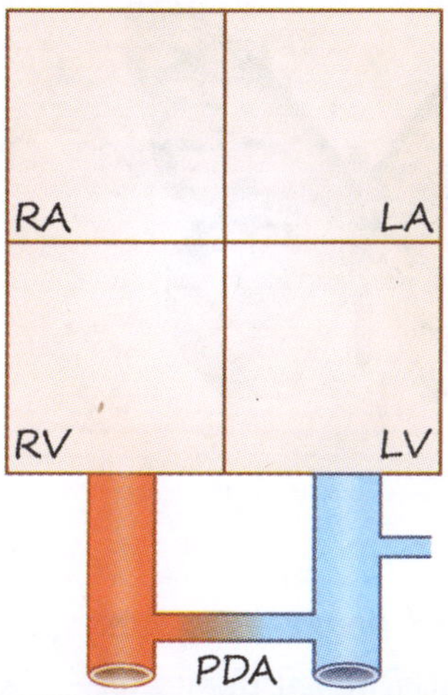

- **Tetralogy of Fallot (boot shape) components:**
  - Right ventricular hypertrophy
  - Ventricular septal defect
  - Overriding of aorta
  - Progressive pulmonary stenosis
- **Pentalogy:** Components of TOF + ASD

Imp PYQs

Q. Which test is done to rule out CVS cause of cyanosis from respiratory cause of cyanosis?

Ans: Hyperoxia Test

Basic Points

- Best limb to detect the preductal saturation is right upper limb.
- Anterior chest wall overlying the heart is known as precordium.
- Right heart border is formed by SVC + right atrium + IVC.

- Pectus excavatum and carinatum

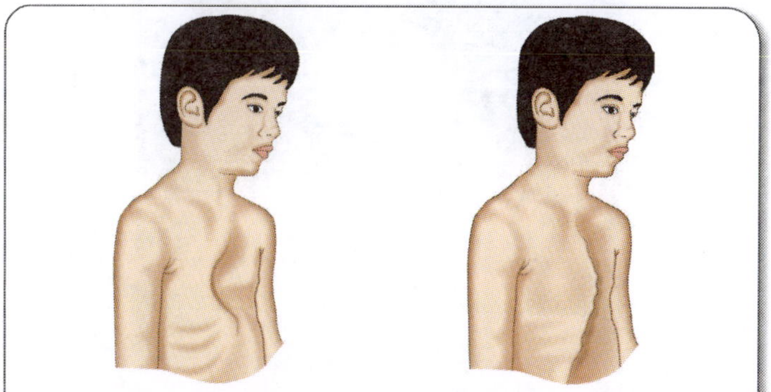

Pectus excavatum Pectus carinatum

Apical Impulse

Definition: It is the outermost and lowermost definitive palpable outward thrust of cardiac impulse in the lower precordium.

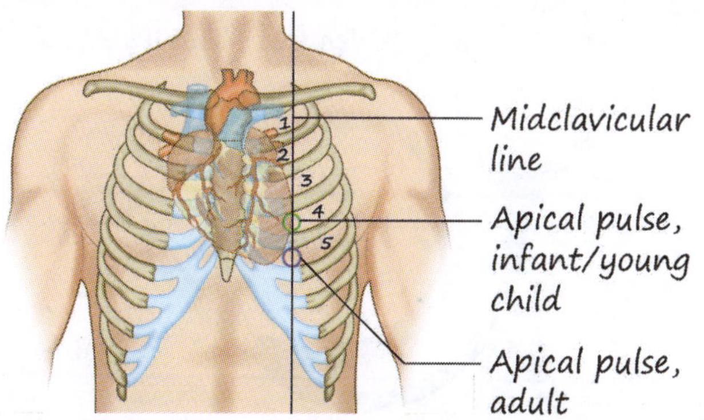

Causes of Shift to Right

- Dextrocardia
- Kartagener syndrome
- Congenital lobar emphysema
- CCAM—Cong. cystic adenomatoid malformation

Types of Apical Impulse

Absent apical impulse is seen in:

- Dextrocardia
- Behind a RIB
- Obesity
- Pericardial effusion
- Dilated cardiomyopathy

Hyperdynamic impulse is seen in:

- Thin chest wall
- High cardiac output states
- PDA, VSD, AR, MR

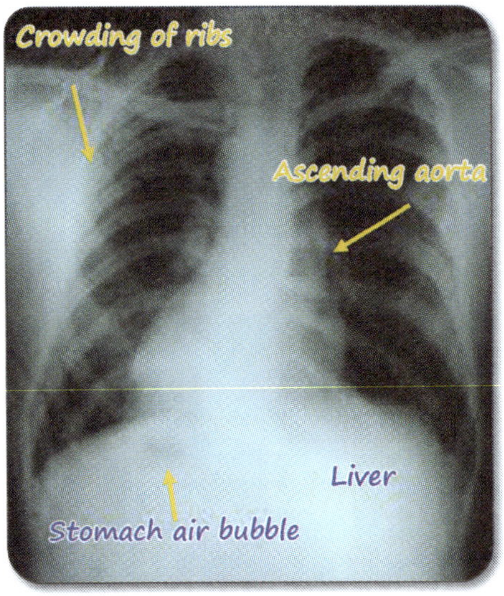

Dextrocardia

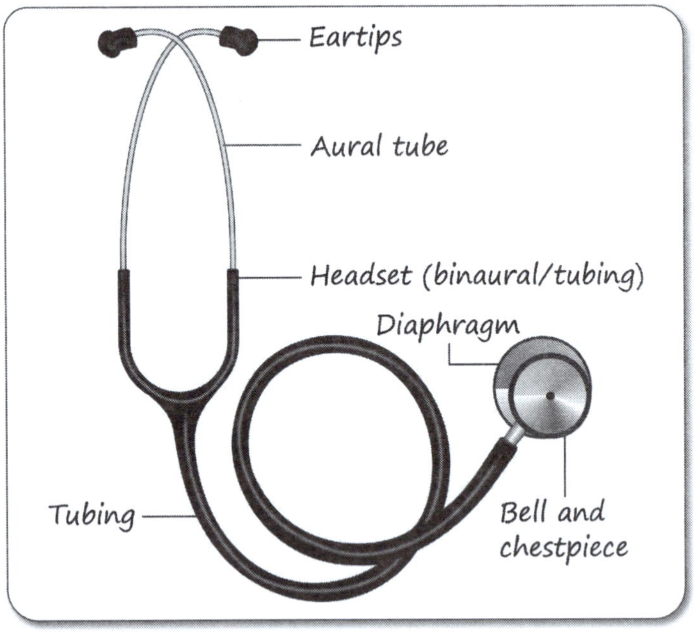

Syndrome	Most common congenital heart disease associated
Down syndrome	Ostium primum ASD
MCC type of ASD	Ostium secundum type of ASD
Holt-Oram	Ostium secundum type of ASD
Lutembacher	Ostium secundum type of ASD
IDM	Ventricular septal defect
Noonan	Pulmonary stenosis
Alagille	Pulmonary stenosis
Rubella	Patent ductus arteriosus
Marfan	Mitral valve prolapse
RHD	Mitral valve—most common
William	Supravalvular aortic stenosis
Turner	Bicuspid aortic valve

ALAGILLE SYNDROME BUTTERFLY-SHAPED VERTEBRAE

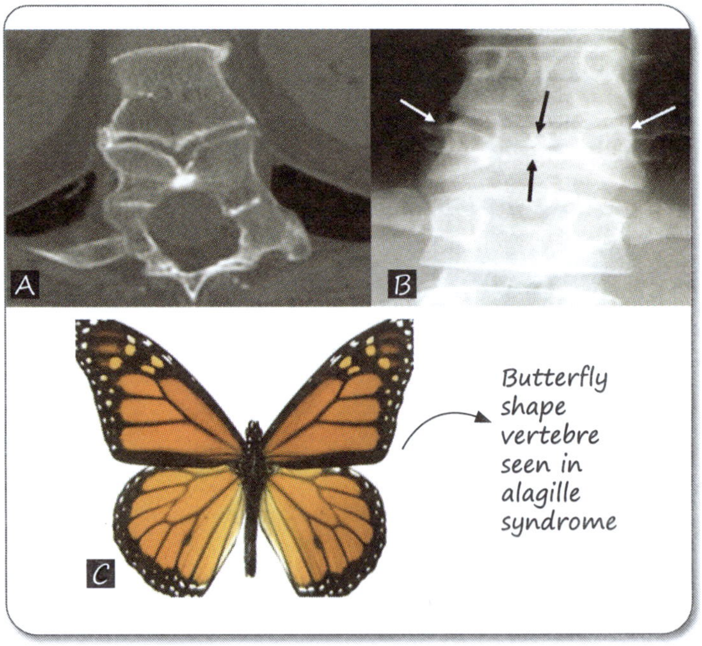

Shape of Heart

- Boot-shaped heart—Tetralogy of Fallot (TOF).
- Egg on string appearance—Transposition of great arteries (TGA)
- Snowman/figure of 8 appearance—supracardiac TAPVC
- Figure of 3—COA** NEET
- Heart condition where you will see white out lung—infracardiac TAPVC (total anomalous pulmonary venous connection)
- Scimitar sign—PAPVC (partial anomalous pulmonary venous connection)
- Box-shaped heart—Ebstein anomaly (Lithium* exposure)
- Goose neck sign—Endocardial Cushion defect
- Water bottle-shaped heart—pericardial effusion

FETAL CIRCULATION

- Umbilical cord has 2 arteries and 1 vein.
- Deoxygenated blood enters from the baby to the placenta through umbilical arteries.

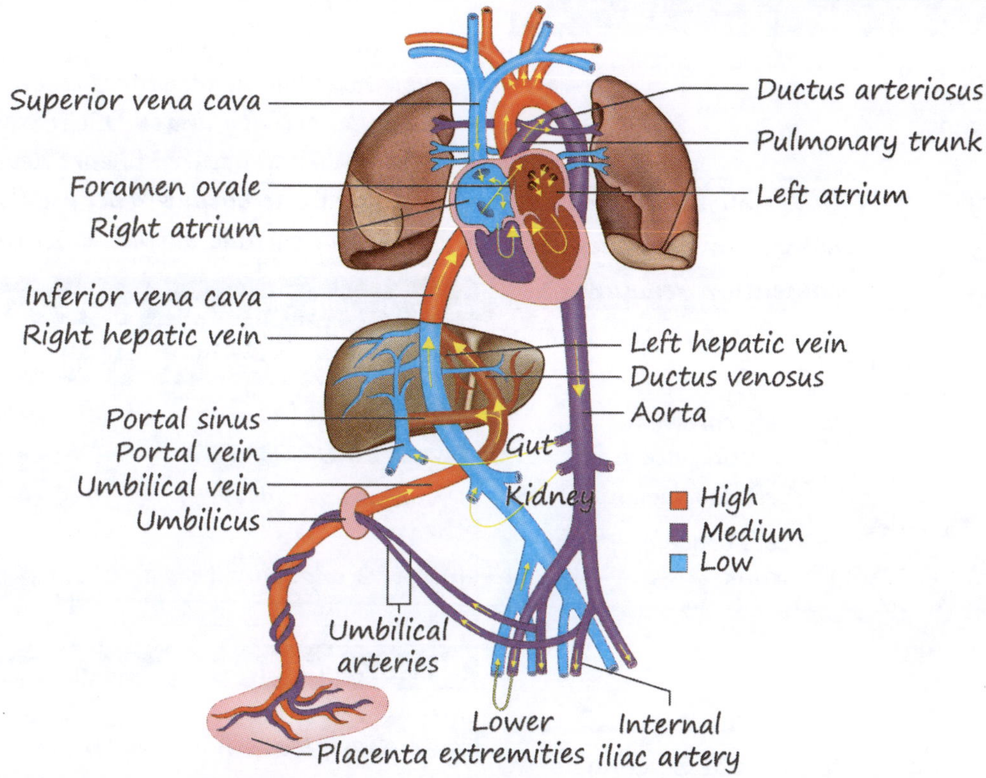

Fetal circulation

- Oxygenated blood enters from the placenta to the baby through umbilical vein.
- Umbilical vein enters the baby and continues as portal vein
- Portal vein continues as ductus venosus followed by IVC
- PVR: Pulmonary vascular resistance increases
- SVR: Systemic vascular resistance decreases
- Flow of ductus arteriosus: Right to left
- IVC blood is more saturated than SVC blood
- Lungs are never working in fetal circulation
- The placenta is the principal site of gas exchange, excretion and acquisition of nutrients
- Factors causing closure of ductus arteriosus: oxygen, bradykinin, cutting of placenta
- If a patient has single artery-single vein we should rule out: Renal agenesis

	Functional closure	Anatomical closure
Ductus venosus	After removal of placenta/ umbilica l cord clamp	7 days
Foramen ovale**	During breastfeeding	Months – years
Ductus arteriosus	10–15 hours	10–21 days

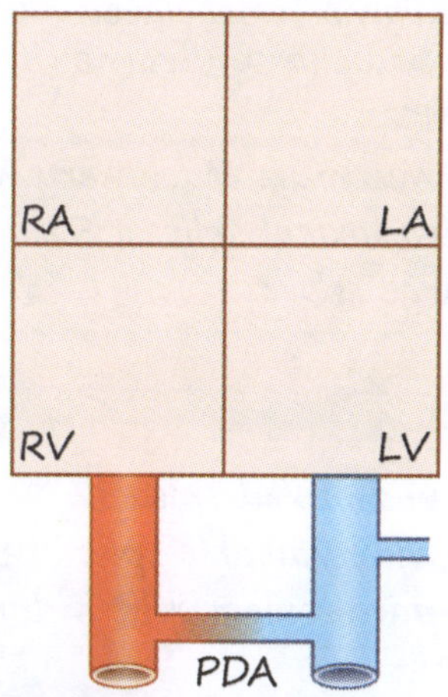

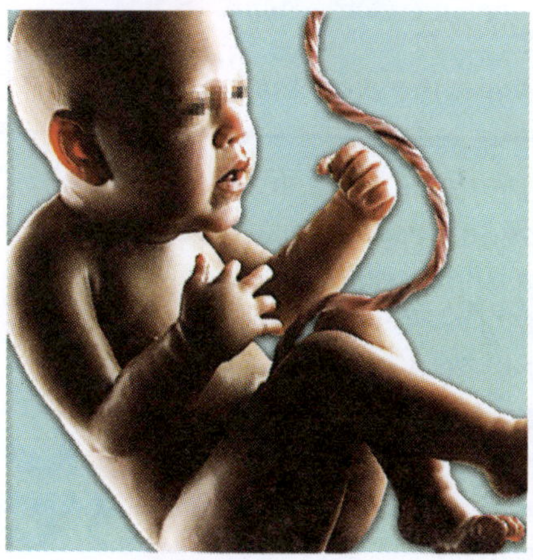

Fetal circulation

Structure	Remnant
Ductus arteriosus function 10–15 hours, anat. 10–21 days	Ligamentum arteriosum
Umbilical artery	Medial umbilical ligament
Umbilical vein	Ligamentum teres hepatis
Ductus venosus	Ligamentum venosum

PATENT DUCTUS ARTERIOSUS

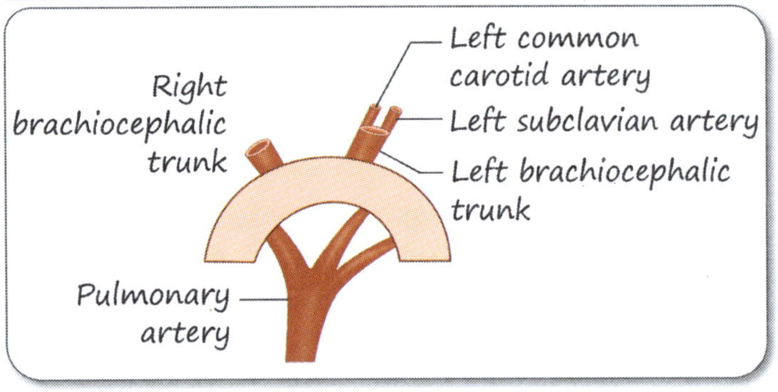

Present with pulmonary artery and descending aorta

Please Note

- More common in females and high altitudes
- One syndrome associated with PDA is Congenital rubella syndrome findings:
    - Loud M1
    - Shunt murmur: Machinery murmur
    - S2: Paradoxical split of S2
    - S3: Large shunt

Crystal Points

- ASD S2—wide fixed split S2
- VSD S2—wide variable split of S2
- PDA S2—paradoxical split in large PDA

Clinical Features

- Hyperdynamic circulation
- Bounding pulses
- Easily palpable dorsalis pedis artery
- Wide pulse pressure >25 mm Hg
- Hyperactive precordium (visible pulsation is >2 rib spaces)
- Ejection systolic murmur
- Persistent tachycardia
- Gold standard IOC: ECHO
- Medical management: Iburprofen/indomethacin/paracetamol
- Surgery: Coil embolization

- I want to keep the PDA open: Alprostadil
- PDA is plethoric lung field condition
- Fetal cardiac heart starts to beat by: 3 weeks
- Cardiac activity under USG is seen by: 6 weeks
- 4 chamber structure of heart develops by: 6 weeks
- Fetal cardiac output: 450 mL/kg/min
- Neonatal cardiac output: 350 mL/kg/min

Left to right shunt–name and clinical features	Right to left shunt–name and clinical features
ASD, VSD, PDA	Pulmonary stenosis
Features: URTI, LRTI	Tricuspid stenosis
Pneumonia, failure to thrive	Ebstein anomaly
Infective endocarditis	Features: Polycythemia + brain abscess

Oligemic lung fields	Plethoric lung fields
Means decreased pulmonary blood flow	Means increased pulmonary blood flow
	For example: ASD, VSD, PDA

GRADES OF MURMUR

Grade	Description
Grade I	Very faint, may only be heard by an expert, not heard in all positions, no thrill
Grade II	Soft, heard in all positions, no thrill
Grade III	Moderately loud, no thrill
Grade IV	Loud and associated with a palpable thrill
Grade V	Very loud, with thrill, heard with the stethoscope partly off the chest
Grade VI	Loudest, with thrill, heard with the stethoscope entirely off the chest (just above the precordium, not touching the skin)

BASIC CONCEPTS OF LEFT TO RIGHT SHUNT

- Common in females.
- They present with features of CCF @ 6 weeks of life.
- Left to right shunt means plethoric lung fields.
- Means more signs of URTI/LRTI leading to infective endocarditis.
- Complication: Reversal of shunt, pulmonary hypertension, Eisenmenger syndrome.

- Reversal of shunt is most commonly associated with PDA F/B VSD and very less likely in the case of ASD

ASD—ATRIAL SEPTAL DEFECT

Most common type is: Ostium secundum
Type Findings:
Loud M1

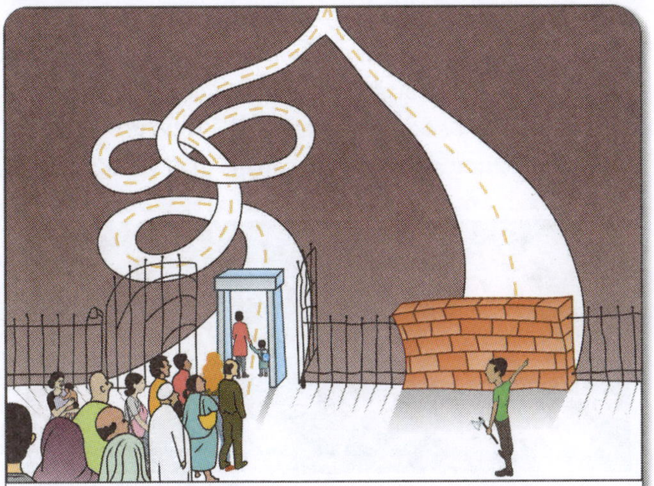

"An idea can change your life."

Parasternal Heave

- Primary murmur—Pulmonary—ejection systolic
- Secondary murmur—Tricuspid—delayed diastolic
- Shunt murmur: Absent
- Wide fixed split of S2

Please Note
It is rare to see failure in ASD

Treatment

- **Rx:** Asymptomatic cases—Rx not required
- **Indication for surgery:** All symptomatic and asymptomatic with a (Qp:Qs) ratio of at least 2:1 (Pulmonary blood: Systemic blood ratio)
- **Pearls:**
  - Ostium primum—left axis deviation
  - Ostium secundum* (most common)—right axis deviation

SYNDROMES ASSOCIATED WITH RADIAL DEFICIENCY

- **H** : Holt-Oram syndrome
- **T** : TAR syndrome (thrombocytopenia absent radius)
- **V** : VACTERL anomalies
- **F** : Fanconi anemia

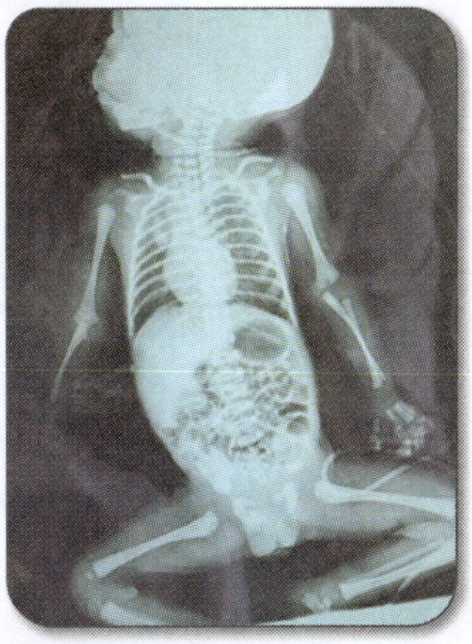

Holt-Oram Syndrome

- Thumb absent, TBX 5 gene mutation
- Ostium secundum ASD present
- Autosomal dominant
- Surgery for the absent thumb: Pollicization

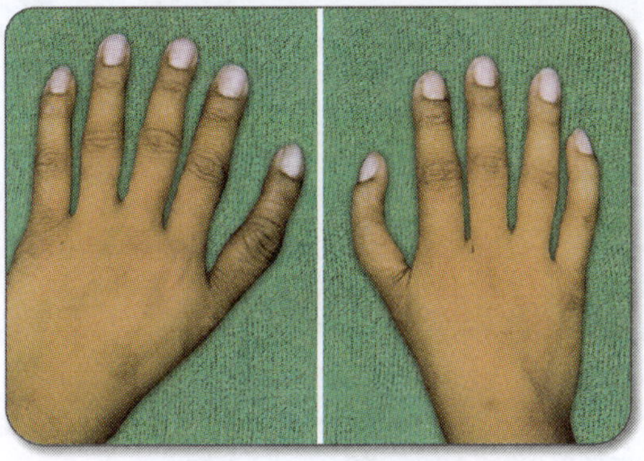

Holt-Oram syndrome

TAR Syndrome

- Thrombocytopenia-absent radius syndrome
- ASD present
- Autosomal recessive

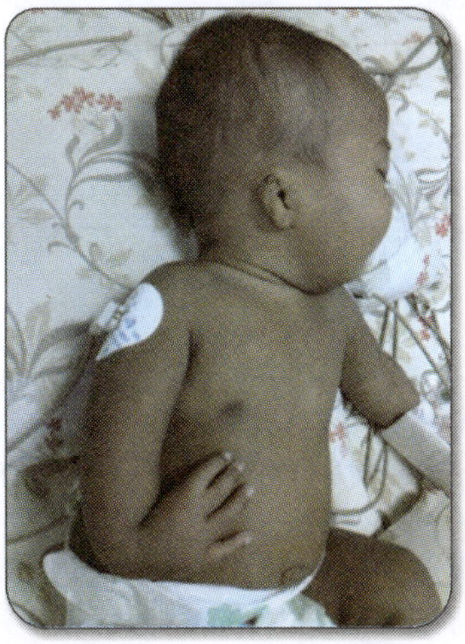

TAR syndrome

Fanconi Anemia

- **F** : Fanconi anemia
- **A** : Absent thumb/abnormality of upper limb
- **N C** : Horseshoe kidney (image)
- **O** : Macrocytic anemia
- **N** : No cells/pancytopenia
- **I** : Intellectual disability
- **S** : Short stature/skin abnormalities

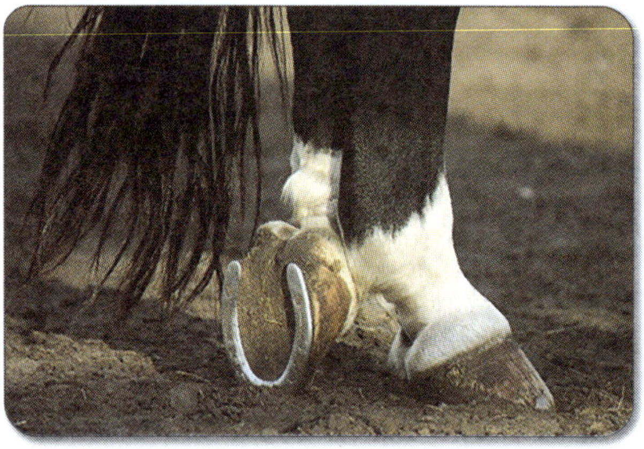

VENTRICULAR SEPTAL DEFECT (VSD)

"Give energy to your dreams."

- **Which is the most common congenital heart disease in cardiology?** VSD
- **Most common type of VSD:** Perimembranous f/b muscular
- **Most common congenital heart disease affected by infective endocarditis is:** VSD
- Patients of VSD becomes symptomatic by 6–10 weeks
- **Clinical features:**
    - URTI
    - LRTI
    - Dyspnea on exertion
    - Palpitations
    - Not gaining weight/height
    - FTT
    - Infective endocarditis
- Shunt murmur: Pansystolic murmur
- Flow murmur @ pulmonary: Ejection systolic
- S2: Wide variable split of S2

Quick Points

- ASD: delayed diastolic murmur in tricuspid valve
- VSD: delayed diastolic murmur in mitral valve

Indication of surgery

Patients >2 years with Qp:Qs ratio is >2:1

TRANSPOSITION OF GREAT ARTERIES (TGA)

"You don't need a new year to make a change, you only need a Monday."

- MC cyanotic congenital heart disease.
- TGA is associated with uncontrolled phenylketonuria in mother.*
- Parallel circulation.
- X-ray: Egg on string appearance.
- Medical treatment: Alprostadil.
- Emergency procedure: Balloon atrial septostomy.
- Definite treatment: Jatene repair.
- Rashkind procedure is done in: Dextro-TGA.
- TGA is a duct dependent congenital heart disease.

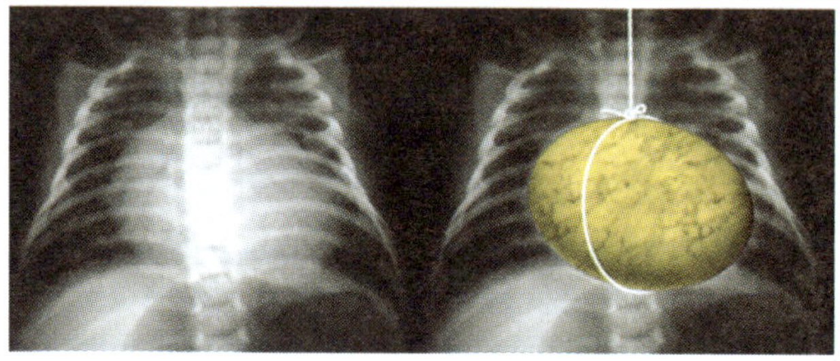
Egg on string appearance — TGA

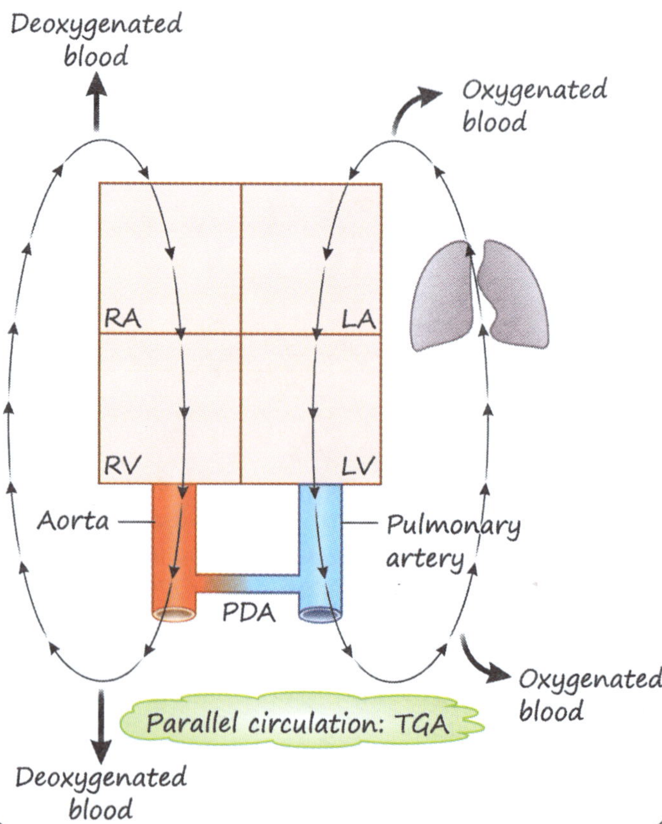

Golden Points

- Norwood procedure is done in: HLHS (hypoplastic left heart syndrome)
- Lutembacher's syndrome: ASD, which is complicated by MS (mitral stenosis)

Differential Cyanosis

- Means lower limbs are > cyanosed than upper limbs.
- For example: PDA with reversal of shunt.

Reverse Differential Cyanosis

- Means upper limbs are > cyanosed than lower limbs.
- For example: TGA with pulmonary hypertension.

Imp PYQs

Q. Calculate the heart rate of the patient.

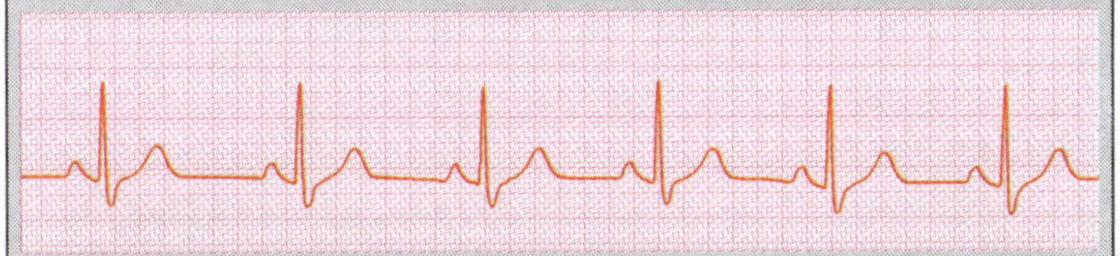

Ans: 1500/no. of small square B/W RR interval.

Ebstein Anomaly

There is downward displacement of tricuspid valve (image)

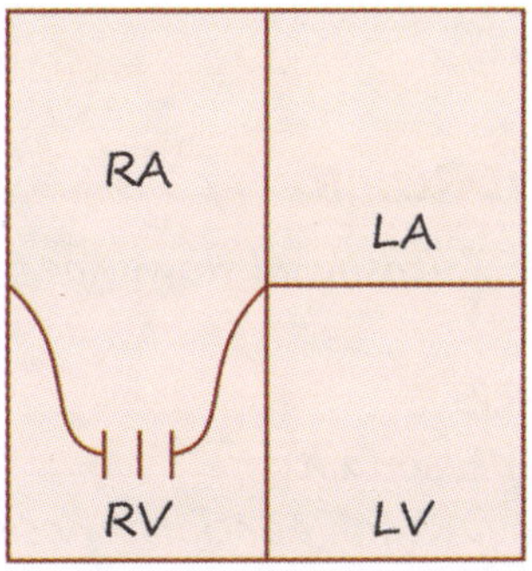

Downward displacement of tricuspid valve: Ebstein anomaly

Therefore RA becomes bigger than the RV.

So, RV will not have that much pressure to push the blood into the pulmonary artery.

That leads to decrease pulmonary blood flow which is also known as Oligemic lung fields (means lung fields with decrease pulmonary blood flow).

As the RA is bigger than RV, if we see ECG: P wave causes atrial contraction, QRS wave causes ventricular contraction

Therefore, we will see tall P waves or HIMALYAN P WAVES.

If the mother has taken LITHIUM during pregnancy, baby can have Ebstain anomaly

Chest X ray: BOX shape heart (image)

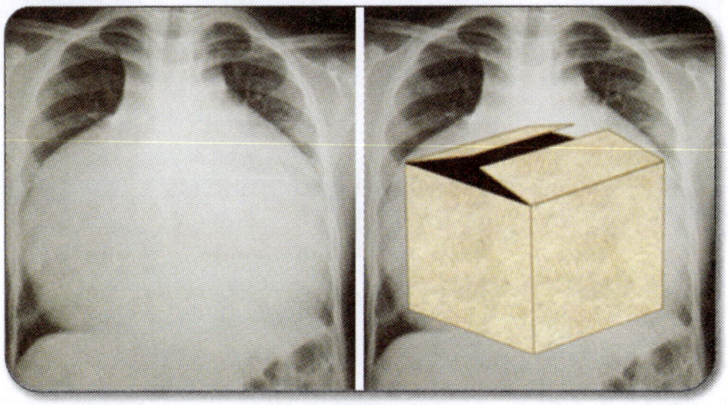

Box shape heart

TAPVC: Total Anomalous Pulmonary Venous Connection

Pulmonary veins instead of joining into left atrium, they get connected into the right side of the heart.

- If the pulmonary veins get connected to the superior vena cava (SVC) that is known as supra cardiac TAPVC (image).

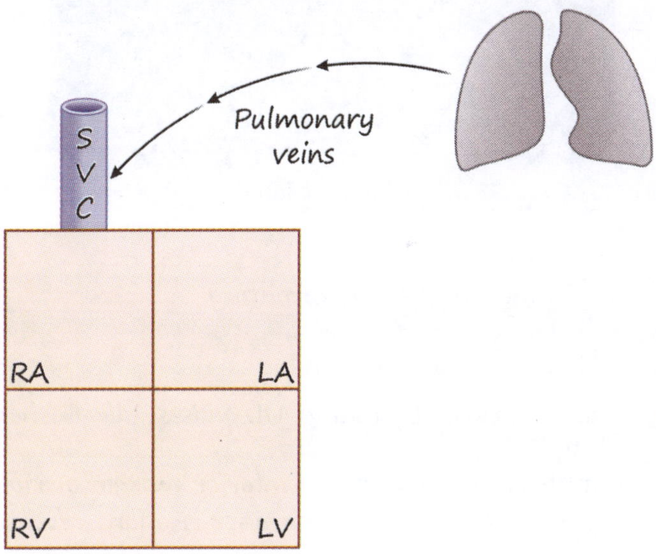

Supracardiac TAPVC

- If the pulmonary veins get connected to the right atrium then that is known as Cardiac TAPVC
- If the pulmonary veins get connected to the inferior vena cava (IVC) that is known as infra cardiac TAPVC

Chest x ray: figure of 8 appearance which is only seen in supra cardiac TAPVC (image attached)

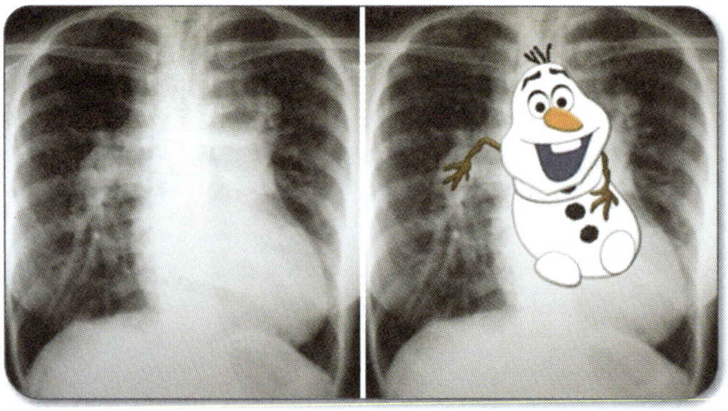

Figure of 8 appearance

Infracardiac TAPVC will present as white out lung on chest x ray.

White out lung is also seen in neonatal respiratory condition known as HMD (hyaline membrane disease) also know as RDS (respiratory distress syndrome) (image attached)

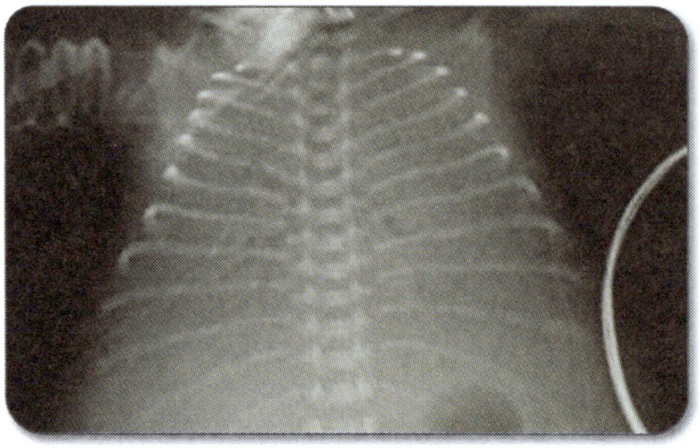

White out lung

- Treatment:
    - Pulmonary venous rerouting

COA: Coarctation of Aorta

- Early feature: Bounding UL pulses, diminished LL pulses.
- Late feature: Notching of inferior margin of ribs.
- X-ray: Figure of 3 appearance, E sign, reverse 3 sign.

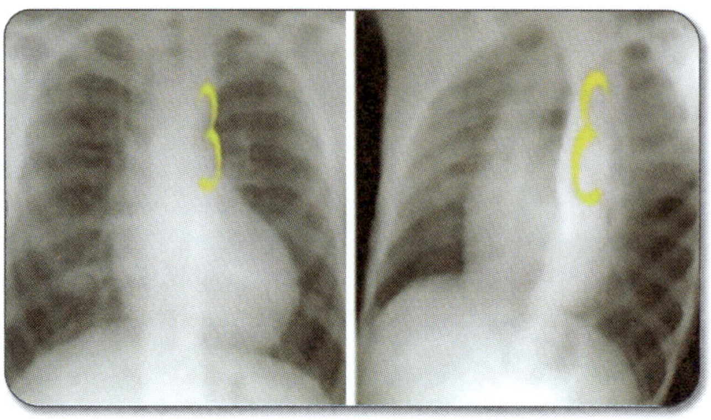

Figure of 3 Coarctation of aorta

NADAS CRITERIA

Major	Minor
Systolic murmur grade 3 or more	Systolic murmur grade <3
Any diastolic murmur	Abnormal S2
Cyanosis	Abnormal ECG
Congestive heart failure	Abnormal chest X-ray, BP

- Criteria to diagnose a congenital heart: NADAS criteria.
- 1 major + 2 minor should be present

Golden Points

- Heart: White out lung: Infracardiac TAPVC.
- Scimitar sign: PAPVC (partial anomalous pulmonary venous connection).
- Goose neck sign: Endocardial cushion defect.
- Water bottle-shaped heart: Pericardial effusion.
- Duct indepndent congenital heart: Truncus arteriosus.
- Name of the classifications of truncus arteriosus: Collett and Edwards classification.
- Biventricular hypertrophy is seen in truncus arteriosus.

WILLIAM SYNDROME

- Inheritance: Autosomal dominant
- Elfin facies
- Starburst IRIS
- Gregarious personality
- CHD: Supravalvular aortic stenosis

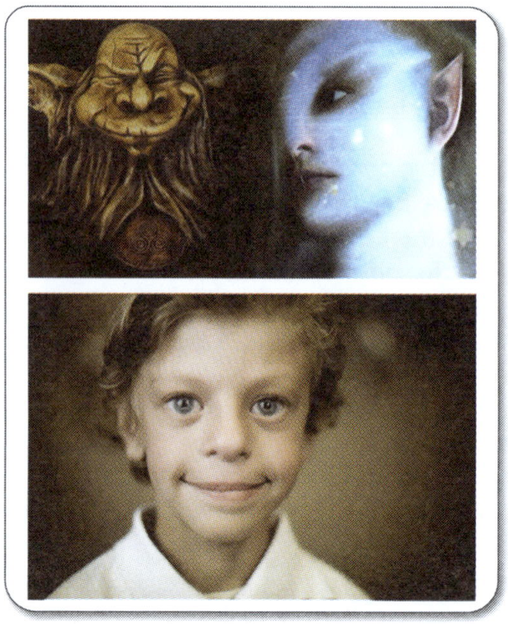

William syndrome

- Hypercalcemia is present
- MC – CHD: Supravalvular aortic stenosis

Examples of autosomal dominant inheritance:

D : Dystrophia myotonica
O : Osteogenesis Imperfecta
M : Marfan syndrome
I : Intermittent porphyria
N : Noonan syndrome
A : Achondroplasia
N : Neurofibromatosis
T : Tuberous sclerosis/Treacher Collins syndrome

Examples of autosomal recessive:

A : Albinism/alkaptonuria
B : Beta thalassemia
C : CAH, cystic fibrosis
D : Deafness
E : Emphysema
F : Friedreich's ataxia
G : Galactosemia, Gaucher disease
H : Homocystinuria

DIGEORGE SYNDROME

C : Cleft lip
A : Abnormal facies
T : Thymic aplasia
C : Cardiac outflow tract defects
H : Hypocalcemia
22 : 22q11 deletion

Extra features: Antimongoloid slant, hypertelorism

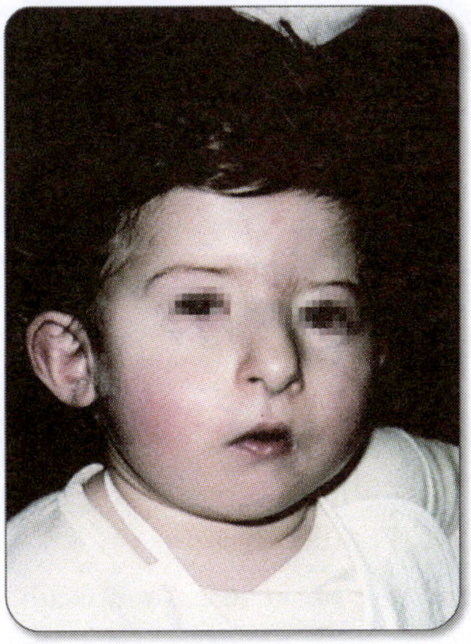

Digeorge syndrome

TETRALOGY OF FALLOT (TOF)

Components

- Right ventricular hypertrophy
- Peripheral pulmonary stenosis
- Ventricular septal defect
- Overriding of aorta

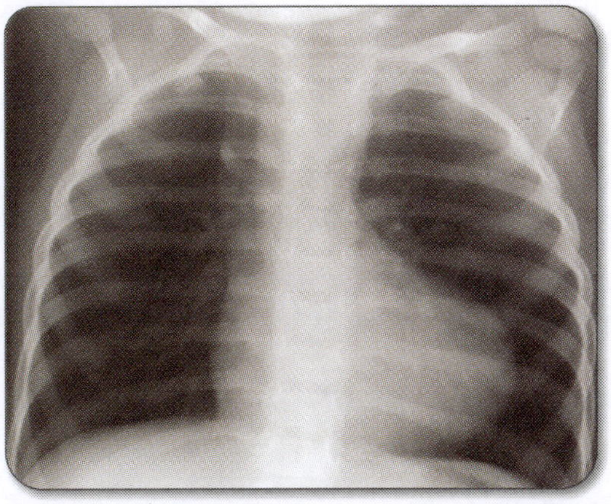

Boot shape heart—TOF

- There is no cardiac enlargement in TOF
- There is concentric right ventricular hypertrophy due to pulmonary stenosis

  Heart sounds:

  S1—normal

  S2—single, only A2 is heard

  P2—soft or inaudible as the pulmonary artery pressure is reduced

Extra Point

TOF patient don't go into failure because the VSD of the TOF is always large enough to allow free exit from the right to left shunt.

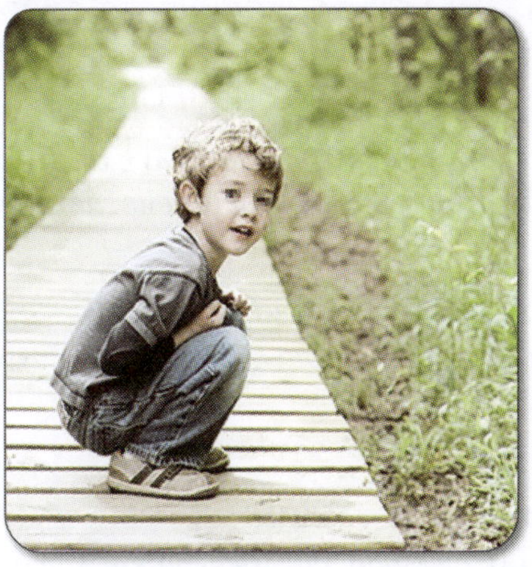

Knee chest position—TOF

TET spell/cyanotic spell in TOF—when baby cries

- There will be infundibular spasm
- Leading to cyanosis
- Leading to more right to left shunt

Treatment

- Knee-chest position.
- It will decrease the venous return from lower limbs to upper limbs.
- That will decrease the blood entering the right side of heart.
- Therefore reducing the infundibular spasm and the right to left shunting.

Treatment of cyanotic spell	
Knee-chest position*	• Increases systemic vascular resistance • Decreases venous return
100% oxygen	Combats hypoxia
IV/SC morphine* 0.1–0.2 mg/kg	Depresses respiratory center
Sodium bicarbonate	Neutralizes acidosis
Beta blocker propranolol 0.5–1.5 mg/kg/dose	Causes vasoconstriction
Methoxamine/ phenylephrine	Alpha agonist-causes vasoconstriction

Shunt surgeries for TOF:

- **Blalock-Taussig shunt:** It connect pulmonary artery to subclavian artery.
- **Waterston shunt:** Pulmonary artery to ascending aorta.
- **Potts shunt:** Pulmonary artery to descending aorta.

CONGESTIVE CARDIAC FAILURE

- **Definition:** Inability of the heart to supply cardiac output to meet the metabolic demands of the body.
- **What is cardiac output?**
  Amount of blood pumped by each ventricle per minute.
- CO = Heart rate* stroke volume.
- **What is stroke volume?**
  Amount of blood pumped by each ventricle with each contraction.

Causes of CCF in Children

- Rheumatic fever (beyond 5 years)
- Rheumatic heart disease
- Systemic hypertension
- Myocarditis

Features of Right Heart Failure

- Periorbital swelling
- Facial puffiness
- Raised JVP
- Tender hepatomegaly
- Ascites/effusion
- Scrotal edema
- Bilateral pitting edema

Features of Left Heart Failure

- Tachycardia
- Tachypnea
- Cough
- Wheezing
- Rales in chest

Features of Either Side

- Cardiac enlargement
- Peripheral cyanosis
- Not gaining weight
- Small volume pulse

Treatment

Reducing the Cardiac Work

1. : Restricting pt activities
2. : Sedatives
3. : Treat fever/anemia/obesity
4. : Mechanical ventilation
5. : Propped up to 30°
6. : Digoxin

Dose of digoxin in a child is?
A. 0.02–0.04 mg/kg
B. 0.04–0.06 mg/kg
C. 0.06–0.08 mg/kg
D. 0.1–0.4 mg/kg

RHEUMATIC FEVER

- Most common heart disease in India
- Rheumatic heart disease (MS is more common than MR)

- *Caused by: Group A beta hemolytic streptococci (GABHS)*
- *Age group: 5–15 years*

Revised Jones Criteria

Major Criteria

Low-risk	Moderate-High-risk
Carditis: Clinical or subclinical	Carditis: Clinical or subclinical
Arthritis: Polyarthritis only	Arthritis: Monoarthritis, polyarthritis, polyarthralgia
Chorea	Chorea
Erythema marginatum Subcutaneous nodules	Erythema marginatum Subcutaneous nodules

Minor Criteria

Low-risk	Moderate-High-risk
Polyarthralgia	Monoarthralgia
Fever (>38.5°C)	Fever (>38.0°C)
ESR > equal to 60 mm in the first hour; CRP > equal to 3.0 mg/dL	ESR > equal to 30 mm in the first hour; CRP > equal to 3.0 mg/dL
Prolonged PR interval, (unless carditis is a major criterion)	Prolonged PR interval, (unless carditis is a major criterion)

Treatment

Carditis with congestive cardiac failure:	Corticosteroids 2 mg/kg/day for 3 weeks** then taper next 9 weeks
Carditis without congestive cardiac failure	Steroids (better) or aspirin
No carditis	Aspirin 90–120 mg/kg/day for 10 weeks then taper next 2 weeks

TRUNCUS ARTERIOSUS

- Instead of 2 main vessels—pulmonary artery and aorta. We have 1 single vessel
- Keeping the PDA open in this case will not be useful

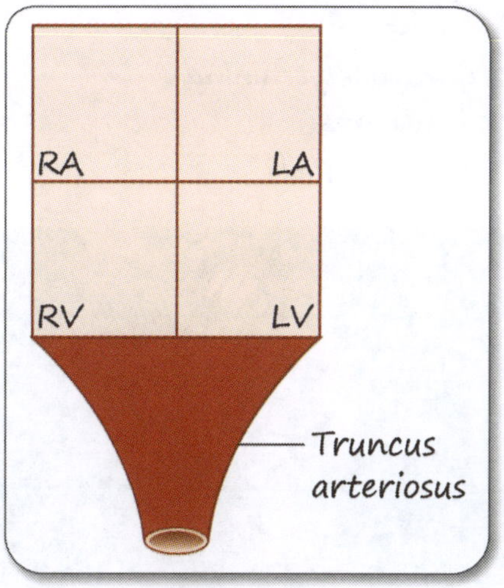

Therefore, truncus arteriosus is a duct independent congenital heart disease

- Mixing of blood is present
- Name of the classification: Collett and Edwards classification
- **Clinical features:**
  - Cyanosis
  - Features of CHF
  - Distress after feeding
  - Failure to thrive
  - Frequent respiratory infections

Extra Points

- Biventricular hypertrophy is seen in truncus arteriosus
- Surgery: Rastelli repair

"If you are not willing for it, then don't complain of not having it."

5. BEHAVIORAL DISORDERS

- Pica
- Bruxism
- Anorexia nervosa
- Bulimia
- Food fussiness
- Difficulty in toilet training
- Temper tantrums
- Breath-holding spells

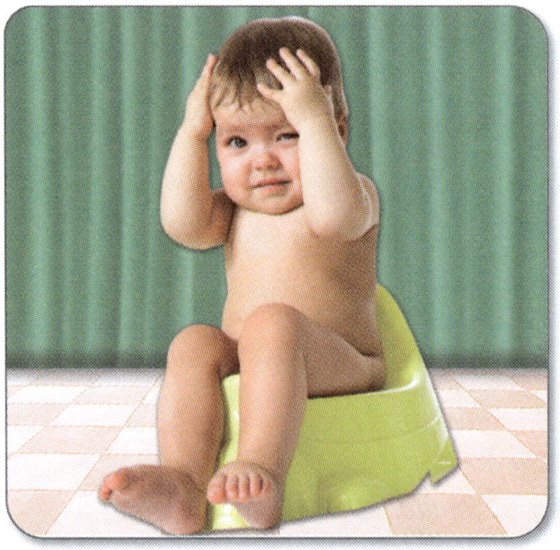

HABIT DISORDER

- Nail biting
- Thumb sucking
- Tics

PICA

Definition: Persistent eating of non-nutritive substances such as Wood, charcoal, paint, lead, earth for at least 1 month in a manner that is inappropriate for the developmental level.

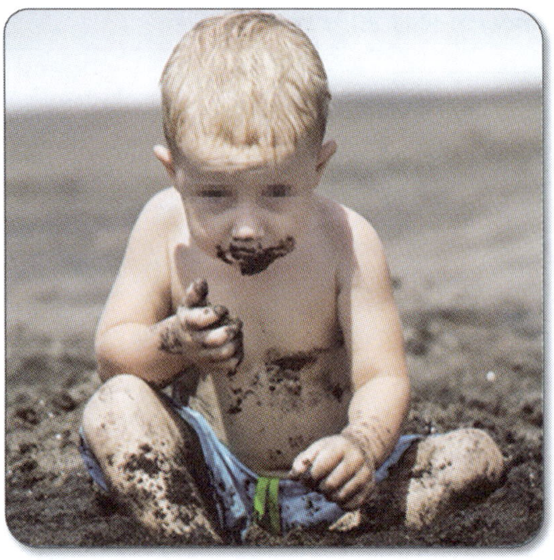

PICA

Common in <5 years

- They are at increased risk of lead poisoning and parasitic infections.
- Treatment:
  - Behavioral modification
  - Deworm the child—albendazole <2 years: 200 mg, >2 years: 400 mg
  - Screen for lead poisoning + give iron.

THUMB SUCKING

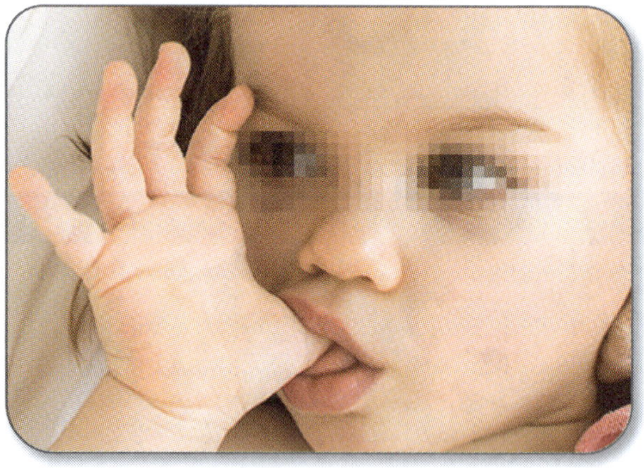

Thumb sucking

- Self-soothing behavior + discharges tension
- Peaks at 18–21 months and disappears by 4 years

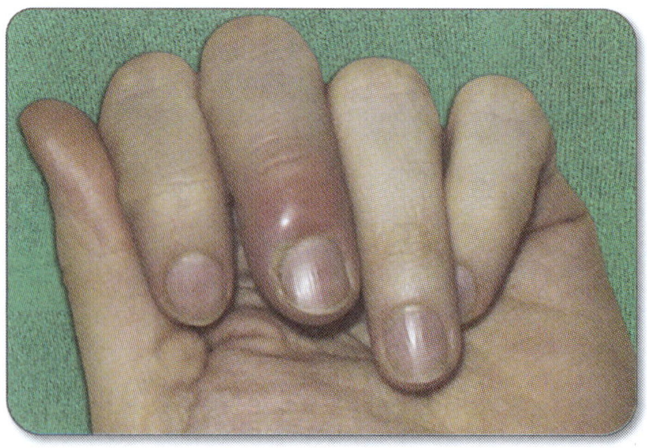

Paronychia

- It can lead to paronychia: Bacterial or fungal infection of the nail

BRUXISM/TEETH GRINDING

Can begin in the 1st 5 years of life associated with day time anxiety can lead to TM joint pain

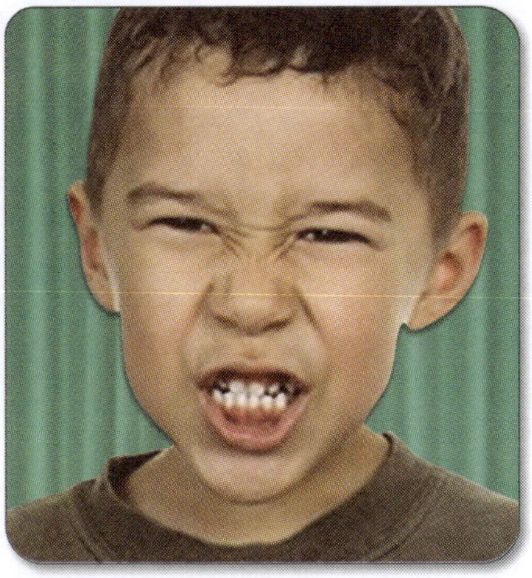

Bruxism

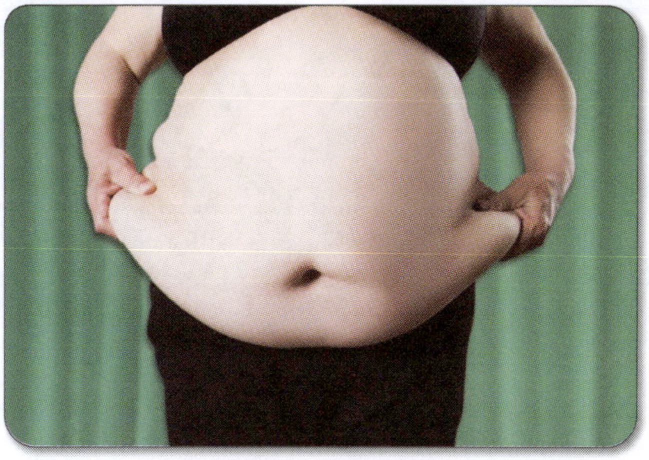

TICS

- Tics are:
  - Abrupt
  - Fast
  - Paroxysmal
  - Nonrhythmic
  - Motor or vocal manifestations

Types

Motor Tics

- Simple motor: Eye blinking, neck jerking, shoulder shrugging
- Complex motor:
  - Foot tapping
  - Echopraxia (imitating others)
  - Copropraxia: Obscene gestures

Vocal Tics

- Simple vocal: Throat clearing, sniffing, coughing
- Complex vocal:
  - Coprolalia—obscene words
  - Echolalia—repeating heard phrases or words
  - Palilalia—repeating own words or phrases
- Rx: Behavior therapy

ANOREXIA NERVOSA

- Age group: 15–19 years/females
- Characteristic features:
  - Intense fear of becoming fat even though the child is underweight
  - Restricted eating
  - Increased physical activity
  - Induced vomiting
  - Use of laxatives

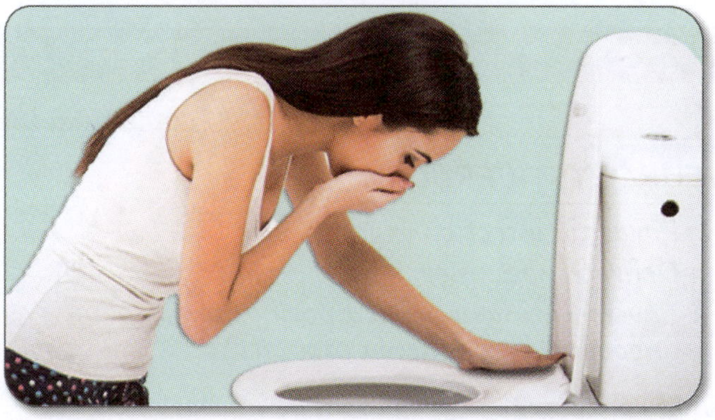

- Complications
  - Secondary amenorrhea
  - Malnutrition

BREATH HOLDING SPELLS

- Reflex events
- Triggered by provocation, anger, pain, frustration
- When the child cries—at full expiration child becomes apneic, cyanotic, becomes pale, f/b loss of consciousness, GTCS.
- Age group: Rare before 6 months, peak at 2 years and stops by 5 years.
- Treatment: Reassurance.
- Tell the family to remain calm during the event.

NOCTURNAL ENURESIS

- **Definition:** Enuresis is defined as normal, nearly complete evacuation of the bladder at the wrong place and time at least twice a month after 5 years of age.
  - **Types:**
    - Primary: Patient was never dry by night
    - Secondary: Loss of control after initial bladder control for 6 months or more
  - If 1 parent has +ve, then each child has 44% risk of nocturnal enuresis

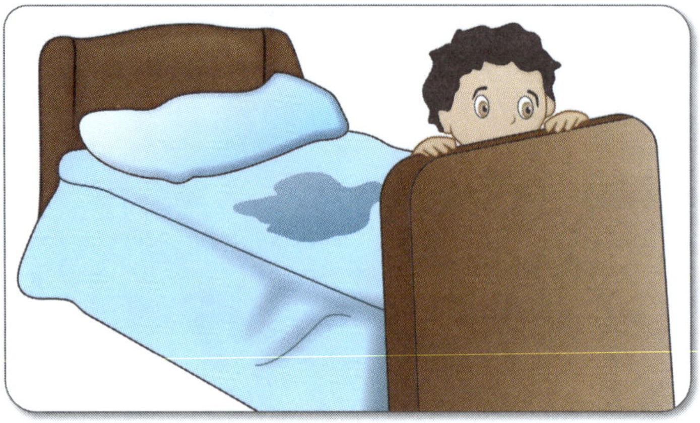

Nocturnal enuresis

- If both parents are +ve: each child has 77% risk of nocturnal enuresis
- Rx: Reassurance
- Fluid intake restricted after 6 am
- Caffeine, sugar avoid after 4 am
- Void bedtime
- Toc: Motivation/alarm therapy
- Doc: Desmopressin

6. CENTRAL NERVOUS SYSTEM

"People who hate me, motivate me."

NEUROCYSTICERCOSIS

- Parasitic infection
- Definite host: Man
- Cause: Eating uncooked pork (Taenia solium) and uncooked beef (Taenia saginata)

What is scolex?

- Head of the tapeworm
- Hallmark of NCC: Starry sky appearance on imaging
- Treatment: Prednisolone 2 mg/kg/day f/b albendazole

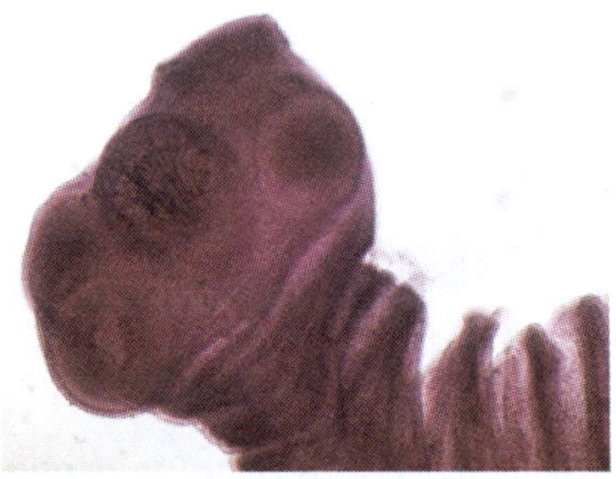

Head of tape worm

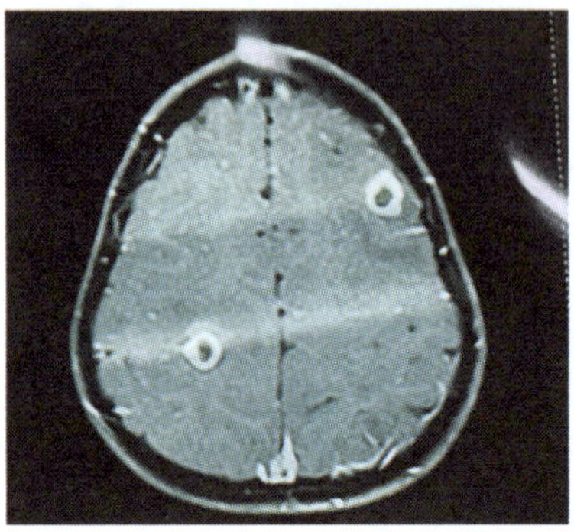

Starry sky appearance

Features	Neurocysticercosis	Tuberculoma
Size	<20 mm	>20 mm
Site	Supratentorial	Infratentorial
Perilesional edema	Mild	Mod/Sev
Midline shift	Less common	More common
Cyst wall	Thin	Thick
Scolex	Present	Absent
Raised ICT	Uncommon	Common
Focal deficit	Uncommon	Common

NEURAL TUBE DEFECT (NTD)

- Neural tube is a hollow structure from which the brain and spinal cord form.
- Incomplete closure of the neural tube results in NTD.
- Most common neurological abnormality in neurology: NTD.
- NTD – multifactorial inheritance.
- Which NTD has best prognosis: Spina bifida.
- Which NTD has worst prognosis: Craniorachischisis.
- Sensitive marker for screening—alpha fetoprotein.
- Specific—acetylcholine esterase level @ 16–18th weeks of POG.
- Treatment: Folic acid to the mother.
  400 µg in the first pregnancy.
  4000 µg if there is previous history of NTD.

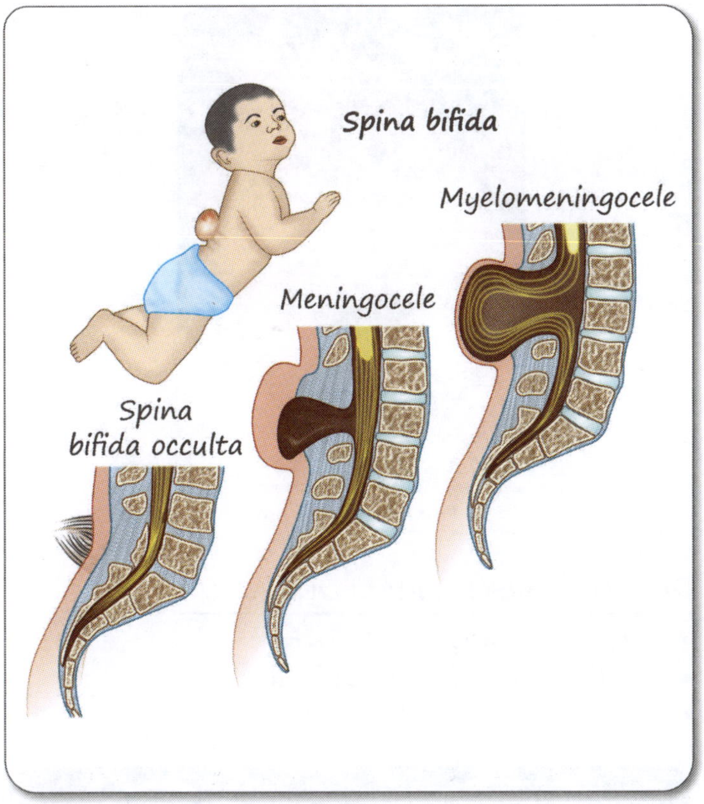

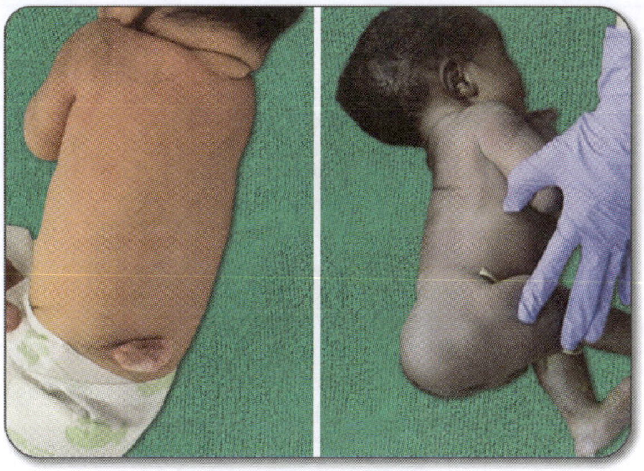

Spina bifida cystica

SPINA BIFIDA OCCULTA

- Spinal cord is normal
- A fluctuant midline mass that might transilluminate

SPINA BIFIDA CYSTICA

- Location: Lumbosacral region*
- Protrusion of both meninges and spinal cord protrude into the skin of back
- Risk of developing: Hydrocephalus
- Banana sign* and lemon sign seen on USG

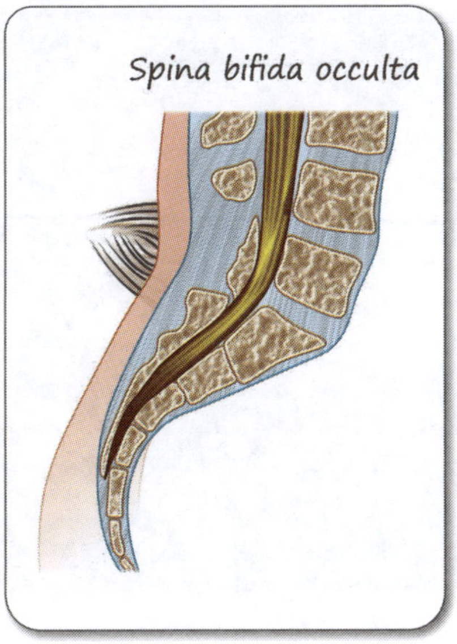

Extra Point

An open abdominal defect should always be covered with gauze piece soaked in normal saline.

Encephalocele

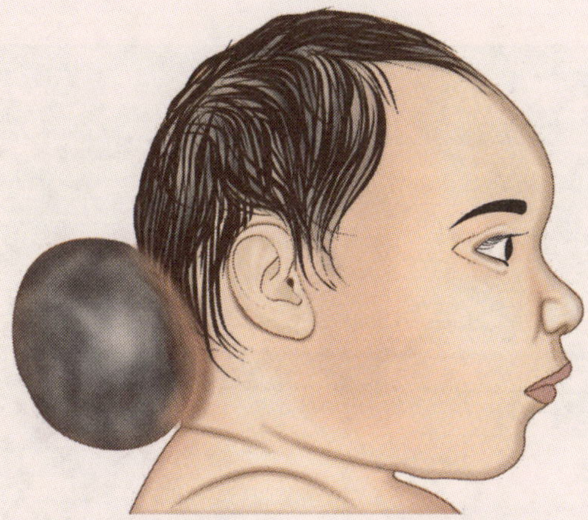

Iniencephaly

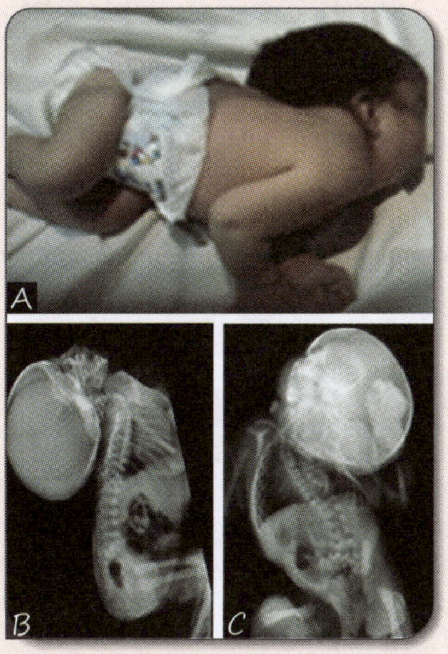

Craniorachischisis

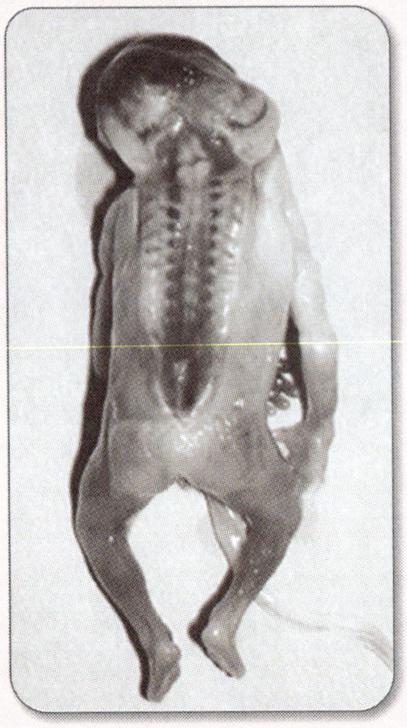

Anencephaly

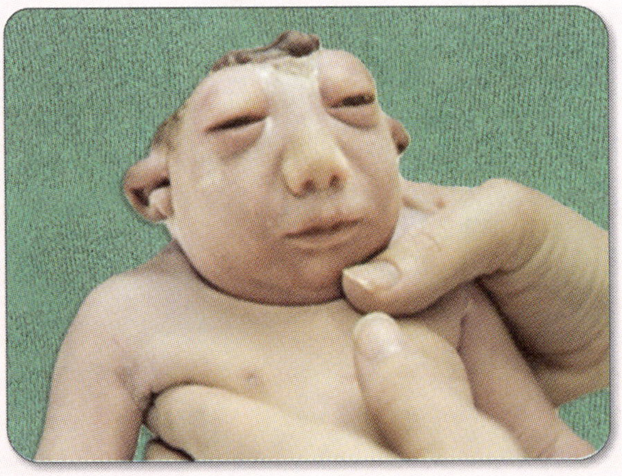

HOLOPROSENCEPHALY/CYCLOPIA/ CYCLOCEPHALY

- It is NOT an NTD
- It is a forebrain anomaly
- Failure of the forebrain to divide into two cerebral hemisphere
- Synophthalmia: Two eyes fused (forming a single eye)
- Single nostril
- Choanal atresia
- Solitary central incisor tooth
- Association with trisomy 18, 13 CHARGE syndrome
- Prenatal diagnosis by USG after 10 weeks POG and fetal MRI gives diagnostic precision
- Syndromes associated: CHARGE syndrome, fetal alcohol syndrome, trisomy 13, 18

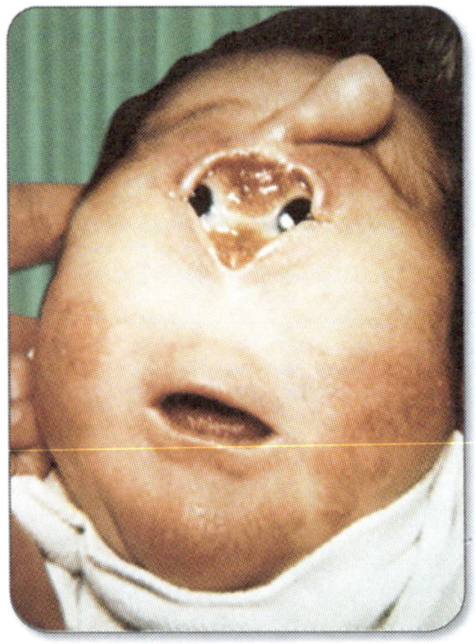

Holoprosencephaly

DANDY-WALKER MALFORMATION

- Cystic expansion of the 4th ventricle
- Midline cerebellar hypoplasia
- 90%—hydrocephalus

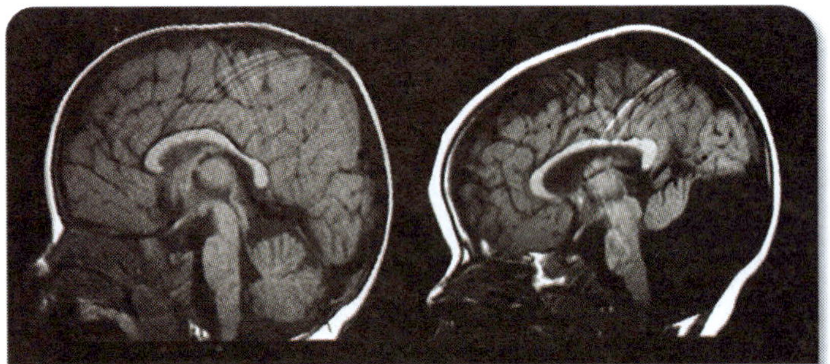

Dandy walker Malformation

VEIN OF GALEN MALFORMATION

Open anterior fontanel and bruit and midline lesion on USG with macrocephaly*

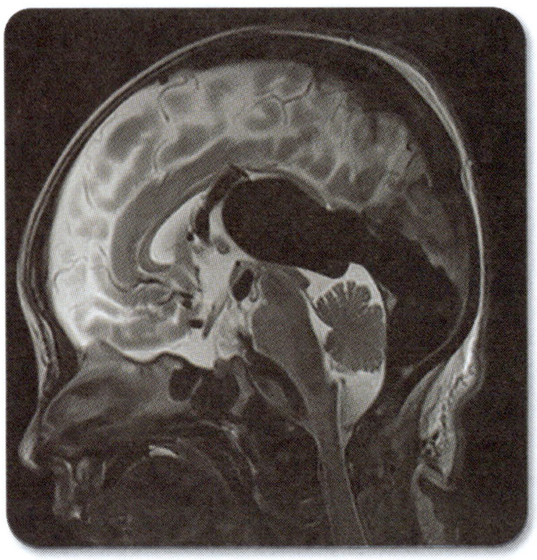

Vein of Galen malformation

ARNOLD-CHIARI MALFORMATION

- In type 1 only cerebellar tonsil extends into the foramen magnum.
- Type 1 produces symptoms during adolescent or adult life and is not associated with hydrocephalus, it is associated with Syringomyelia.
- In type 2 (classic) both cerebellum and brain stem extend into the foramen magnum.
- Type 2 causes progressive hydrocephalus with meningomyelocele.

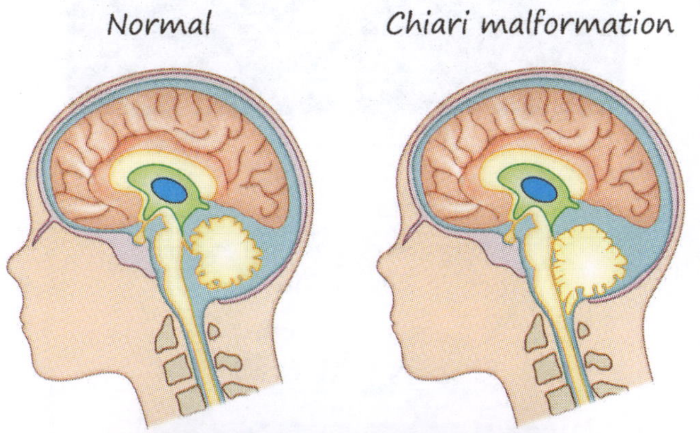

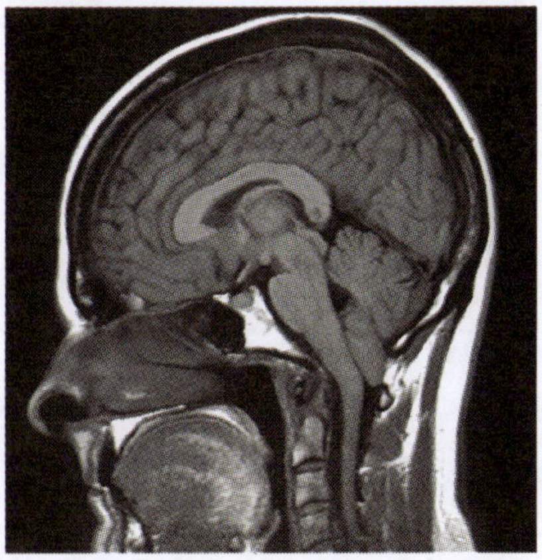

Extra Points

There is no hypoplasia of cerebellar vermis in Arnold-Chiari

- There is herniation of cerebellum
- There is flattened base of skull with small posterior fossa
- Causes of macrocephaly: Mnemonic: ARO water SAVES MY HEALTH

  A : Anemia
  R : Rickets
  O : Osteogenesis imperfecta
  S : Subdural hematoma
  M : Megalencephaly
  H : Hydranencephaly
  H : Hydrocephalus

HYDROCEPHALUS

- There is impaired absorption or circulation of CSF.
- CSF is a clear colorless bodily fluid formed in the ventricular system by the choroid plexus.

Types

Communicating

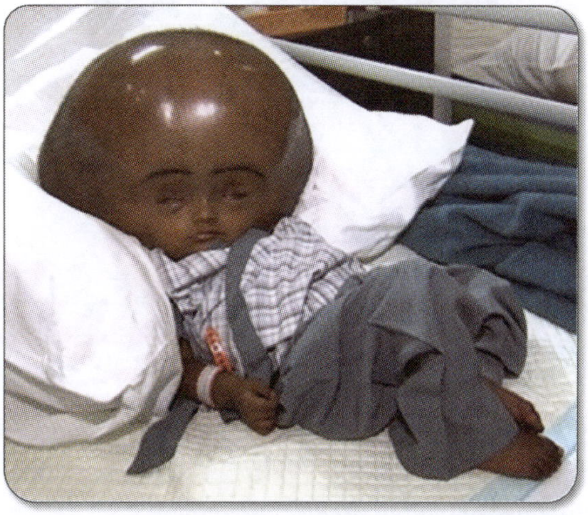

Hydrocephalus

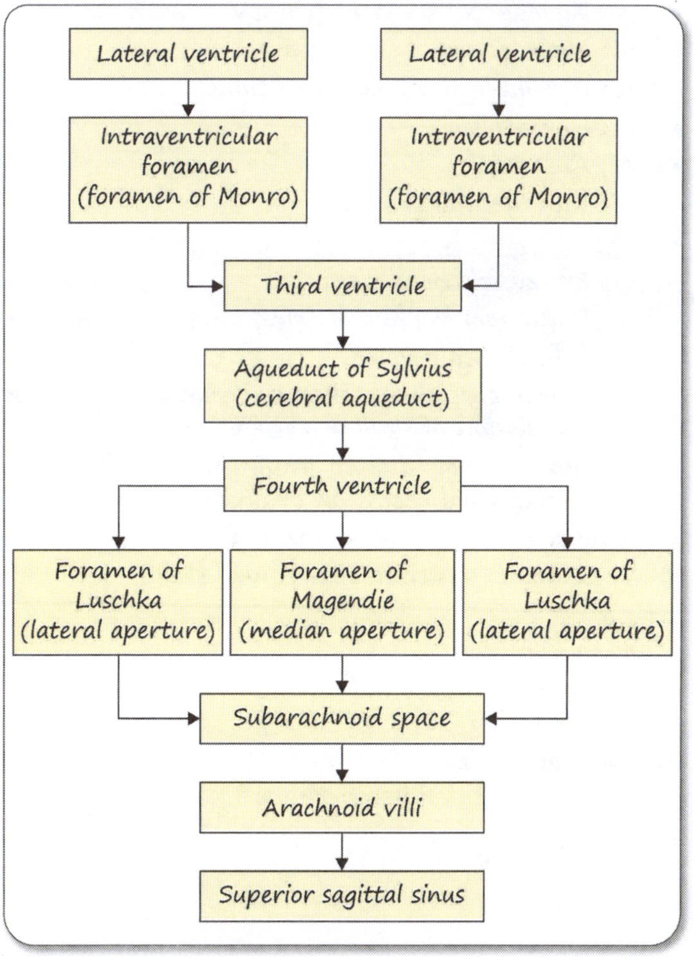

Pathway of CSF flow

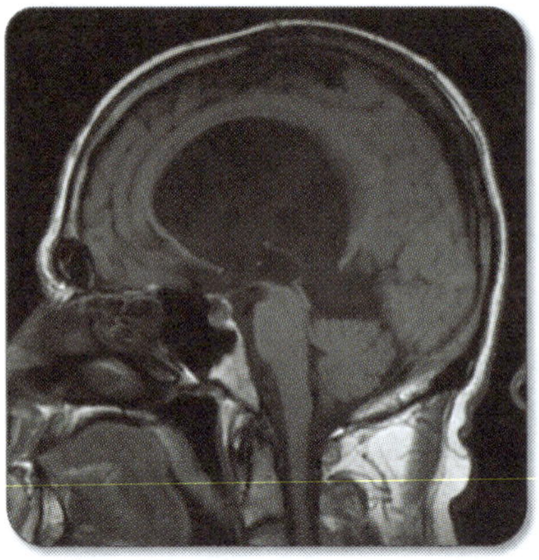

Hydrocephalus

Causes: Mnemonic—CAMP

- C : Choroid plexus papilloma
- A : Achondroplasia
- M : Meningeal malignancy
- P : Posthemorrhagic (most common)

Noncommunicating: Causes—Mnemonic—via Mahad (Mahad is a place in Mumbai)

- V : Vein of Galen malformation
- I : Infection (toxop.)
- A : Aqueductal stenosis* (most common cause)
- M : Mass lesions
- A : Arnold-Chiari malformations
- H : Hematoma
- A : Abscess
- D : Dandy-Walker
- C/f:
  - Increasing head size
  - Wide opening and bulging anteroir. Fontanel
  - Dilated scalp veins
  - Macewen sign/cracked pot sign produced on percussion of skull in raised ICT
  - Sun set sign due to impingement of dilated suprapineal recess on brainstem tectum
- Investigation of choice: Transcranial ultrasound
- Treatment: Ventriculoperitoneal shunt

> **Golden Points**
>
> Transcranial ultrasound is also the investigation of choice in
> - Neonatal seizure
> - Intraventricular hemorrhage

HYDRANENCEPHALY

Cerebral cortex is deficient/hypoplastic in hydranencephaly.

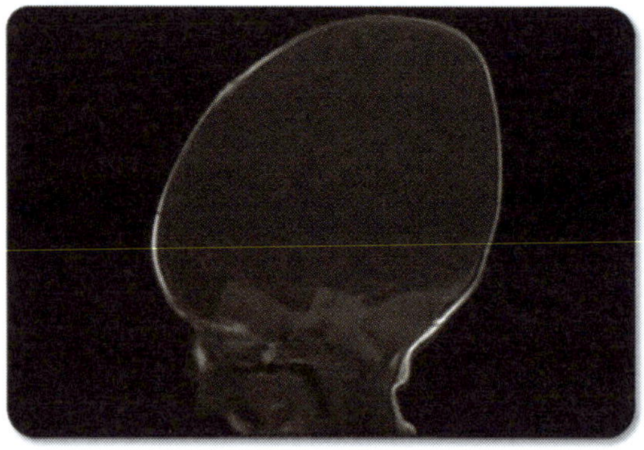

Hydranencephaly

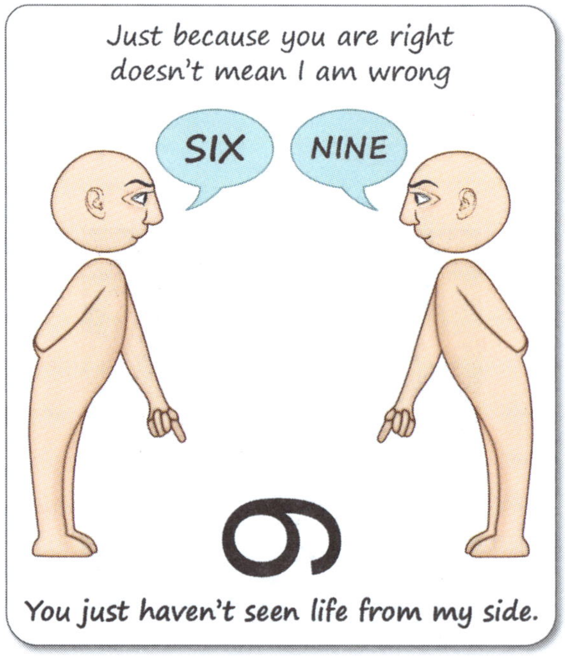
Just because you are right
doesn't mean I am wrong
SIX
NINE
You just haven't seen life from my side.

GLASGO COMA SCALE

Behavior	Response	Score
Eye opening response	Spontaneously	4
	To speech	3
	To pain	2
	No response	1
Best verbal response	Oriented to time, place, and person	5
	Confused	4
	Inappropriate words	3
	Incomprehensible sounds	2
	No response	1

Contd...

Behavior	Response	Score
Best motor response	Obeys commands	6
	Moves to localized pain	5
	Flexion withdrawal from pain	4
	Abnormal flexion (decorticate)	3
	Abnormal extension (decerebrate)	2
	No response	1
Total score:	Best response	15
	Comatose client	8 or <3
	Totally unresponsive	3

Imp PYQs

Q. You are the Doctor in the internal ward at Rajagiri Hospital and you meet Mr Bharath. He responds to strong pain and withdraws his hand, incomprehensible word. GCS:

A. 6 B. 7
C. 8 D. 9

Ans: C. 8

TORCH PROFILE

T : Toxoplasmosis
O : Others
R : Rubella
C : CMV (most common)
H : Herpes

- Which is the most common among all? CMV
- Which one causes recurrent abortions: Syphilis
- Which is the most severe form of intrauterine infection? Rubella
- Which is dangerous in first trimester? Rubella
- Trimester-wise severity of infection:
  - First trimester: Rubella
  - Second trimester: Parvovirus
  - Third trimester: Syphilis, CMV, toxoplasmosis

Congenital Toxoplasmosis

- Triad
  1. Hydrocephalus
  2. Intra cranial calcification (diffuse)
  3. Chorioretinitis* Most common
- Confirmatory test: +ve toxoplasma IgM in serum.
- Maternal RX with spiramycin during pregnancy reduces the risk of transmission significantly.

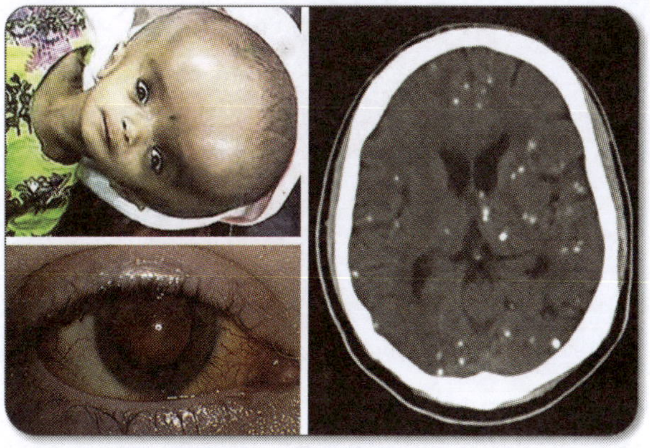

Congenital toxoplasmosis

Imp PYQs

Q. Which of the following agents is likely to cause Cerebral calcification and hydrocephalus in a newborn whose mother has history of taking spiramycin but was not compliant with therapy:

A. Rubella B. Toxoplasmosis
C. CMV D. Herpes

Ans: B. Toxoplasmosis

Congenital Syphilis

- **Early feature:** Syphilitic rhinitis (bloody rhinorrhea)
- **Late feature:** Hutchinson's triad*
  1. Hutchinson teeth
  2. Interstitial keratitis
  3. 8th nerve deafness (sensorineural hearing loss)

Other Features

- Mulberry molars: Multiple rounded rudimentary enamel cusps on the permanent first.
- Clutton's joint, painless joint, swelling-knee

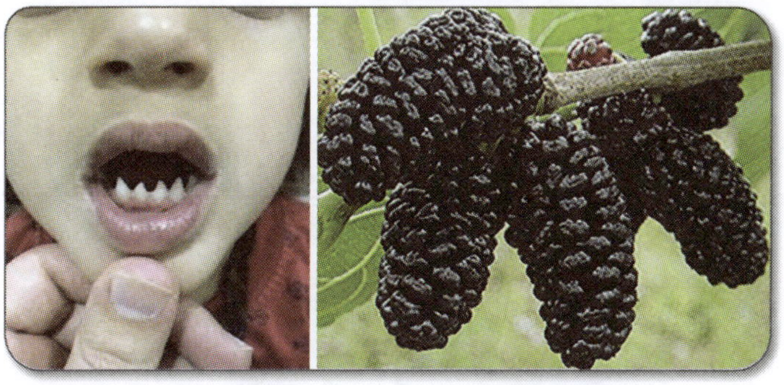

Hutchinson teeth   Mulberry molars

- Higoumenaki's Sign: Thickening of the medial portion of the clavicle
- Diagnosis: IgM-FTA-ABS* NEET

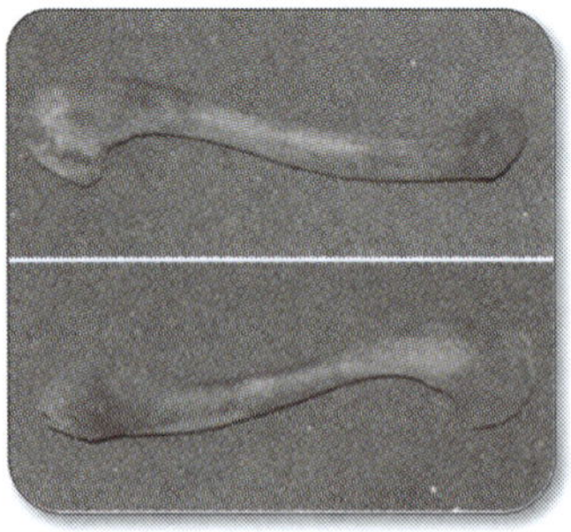

Higoumenaki's sign

Immunoglobulin Flourescent Treponemal Antibody Absorption

- RX: Parenteral penicillin G
- Prenatal screening for syphilis
- Untreated—100% mortality

CONGENITAL VARICELLA SYNDROME

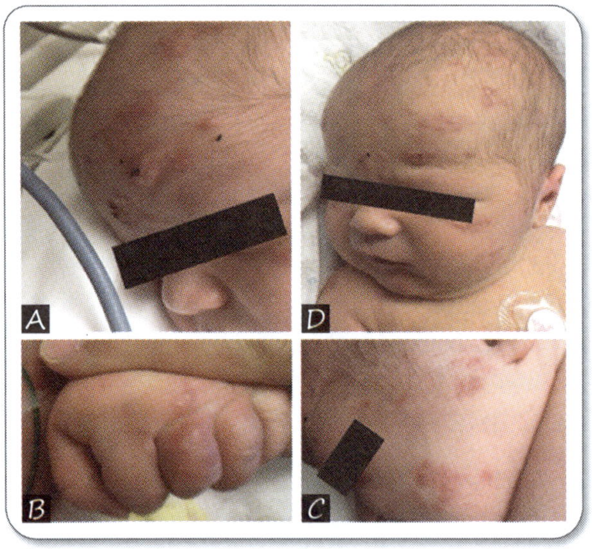

Cicatricial skin lesions

Triad

- Limb hypoplasia
- Cicatricial skin lesions
- H/o fever with rash in end of 1st/2nd trimester
- How to confirm: Anti VZV antibody

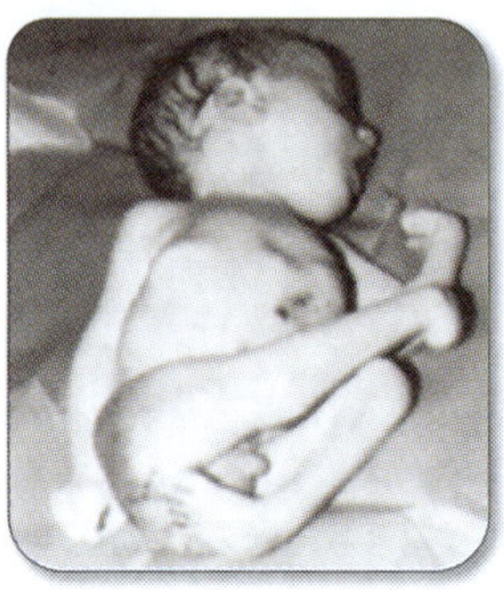

Hypoplasia of lower limb

CONGENITAL RUBELLA SYNDROME/GREGG SYNDROME

Very severe in first trimester

- <11 weeks POG—90% defects
  Triad : MNEMONIC—café coffee day
  - C : Congenital heart disease (PDA*)
  - C : Cataract
  - D : Deafness (most common component)
- Which is the most common cong. Heart in congenital rubella? → PDA
- Least common? → ASD*

Extra Points

- Microcephaly
- Blueberry muffin rash
- Salt and pepper retinopathy
- How do you diagnose congenital rubella?
- IgM antibody in fetal blood**

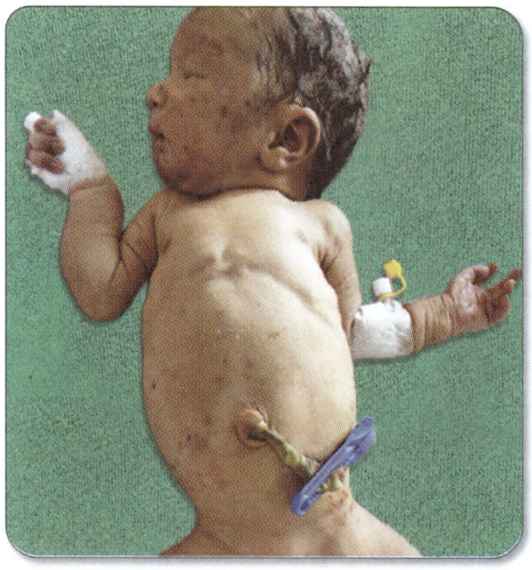

Blueberry muffin rash

CYTOMEGALOVIRUS

- Most common congenital infection among TORCH
- What is its characteristic?
- Periventricular calcification* is characteristic.
- Most common long-term sequelae associated with congenital CMV infection
- Hearing loss
- How to diagnose?
- CMV PCR—best sample is urine**
- Saliva is used in newborn screening test*
- Rx: Ganciclovir or Valganciclovir

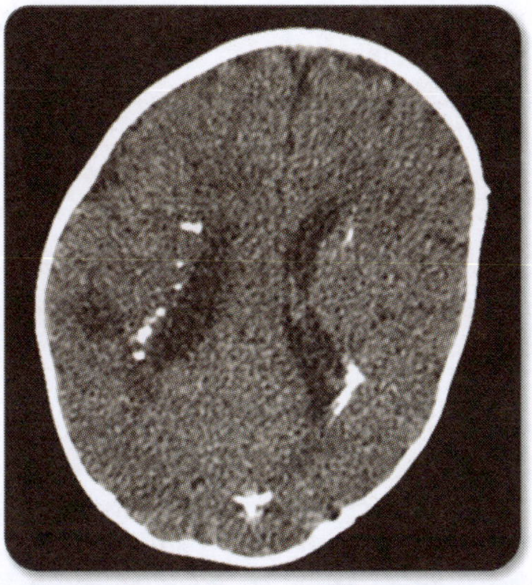

Periventricular calcifications

NEUROCUTANEOUS SYNDROME

"You did not come this far, to go only this far!."

- Neurofibromatosis
- Sturge-Weber syndrome (SWS)
- Tuberous sclerosis complex (TSC)

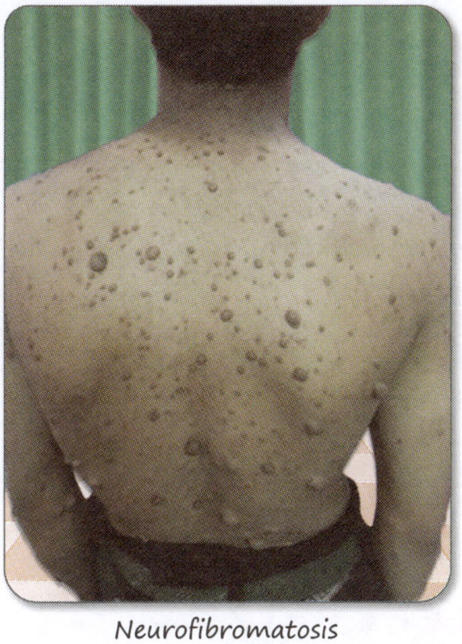

Neurofibromatosis

Neurofibromatosis/von Recklinghausen's Disease

Two or > of the following should present:

- Six or more café au lait spots each of >5 mm before puberty or >15 mm in older persons
- Two or more neurofibromas or one plexiform neuroma
- Freckling in axillary or inguinal regions
- Two or > Lisch nodules: Lisch nodules are dome-shaped gelatinous masses developing on the surface of the iris

Cafe au lait spots

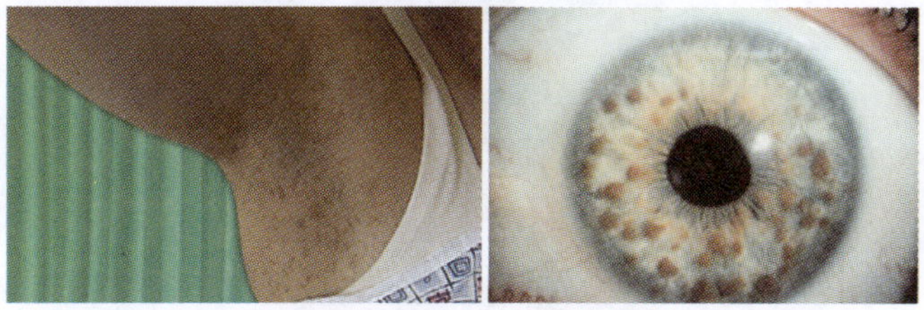

Axillary freckling Lisch nodules

STURGE-WEBER SYNDROME

- Angiomas involving typically in the ophthalmic and maxillary division of trigeminal nerve.

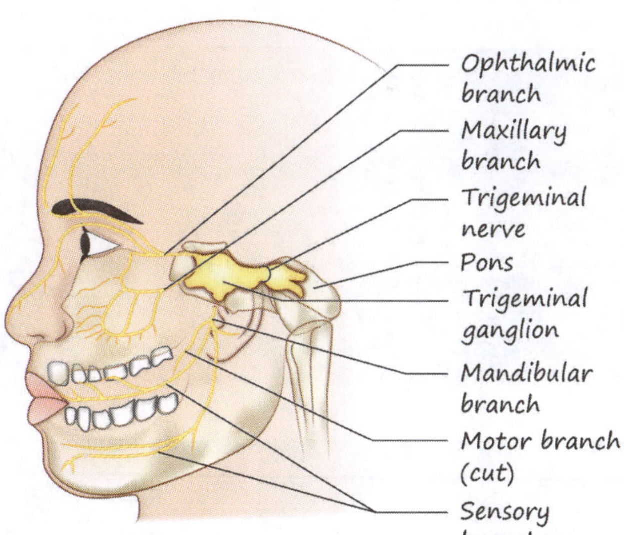

- Seizure + Port-wine stain, intracranial calcification, glaucoma on same side

Tuberous Sclerosis/Epiloia/Bourneville-Pringle Disease

- TSC1 gene: Located on 9q34 (encoding protein hamartin)
- TSC2 gene: Located on chromosome 16q13 (encoding protein tuberin)

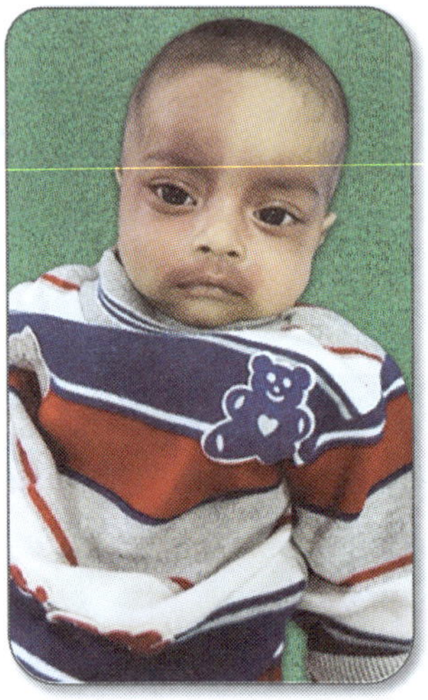

Portwine stain

SKIN LESIONS

- Adenoma sebaceum (image 1)
- Shagreen patches (image 2)
- Subungual fibromas/Koenen's tumors (image 3)
- Hypomelanotic macules (image 4)

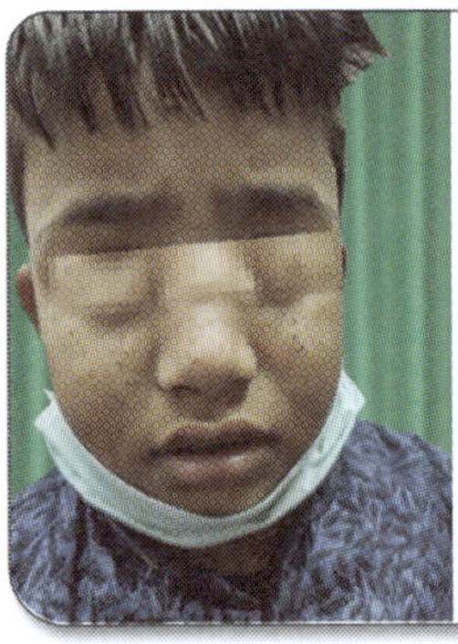

Image 1

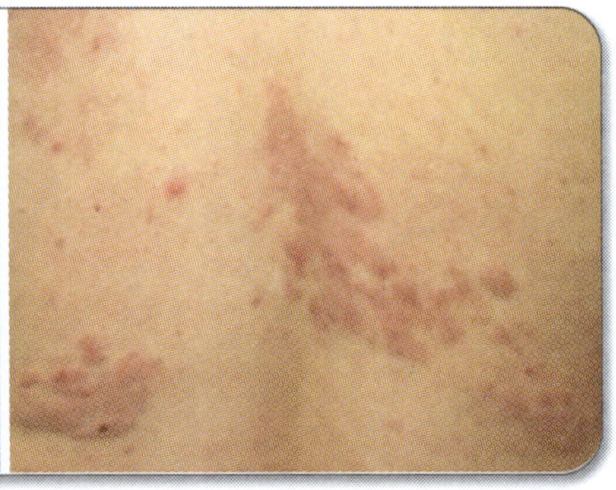

Image 2

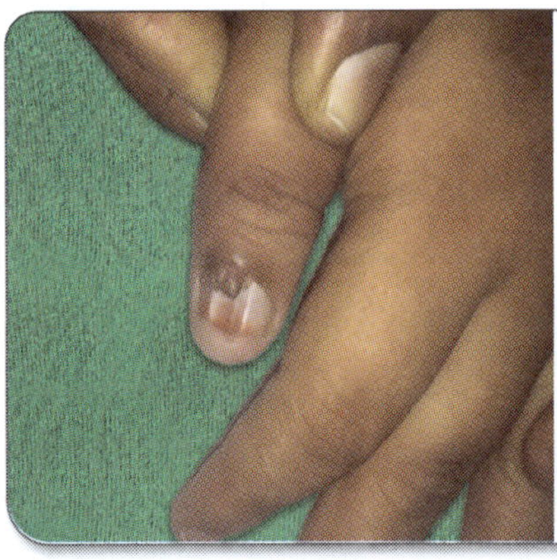

Image 3

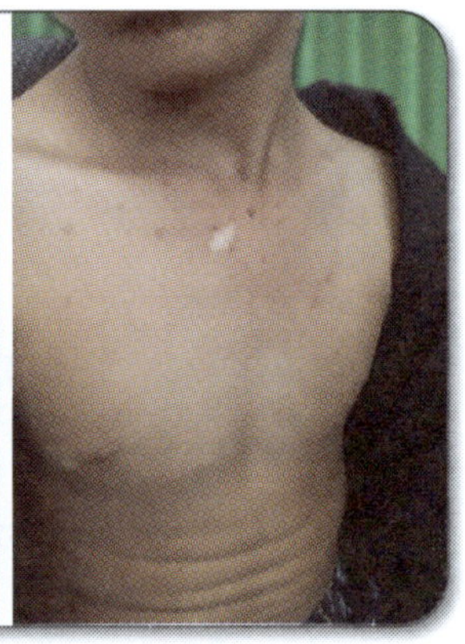

Image 4

- Drug of choice: Vigabatrin* for infantile spasms in tuberous sclerosis
- Drug of choice: Adrenocorticotropic hormone* for infantile spasms in West syndrome

FEBRILE SEIZURES

- MCC of seizure in a newborn: Hypoxia
- MCC of seizure in a child: Febrile seizure
- MC type of seizure in a newborn: Subtle
- Types:
  - Simple febrile: Duration <15 minutes, once in 24 hours, GTCS
  - Complex febrile: >15 minutes, multiple episodes in 24 hours, focal

Occurrence of epilepsy	Risk
Simple febrile seizure	1%*
Neurodevlopment abnormal	33%*
Focal complex febrile seizures	29%*

Major Criteria

- Age <1 year
- Duration of fever <24 hours
- Fever 38°–39°C

Minor Criteria

- Family history of febrile seizure
- Family history of epilepsy
- Complex febrile seizures
- Male gender
- Treatment of choice: Rectal diazepam or intranasal midazolam
- Febrile seizure does not cause developmental delay*

TUBERCULOUS MENINGITIS

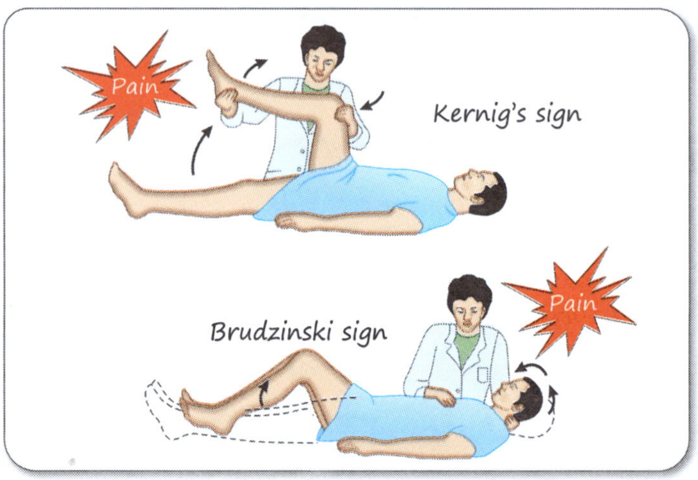

Meningeal signs

Stages of TBM

- **Stage 1:** Fever + headache + loss of appetite + photophobia
- **Stage 2:** Meningeal signs (image attached), seizures, neurological deficit
- **Stage 3:** Decorticate, decerebrate posturing

Diagnosis: CSF: Low sugar, high protein, lymphocytic predominant + cobweb formation
Treatment: Dexamethasone + antitubercular therapy

CSF FINDINGS IN MENINGITIS

	Pressure (40–80 mm H_2O)	Leukocytes (2–4 mm^3)	Protein (20–40 mg/dL)	Glucose (40–80 mg/dL)
Bacterial meningitis	Increased	100–50000 PMN	100–500 (high)	Low <40
Viral meningitis	N or increased	<1000 mononuclear	50–200 (high)	N or high
Viral encephalitis	N or increased	<1000 PMN early, then mononuclear	50–200 (high)	N or high
TB meningitis	Increased	10–500 lymphocytes	100–500 (high)	Low <40
Brain abscess	Increased	10–200 lymphocytes	100–500	Normal

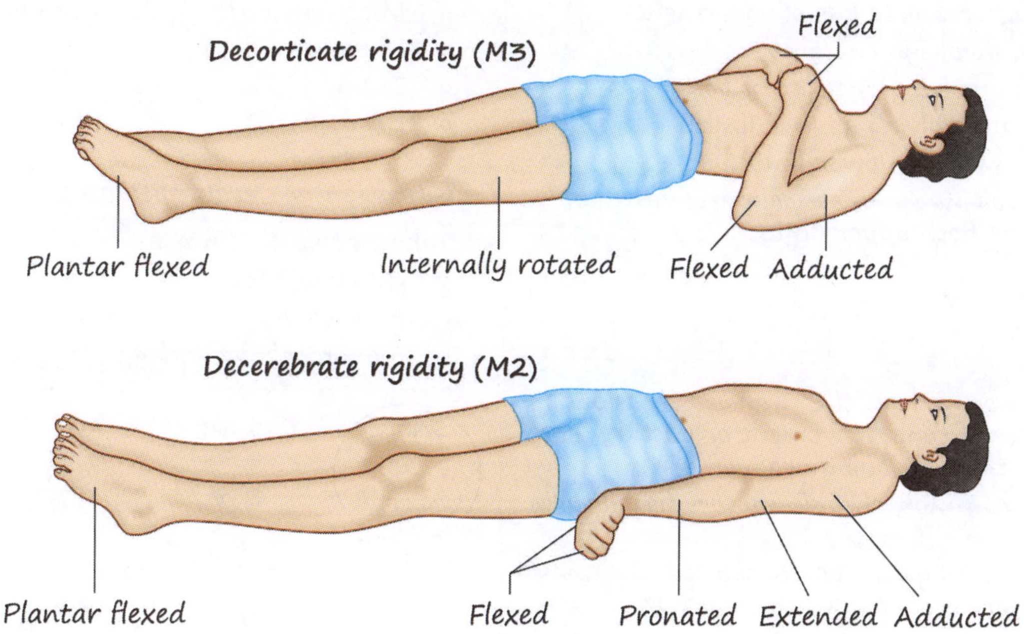

Extra Points

- Acute flaccid paralysis is not a feature of cerebral palsy*
- Prolong fasting followed by seizure = hypoglycemia
- Seizure provoked by fever = febrile seizure
- Diarrhea followed by seizure = dyselectrolytemia
- Meningeal signs f/b seizure = meningitis
- Altered sensorium f/b seizure = encephalitis
- Fever + seizure + café-au-lait macules = neurofibromatosis

BASIC TERMS

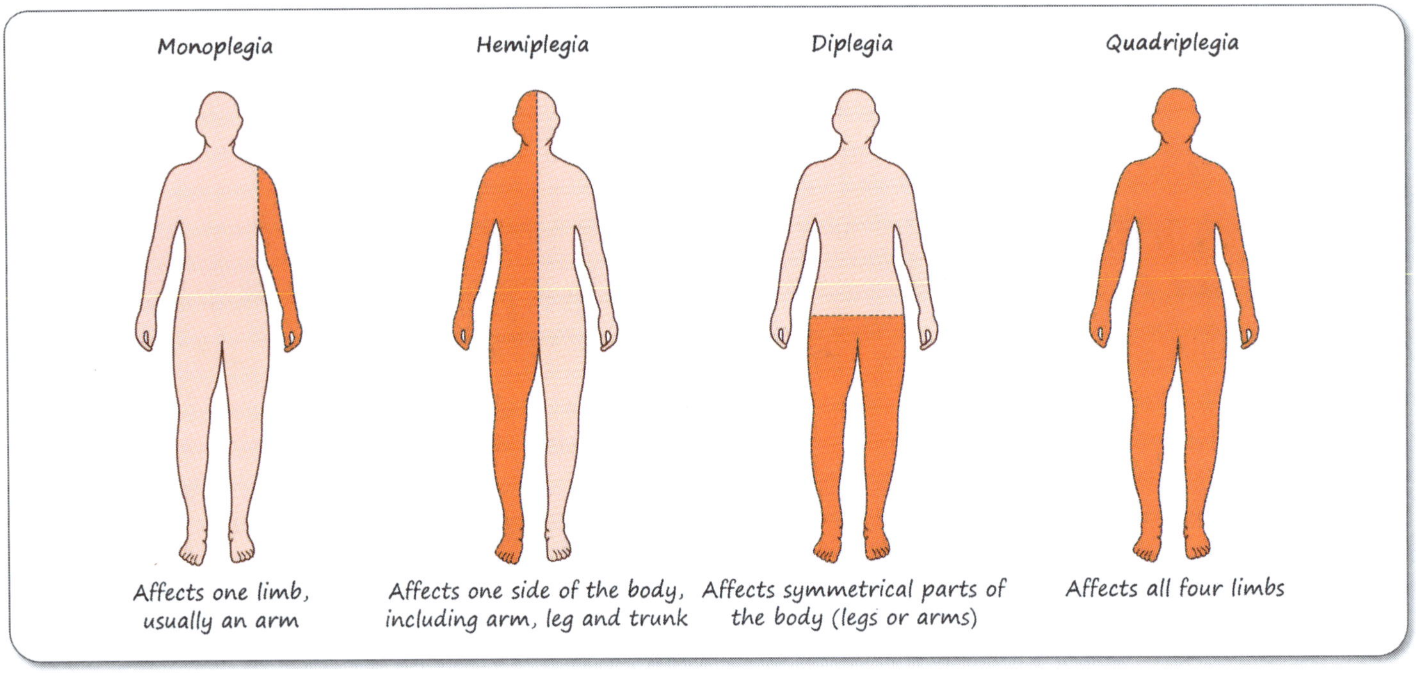

- Paresis means weakness.
- Plegia means complete loss of movement.
- Monoplegia: Involving one limb.
- Hemiplegia: Involving one side of body.
- Quadriplegia: Involving all four limbs.
- Paraplegia: Involving lower limbs.
- Diplegia: Involving symmetrical parts either both lower limb or both upper limbs.

CEREBRAL PALSY

Definition

Permanent, non-progressive and occasionally evolving disorder of tone, movement or posture, cost by an insult to the developing brain..

It is the most common chronic motor disability in childhood.

While perinatal asphyxia was considered the most common cause, it accounts for less than 10% of cases.

Causes

- Perinatal causes
    - Birth asphyxia
    - Prematurity
    - Low birthweight
    - Birth trauma
    - Neonatal infections
    - Neonatal seizures
    - Neonatal hypoglycaemia
- Postnatal causes
    - Infections of the CNS: meningitis
    - Hypoxia
    - Trauma
    - Drug

Classification of Cerebral Palsy

- Topographically (image)
    - Quadriplegic
    - Hemiplegic
    - Monoplegic or diplegic

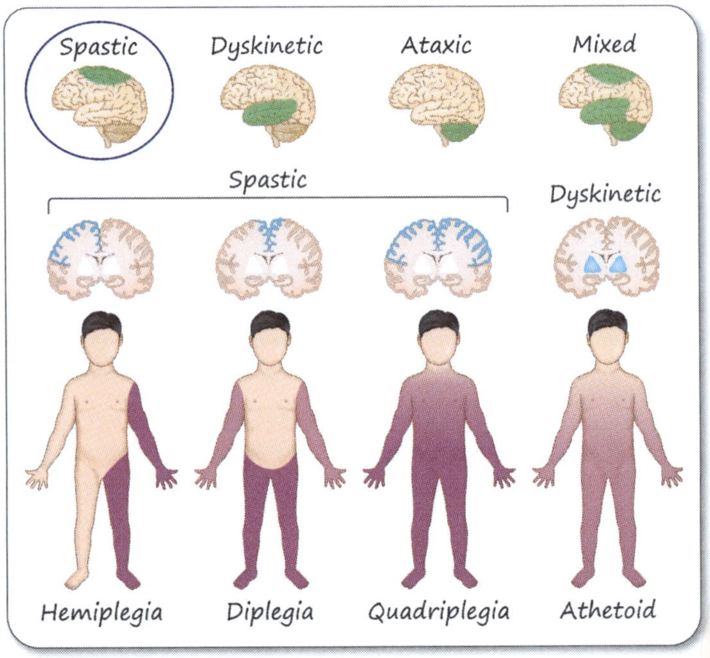

- Physiologically
  - Spastic: Most common
  - Dyskinetic: Second, most common
  - Ataxic or mixed

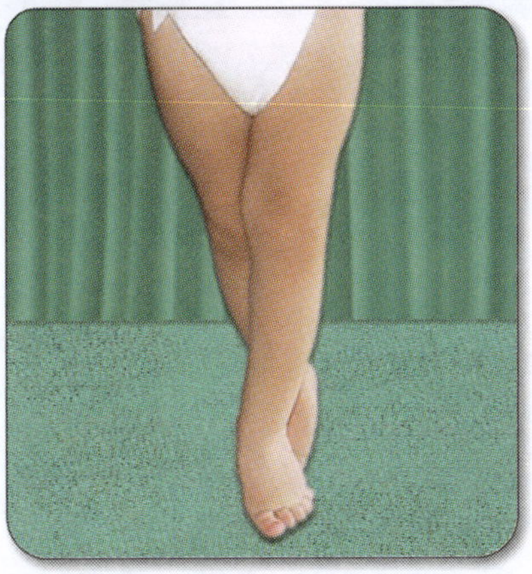

Scissoring gait

Management

- Multidisciplinary approach
- Orthopedic surgeon
- Speech therapist
- Ophthalmologist
- ENT specialist
- Social worker
- Special educator

How to Manage Spasticity?

- Diazepam
- Baclofen
- Tinazidine
- Dantrolene

Manage localized spasticity by Injection of botulinum a toxin

Muscle relaxant: Intrathecal baclofen therapy manage dystonia by:

- Trihexiphenidyl
- Levodopa
- Botulinum toxin injections

> **Extra Points**
>
> Flaccid paralysis is not a feature of cerebral palsy.

GUILLAIN-BARRÉ SYNDROME

- This is one of the common cause of acute flaccid paralysis (AFP) in children.
- Rapid course and predominantly motor symmetric polyradiculoneuropathy.
- Leads to bulbar and respiratory compromise.

> **Extra Points**
>
> **What is Radiculopathy?**
>
> Commonly referred to as a pinched nerve, radiculopathy is injury or damage to nerve roots in the area where they leave the spine.

Subtypes

- AIDP—acute inflammatory demyelinating polyneuropathy* most common.
- AMAN—acute motor axonal polyneuropathy* most common in pediatrics.
- AMSAN—acute motor and sensory axonal neuropathy.
- Miller Fischer syndrome—Triad: Ophthalmological, abnormalities, ataxia, and areflexia.

GBS	Age group
AIDP	Adults
AMAN	• Children • Young adults
AMSAN	Mostly adults
Miller Fischer syndrome	• Adults • Children

Antibodies seen in GBS	Antibody
AIDP	Anti GM1
AMAN	Anti GD1a
AMSAN	Anti GD1a
Miller Fischer syndrome	Anti GQ1b

Clinical Features

- URTI or gastrointestinal infection 1–6 weeks prior to onset of symptoms (history of bloody diarrhea).

- Acute onset of bilateral symmetrical ascending weakness without any features of CNS involvement.
- Weakness of lower limb followed by not able to stand.
- Nadir of the disease comes at 2 weeks.

Imp PYQs*

Recent Questions

If there is early bowel and bladder involvement, it goes against the diagnosis of GBS.

Golden Points

- If the maximum disability is reached within 24 hours or continues to progress beyond 4 weeks—it goes against the diagnosis of GBS.
- Sensory deficit severely affected in GBS is proprioception: Your body's ability to sense movement, action, and location.

Diagnostic Criteria

Diagnostic criteria for Guillain-Barré syndrome

Features required for diagnosis

- Progressive weakness in >1 limb (usually starts in legs).
- Areflexia (or decreased tendon reflexes) in weak limbs.

Features that strongly support diagnosis

- Progression of symptoms over days to 4 weeks.
- Relative symmetry of symptoms.
- Mild sensory symptoms or signs.
- Autonomic dysfunction.
- Cranial nerve involvement, most common bilateral weakness of facial muscles.
- Absence of fever at the onset of neurological symptom.
- Typical electrophysiological findings:
  - Abnormal or absent F-wave, and H-reflex.
  - Reduced motor with or without sensory nerve action potentials (axonal variant: AMAN).
  - Prolonged distal latencies, reduced conduction velocities, presence of conduction block or increased temporal dispersion (demyelinating variant: AIDP).
- Albuminocytologic dissociation on CSF: High concentration of protein in CSF; mononuclear cell counts <50/mm^3

Features that raised doubt about the diagnosis

- Bladder or bowel dysfunction at onset and/or persistent bladder or bowel dysfunction.
- Fever at onset.
- Sharp sensory level.
- Marked persistent asymmetry of weakness.
- Severe pulmonary dysfunction with limited limb weakness at onset.
- Marked sensory signs with limited weakness at onset.
- CSF showing increased number of mononuclear cells (>50 cells/mm^3) or polymorphonuclear cells.

Investigations

- Lumbar puncture: CSF
  CSF TLC count—Normal
- Albuminocytologic dissociation is present that means:
- Elevation of CSF protein (albumin 100–1000 mg/dL) without an elevation of white blood cells (Characteristic of GBS).

Extra Points

Albuminocytologic dissociation is also seen in spinal tumors.

Treatment

- IVIG 2 g/kg/day for 5 days
- Plasma exchange
- Give second dose of IVIG after 2-4 weeks of 1st dose in patients who do not respond to initial treatment

Supportive Care

- Physical therapy
- Nutritional therapy
- Management of neuropathic pain
- Care of bowel and bladder
- Early rehabilitation

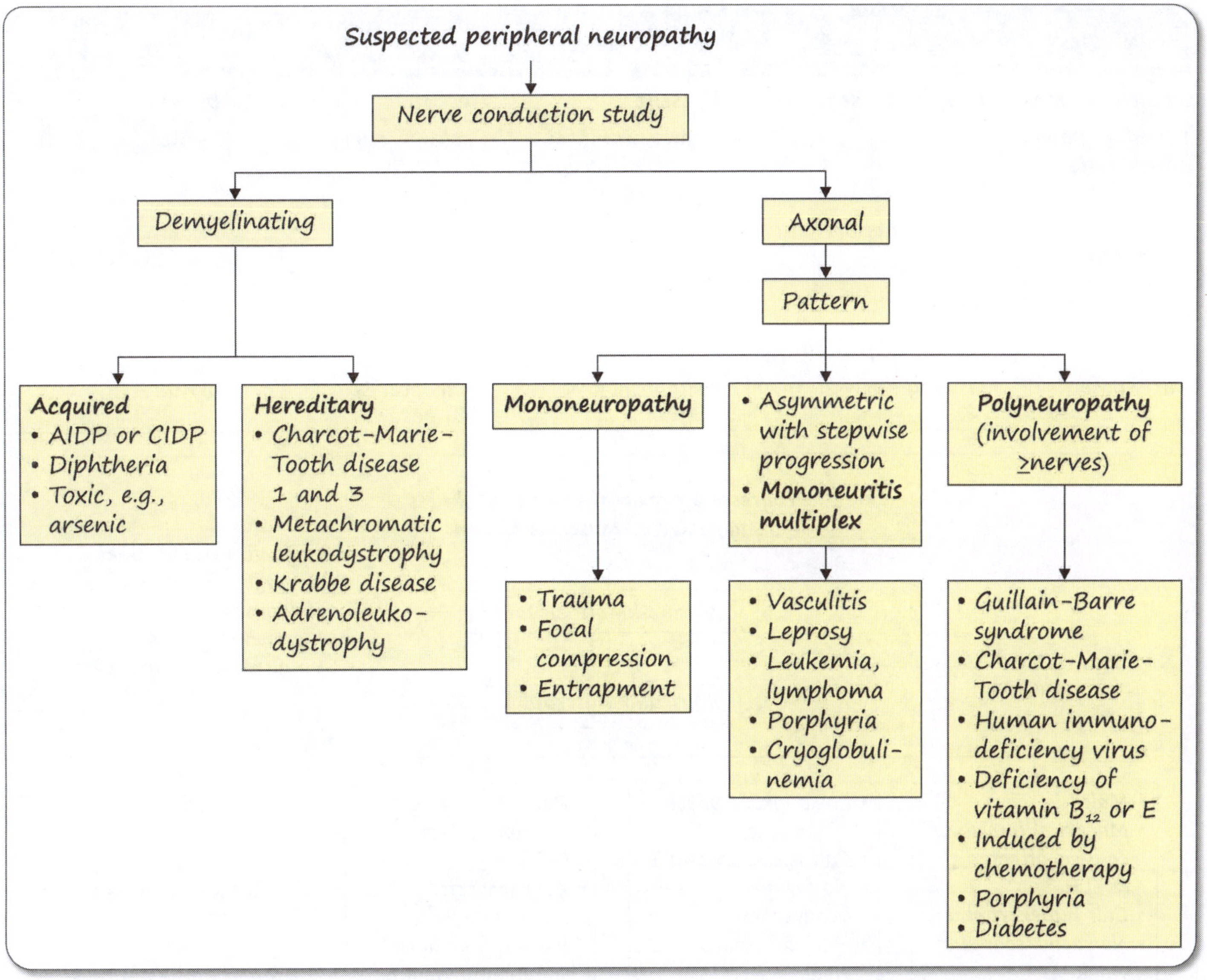

Approach to peripheral neuropathies in childhood. AIDP acute inflammatory demyelinating polyneuropathy; CIDP chronic inflammatory demyelinating polyneuropathy

Differentiating common causes of acute flaccid paralysis

	Poliomyelitis	Guillain-Barré syndrome	Transverse myelitis	Traumatic neuritis
Fever	Present; may be biphasic	May have a prodromal	May have a prodromal illness	Absent
Symmetry	Asymmetric	Symmetrical	Symmetrical	Asymmetric
Sensations	Intact; may have diffuse myalgias	Variable	Impaired below the level of the lesion	Impaired in distribution of the affected nerve
Respiratory insufficiency	May be present	May be present	May be present	Absent
Cranial nerves	Affected in bulbar and bulbospinal variants	Usually affected	Absent	Absent

Contd...

	Poliomyelitis	Guillain-Barré syndrome	Transverse myelitis	Traumatic neuritis
Radicular signs	May be present	Present	Absent	Absent
Bladder, bowel complaints	Absent	Transient, late; due to autonomic dysfunction	Present, early	Absent
Nerve conduction	May be abnormal	Abnormal	Normal	Abnormal
Cerebrospinal fluid	Lymphocytic pleocytosis; normal or increased protein	Albuminocytologic dissociation	Variable	Normal
MRI spine	Usually normal	Usually normal	Characteristic changes	Normal

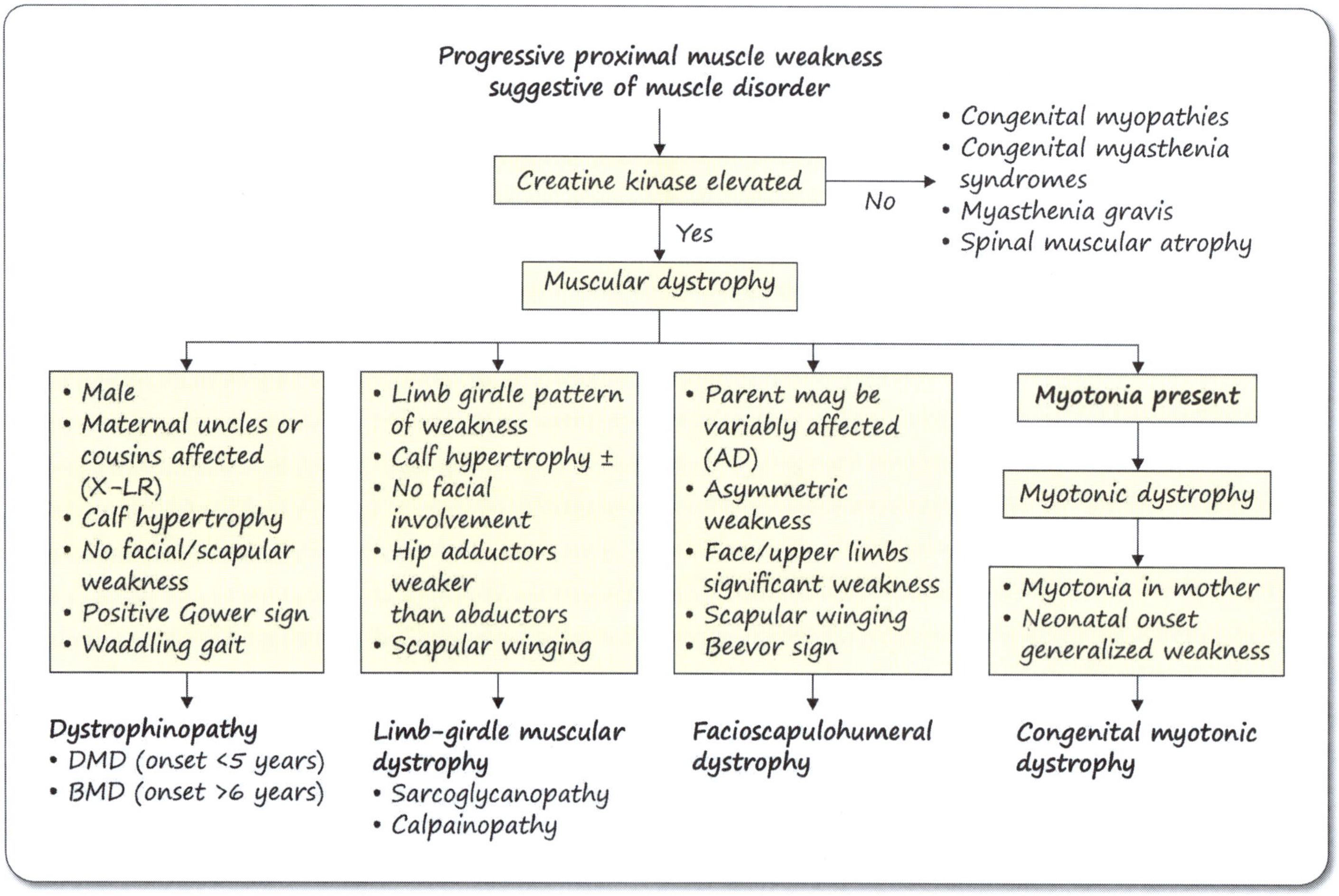

Approach to common childhood muscular dystrophies. DMD Duchenne muscular dystrophy; BMD Becker muscular dystropy; LGMD limb girdle muscular dystrophy

STATUS EPILEPTICUS—APPROACH

Definition: Status epilepticus is defined as continuous or recurrent seizure which lasts for >5 minutes without regaining consciousness

Acute seizures

↓

Maintain airway, breathing, circulation
Administer oxygen

↓ Blood electrolytes; glucose; calcium; magnesium; liver and kidney function tests; blood counts; toxicology (if indicated)

IV Lorazepam (0.1 mg/kg) or Midazolam (0.1 mg/kg); up to 2 doses, 5 minutes apart
Correct metabolic abnormality (e.g., IV glucose, if hypoglycemia)

↓ If seizure continues, administer sequentially

IV Phenytoin or Fosphenytoin 20 mg/kg infusion repeat, if needed, at 10 mg/kg

↓

IV Sodium valproate 20–40 mg/kg infusion

↓

IV Levetiracetam 20–60 mg/kg infusion at 5 mg/kg/min

↓

IV Phenobarbitone 20 mg/kg infusion repeat, if needed, up to twice, at 10 mg/kg

↓

IV Midazolam at 1–30 μg/kg/min infusion

↓

Coma induced by phenobarbitone (or thiopentone and propofol) infusion

↓ Consider

IV ketamine and oral topiramate

In intensive care

Immunotherapy | Dietary therapy
Vagal nerve stimulation | Epilepsy surgery

Sequential drug therapy in the management of status epilepticus

SEIZURE IN A NEWBORN—APPROACH

Neonate with seizures

↓

- Identify and characterize the seizure
- Secure airway and optimize breathing, circulation, and temperature
- Start oxygen, if needed
- Secure IV access and take blood samples for baseline investigations including sugar, calcium, magnesium, sodium, potassium, arterial blood gas, hematocrit, sepsis screen
- If hypoglycemic (blood sugar <40 mg/dL): administer 2 mL/kg of 10% dextrose as bolus followed by a continuous infusion of 6–8 mg/kg/min
- If blood sugar is in normal range, sample for blood calcium should be withdrawn; if abnormal, 2 mL/kg of calcium gluconate (10%) should be given IV under cardiac monitoring

↓ Seizures persist

Administer **phenobarbitone 20 mg*/kg** IV stat over 20 minutes

↓ Seizures continue

Repeat phenobarbitone in 10 mg*/kg/dose aliquots until 40 mg/kg dose is reached

↓ Seizures continue

Administer phenytoin 20 mg/kg IV slowly over 20 minutes under cardiac monitoring*

↓ Seizures continue

Repeat phenytoin 10 mg/kg/dose

↓ Seizures continue

Consider lorazepam/midazolam bolus and midazolam infusion if needed;

↓ Seizures controlled

Wean AED slowly to maintain phenobarbitone

*Levetiracetan or lidocaine may be considered a second-line agent in place of phenytoin

Acute management of neonatal seizures

MYASTHENIA GRAVIS

Neuromuscular junction disorders in children

Immune mediated	Metabolic toxins
• Myasthenia gravis • Lambert-Eaton myasthenic syndrome	• Botulism • Organophosphates • Snake envenomation • Tick paralysis • Hypermagnesemia
Congenital myasthenic syndromes	**Drugs**
• Choline acetyltransferase • Paucity of synaptic vesicles • Endplate acetylcholinesterase deficiency • Acetylcholine receptor defects • Mutations in RAPSN, PLEC1, DOK7	• Aminoglycosides • Erythromycin • Tetracycline • Fluoroquinolones • Neuromuscular blocking agents • Phenytoin • D-penicillamine • Lithium • Interferon α

Introduction: 20% of patients with myasthenia gravis have onset in childhood.

Hallmark: Fatigable weakness as the day progresses.

Clinical Features

Ocular

- Asymmetric ptosis which is variable over time.
- Diplopia (double vision), Ptosis (most common finding) with normal pupillary reflex (pupils are always spared in Myasthenia gravis).
- Ptosis can shift from one eye to another over time.
- **Peep sign:** On attempting to tightly close the eyes, after a few minutes, the cornea may get exposed due to inability to sustain contraction of orbicularis oculi.

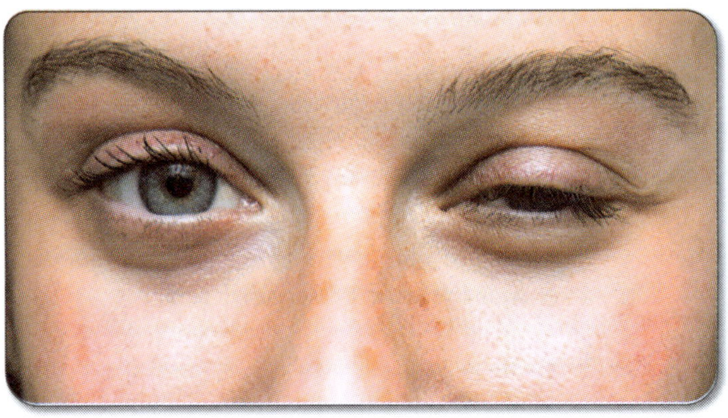

Peep sign

- Patients with ocular findings later develop bulbar or limb girdle weakness which is symmetrical and proximal.
- Normal or reduced deep tension reflexes. (Please note that we don't see absent DTR).
- If respiratory muscles are involved, that is known as myasthenia crisis.

Mechanism

- Myoid cells in the thymus serve as a source of autoantigen in this condition. (PYQ)
- The muscle – like cells in the thymus are known as myoid cells, express AChRs (acetylcholine receptors) on their surface. These cells are known to serve a source of autoantigen and trigger autoimmune reactions within the thymus gland. This stimulates the production of auto antibodies, thus causing myasthenia gravis.
- The thymus is normal in 75% of patients with AChRs antibody positive myasthenia gravis. In these cases, the thymus is hyperplastic. 10% of patients can show symptoms of thymoma.

Investigations

1st Diagnostic Test is Edrophonium Testing

Dose: 0.1–0.2 mg per kg; may be repeated every minute to a total dose of 5 mg (weight <34 kg) or 10 mg (weight >34 kg).

> **Extra Point**
>
> **What is positive edrophonium test? (PYQ)**
>
> Transient resolution of clinical signs (ptosis, ophthalmoplegia, dysarthria) under observation.
>
> Effects are seen within 10 seconds and persist till 120 seconds.

2nd Diagnostic Test is Neostigmine Test

Dose: 0.2 mg per kg in infant and 0.04 mg/kg IM in an older child.

Slower in action, anticipated response comes minimum in 10–15 minutes and maximum in 30 minutes.

3rd Diagnostic Test is Investigation

Nerve stimulation studies: A decrement of >10% is characteristic.

4th Diagnostic Test is Investigation

- Positive acetylcholinesterase antibodies
- Antibodies to muscle specific kinase (anti-MUSK) are seen in 40% seronegative patients.

Imp PYQs

Test for diagnosing myasthenia gravis with highest sensitivity is single fiber electromyography.

Treatment

Cholinesterase inhibitor: (PYQs) first line of drug of choice is Pyridostigmine 1–7 mg/kg/day in 4 divided doses.

Low-dose Prednisolone.

Please Note

Pyridostigmine does not alter the disease process. Drugs like prednisolone or mycophenolate mofetil, are immunosuppressive and they can alter the course of process.

For refractory cases: Steroid-sparing agents are used like azathioprine, cyclosporine, cyclophosphamide, mycophenolate mofetil.

Imp PYQs

- Complete remission is not seen in myasthenia gravis
- Drug of choice in a patient with myasthenia gravis + having Methicillin-resistant Staphylococcus aureus (MRSA) = Daptomycin
- MRSA = Daptomycin

Congenital myasthenia gravis (CMS)

- It is an uncommon cause of neuromuscular junction failure in newborn.
- The common syndromes associated with CMS are:
  - Slow channel congenital myasthenia gravis (SCCMS).
  - Fast channel congenital myasthenia gravis (FCCMS).
  - Primary acetylcholine receptor deficiency.
  - Endplate acetylcholinesterase deficiency.

Imp PYQs

Dysferlin deficiency is not associated with CMS.

7. IMMUNE SYSTEM

"It's going to be hard, but hard does not mean impossible."

VASCULITIS

- **Large vessel:**
  - Takayasu arteritis
  - Giant cell arteritis
- **Medium vessel:**
  - Kawasaki disease
  - Polyarteritis nodosa (PAN)
- **Small vessel**
  - Henoch-Schonlein purpura (HSP)
  - Wegener's granulomatosis
    - Most common vasculitis in pediatric age group: HSP
    - Most common vasculitis in adults: Giant cell arteritis
    - Most common vasculitis causing death in children: Kawasaki disease

TAKAYASU ARTERITIS

- It is the most common cause of renovascular hypertension in India*.
- Also known as pulseless disease.
- Age of onset: 10–40 years.

Pathology

Inflammation of blood vessels by T cells, natural killer cells causing blood vessel dilatation and aneurysm.

Clinical Features

Phase of prepulseless disease

- Fever
- Malaise
- Headache
- Hypertension

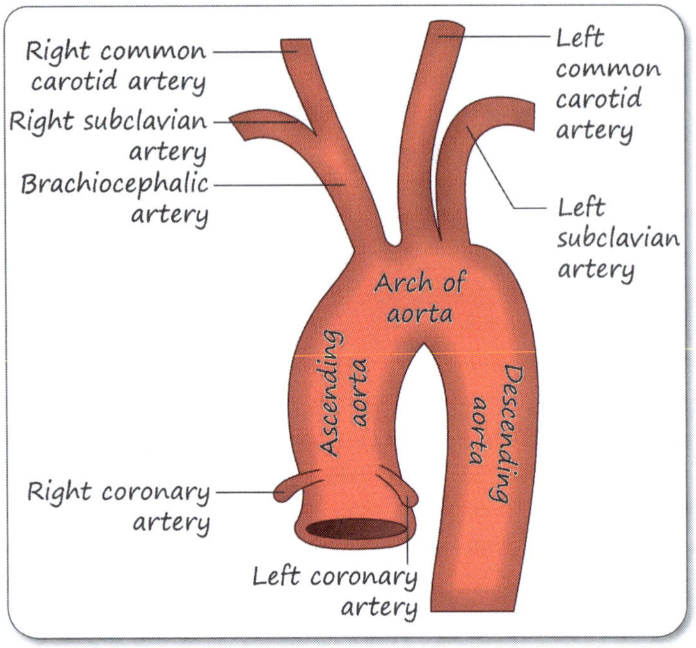

Takayasu arteritis

Late clinical features

- Diminished pulse
- Asymmetric blood pressure
- Claudication
- Raynaud phenomenon
- Valvular insufficiency

Why Hypertension?

- Because of aortic insufficiency—there is less blood reaching kidneys.
- That activates RAAS which leads to sodium, water retention causing hypertension.

How to Diagnose?

- Angiographic abnormalities: CT/MRI of the aorta to look for one or more of the following:
  - Decreased peripheral artery pulse(s) and/or claudication of extremities
  - Blood pressure difference between arms or legs of >10 mm Hg
  - Hypertension
  - Elevated acute phase reactant (ESR/CRP)

Treatment

- Prednisolone @ 1–2 mg/kg/day or same dose of methylprednisolone IV
- If TA persists or reoccurs:
  - Methotrexate/azathioprine
- For severe or refractive disease:
  - Cyclophosphamide

KAWASAKI DISEASE

- It is not seen in adults
- Fever for >5 days with irritability
- With any 4 out of 5 clinical features:
  - R—rash (polymorphous, nonvesicular)
  - E—edema (hands, feet)
  - E—conjunctivitis (nonpurulent)
  - M—mucosal involvement (strawberry tongue, cracked lips)
  - A—adenopathy (cervical/unilateral) + nonsuppurative, nontender

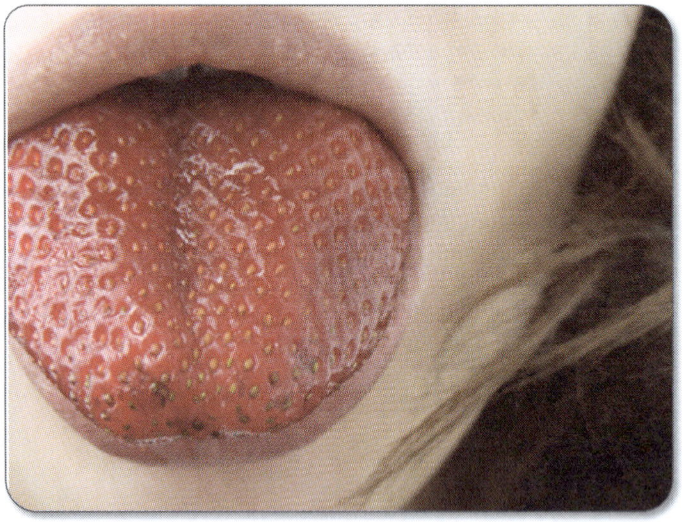

Kawasaki disease

- Inflammatory Marker in Kawasaki is thrombopoietin.
- Complications: Coronary artery aneurysm (seen in 25% cases) → acute myocardial infarction*.

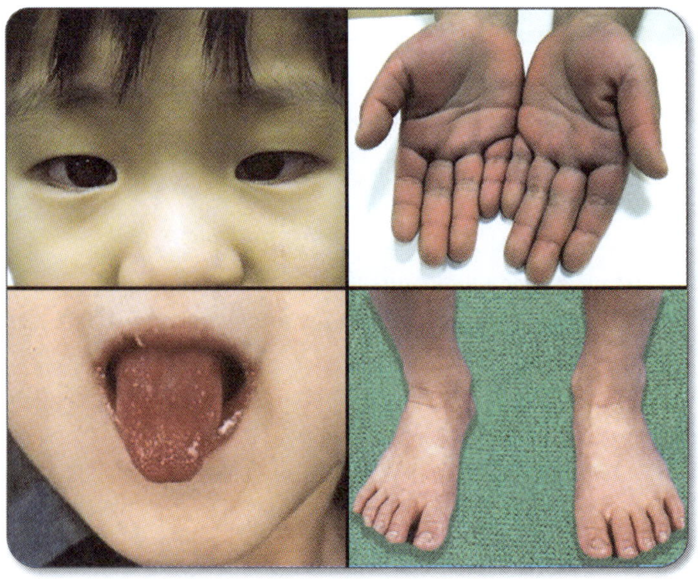

Kawasaki disease

Acute stage	IVIG 2 g/kg over 10–12 hours and aspirin 80–100 mg/kg/day QID until patient is afebrile for at least 48 hours
Convalescent stage 6–8 weeks of illness	Aspirin 3–5 mg/kg/day once daily until 6–8 weeks if normal coronary findings
Long-term therapy with coronary abnormalities	Aspirin 3-5 mg/kg once daily or clopidogrel 1 mg/kg/day (max: 75 mg/day) Warfarin added for pts. at high risk of thrombosis
Acute coronary thrombosis	Fibrinolytic therapy with tissue plasminogen activator

HENOCH-SCHONLEIN PURPURA

- Petechiae–small 1–2 mm, blood filled maculopapular lesion, do not blanch on pressure.

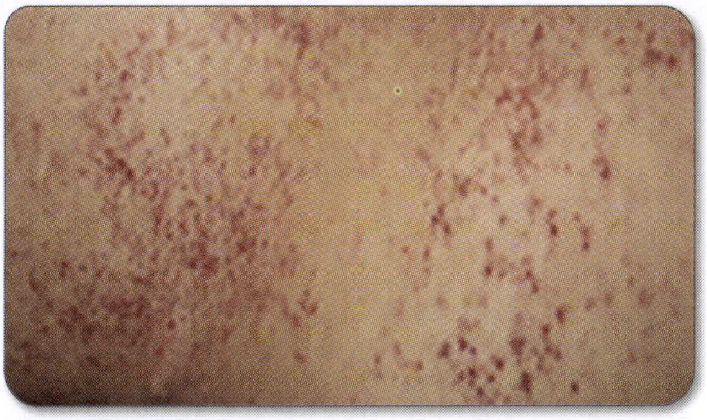

- Purpura: 0.3-1 cm maculopapular rash formed due to subdermal bleed, do not blanch.

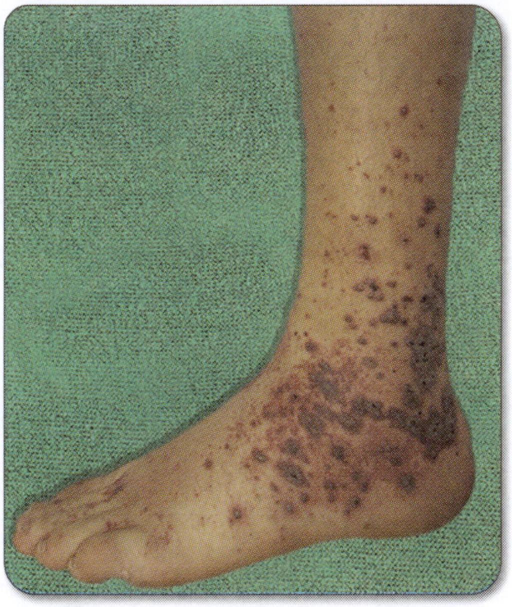

- Ecchymosis: >1 cm subdermal bleed.

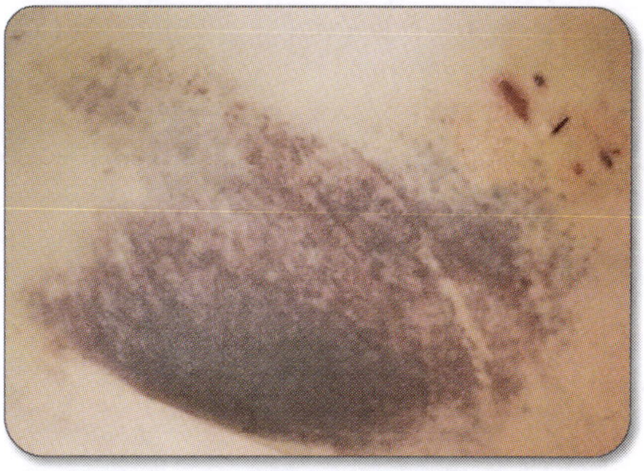

- It is a small vessel vasculitis.
- There is IGA deposition leading to (tetrad).
    - IGA deposition in skin causing: Palpable purpura.
    - Kidney: Hematuria seen in 50% cases in which 2% can go into renal failure.
    - GIT: Postprandial abdominal pain (bowel angina) seen in 80% cases.
    - Joints: Arthritis.
- Remember 3–10
    - Rash stays for 3–10 days
    - And is seen in age group 3–10 years (90%)
- Males > females.

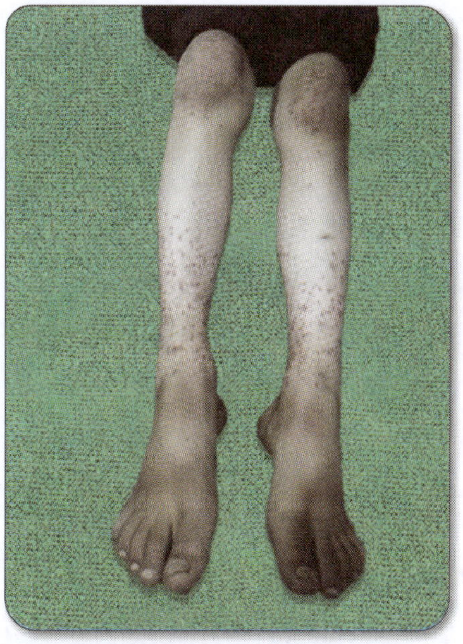

Palpable purpura

- ***Criteria:*** American College of Rheumatology
    - Two of the following:
        - Palpable purpura only in the lower limbs
        - Age of onset <20 years

- Bowel angina (postprandial abdominal pain with bloody diarrhea)
- Biopsy—intramural granulocytes in arterioles/venules.

- Rx: Mild supportive
- Prednisolone 1 mg/kg/day for 1–2 weeks reduces abdominal pain and joint pain
- Prognosis: Self-limiting course lasting around 4 weeks
- Good prognosis

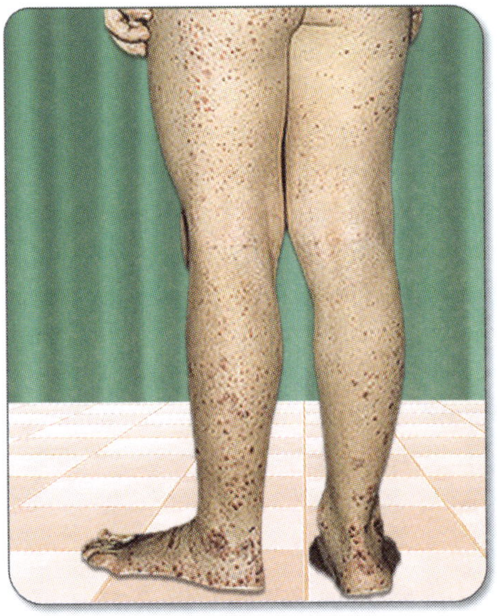

Rash specitically involving lower limbs

Extra Points

- Monoarthritis means single joint involvement: Seen in tubercular, septic arthritis and fracture
- Oligoarthritis: less than or equal to 4 joints involvement: Seen in HSP
- Polyarthriits: >4 joints: Seen in acute rheumatic fever
- Age group: 5–15 years (acute rheumatic fever)

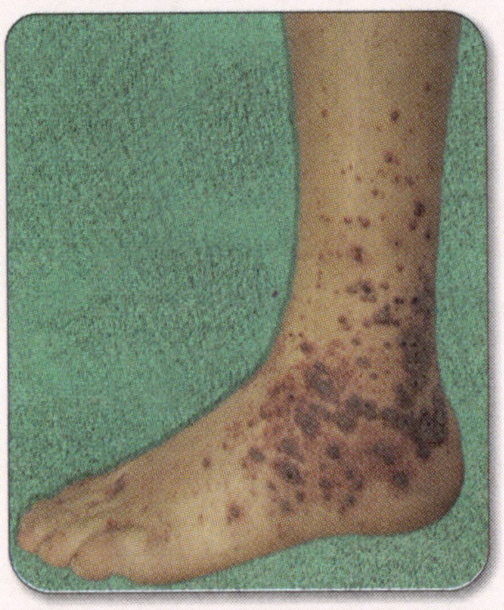

Golden Points

One more condition which mimics HSP is rickettsial infections.

Rickettsia are classified into:

- Typhus group
  - Epidemic typhus
  - Endemic typhus
  - Scrub typhus caused by R. tsutsugamushi
- Spotted fever group
  - Rocky Mountain spotted fever group
  - Indian spotted fever group

Triad:

- Fever
- Headache
- Palpable purpura

CHURG-STRAUSS SYNDROME/EOSINOPHILIC GRANULOMATOSIS WITH POLYANGIITIS/ EGPA SYNDROME

- **Which is the main organ it involves?**

  Lungs: Infiltrates, peripheral hypereosinophilia, extravascular necrotizing granulomata*.
- **If the lung is involved—how will the patient present?**

  Uncontrolled asthma.
- Allergic rhinitis 75% cases it will be present*.
- Eosinophilia.
- Palpable purpura, GI bleeding, renal post-streptococcal glomerulonephritis (PSGN).

WEGENER'S GRANULOMATOSIS (GRANULOMATOSIS WITH POLYANGIITIS)

Triad

1. Acute necrotizing granulomas of respiratory tract (URTI)—chronic sinusitis, rhinitis, epistaxis.
2. Necrotizing granulomas vasculitis affecting vessels in lungs (LRTI)—cough, hemoptysis.
3. Focal necrotizing often crescentic glomerulonephritis (kidney)—hematuria, high BP, renal failure.

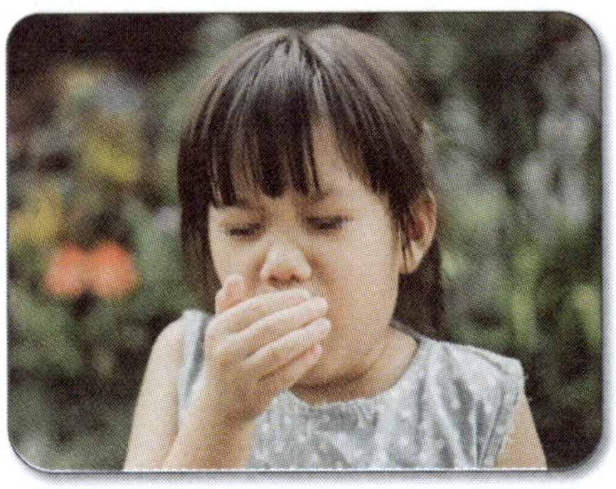

BEHÇET'S DISEASE—SILK ROAD DISEASE*

Triad

1. **Can't see:** Uveitis

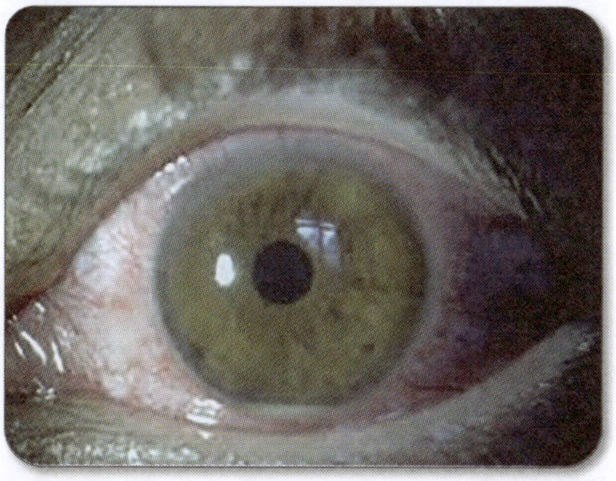

2. **Can't pee:** Genital ulcers

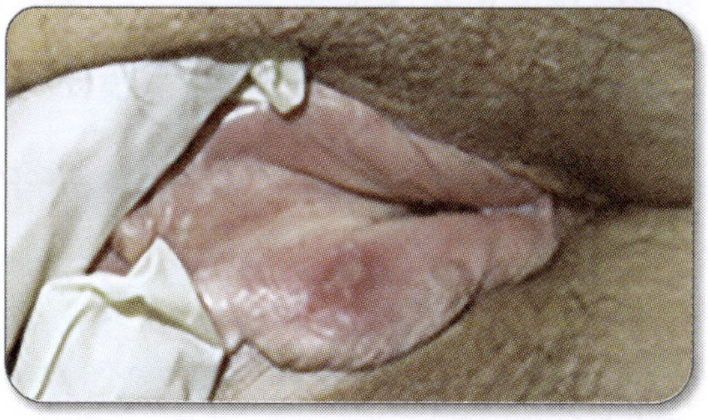

3. **Can't eat:** Recurrent aphthous ulcers
   - Sine qua non for diagnosis: Oral ulceration (hallmark)*
   - Microscopy: Neutrophils infiltrating vessel wall
   - HLA-B51* is associated
   - Steroids and TNF antagonist therapies are effective.

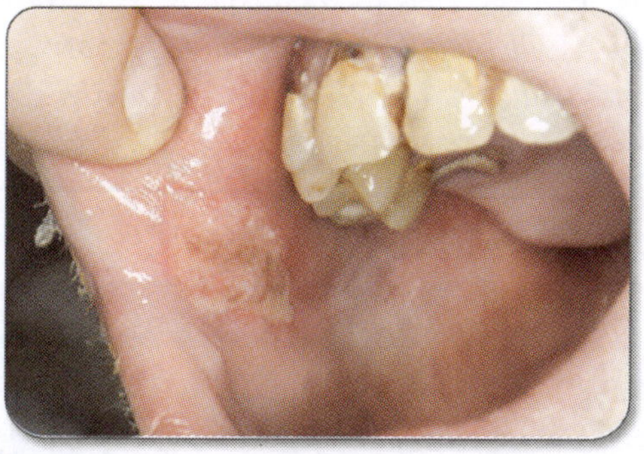

JUVENILE DERMATOMYOSITIS

- **Rash:** Photosensitive erythematous rash:
  - Rash over the neck and upper shoulder known as "v-sign".
  - Rash over the shoulder and upper arm known as "shawl sign".

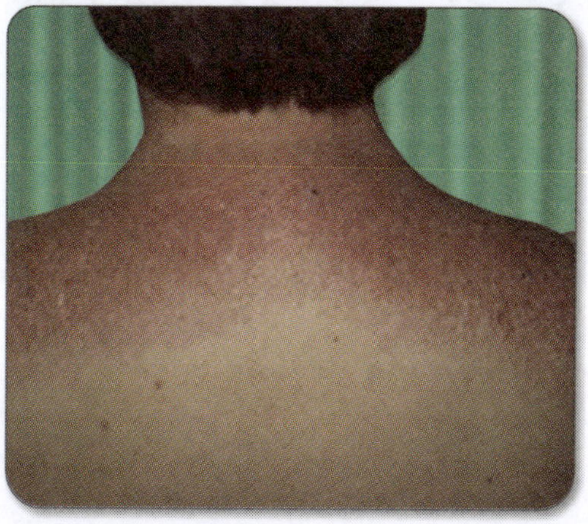

  - Blue/violet discoloration of eyelids: Heliotrope rash.

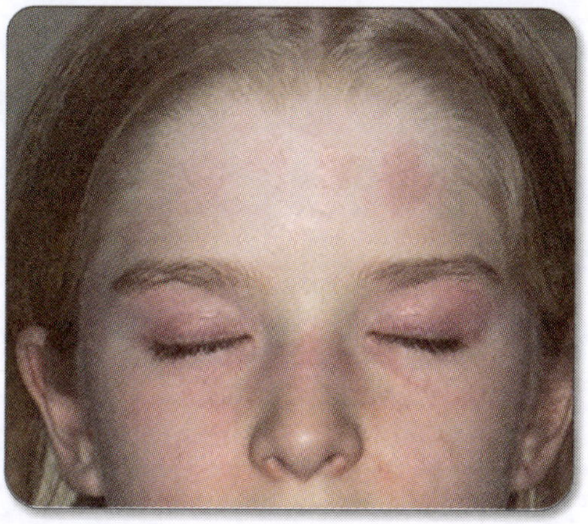

- **Gottron papules**

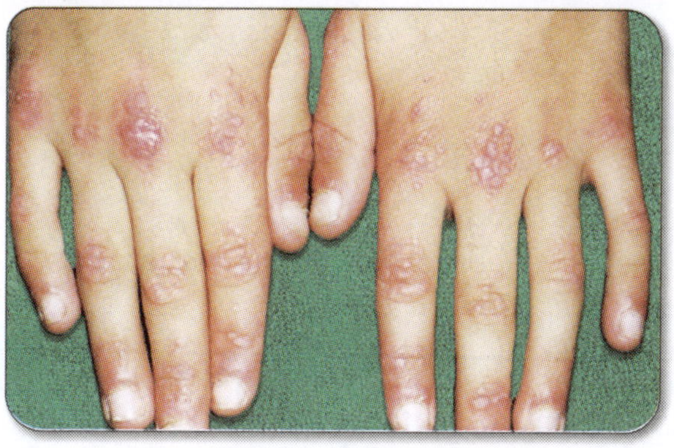

- Nails: Thickened and tortuous capillary loops in nail folds
- **Diagnostic criteria:**
  - **Classic rash:** Heliotrope rash on the eyelids and Gottron papules + three of the following:
    1. SGPT elevated
    2. Weakness—muscles
    3. Muscle enzyme elevation—creatine kinase

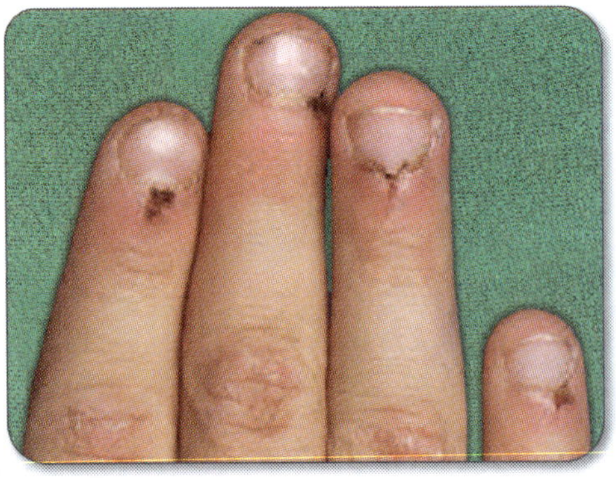

- **Electromyography** changes:** Short small polyphasic potentials
- **Muscle biopsy:** Necrosis and inflammation

- **Investigations:**
  - Blood: Elevated enzymes
  - Alanine aminotransferase
  - ANA is seen in >80% of children in JDM
  - Muscle biposy

8. BREASTFEEDING

"Do it now, sometimes later becomes never."

ALL TO KNOW ABOUT BREASTFEEDING

Exclusive breastfeeding: Till 6 months.

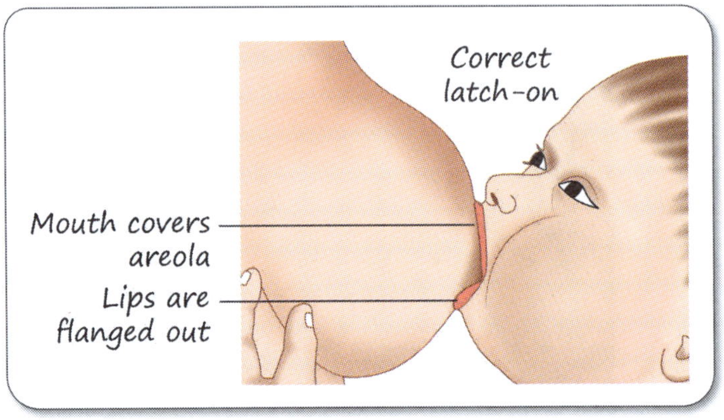

Signs of good attachment

When to Feed?

- In case of normal vaginal delivery (NVD): ASAP.
- LSCS: Within 4 hours.

Signs of Good Attachment

- Chin touching the breast
- Mouth wide open with fullness of cheeks
- Lower lip everted out
- Upper areola exposed out

Signs of Good Positioning

- Body of baby should be well supported
- Baby should be turned toward the mother
- Occiput, shoulder and buttocks of baby should be in a straight line
- Abdomen of baby should touch the abdomen of mother.

Golden Points

- Breastfeeding week: 1—7 August
- Reflexes help in breastfeeding:
  - Remember "P P – O O"
  - Prolactin produces the milk (milk secretion reflex)
  - Oxytocin oozes out the milk (milk ejection reflex)

Storage of Breast Milk

- We can store breast milk at room temp. for 8 hours
- Refrigerate for 1 day
- −20°C for 3 months

Contraindications

- In the baby: Galactosemia, lactose intolerance
- In the mother: Mother on chemo/radiotherapy

Vitamins

- Breast milk is rich in vitamin A, C (pneumonic—mother will feed the child in AC room)
- Breast milk is deficient in Vitamin D, K, B_{12} (if she is a pure veg)

Difference between Breast Milk and Cow's Milk

	Human milk	Cow's milk
Protein	1.1 g*	3.1 g*
Calories	65 Kcal	67 Kcal
Lactose	7.4 g	4.5 g
Fat	3.8 g rich in PUFA*	3.7 g
Sodium/ potassium	7 and 14	25, 35

Extra Points

- *Cow's milk is not good because it is rich in "4C"*
  - *Casein which causes*
  - *Colicky pain*
  - *Constipation*
  - *CMPA—cow milk protein allergy*
- *Breast milk is rich in Whey protein*

One Liners

- Fatty acid present in breast milk which is important for growth and CNS development is (DHA) docosahexaenoic acid
- Component present in the breast milk which prevents the baby from malaria is (PABA) para-aminobenzoic acid
- Human milk contains 2 types of protein: 60% whey and 40% casein helps in quick and easy digestion
- Cow milk: Whey casein ratio is 20:80

COLOSTRUM

- The first immunization of the baby.
- Golden thick yellow milk during first 3 days of life.
- Rich in IgA*, proteins* (as compared to breast milk) and WBCs.
- Ideal first MEAL for the baby.

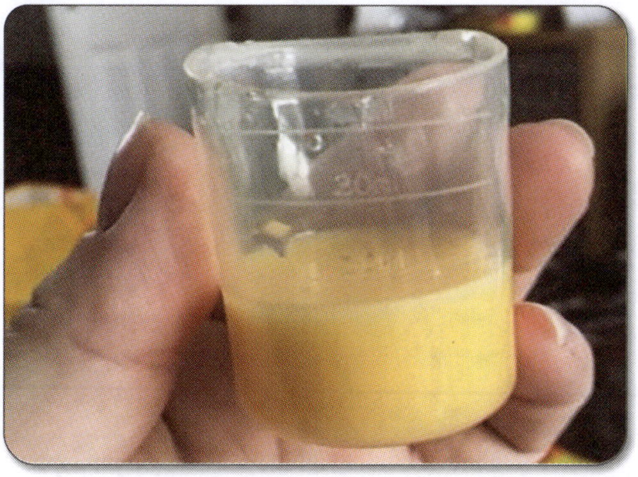

Colostrum

Extra Points

What is nipple confusion?

Answer: Shifting from bottle nipple to mother nipple.

IMPORTANT DATES

- World Autism Day: 2nd April
- World Health Day: 7th April
- World Malaria Day: 25th April
- World Nutrition Day: 28th May
- World Tobacco Day: 31st May
- World Environment Day: 5th June
- World Brain Tumor Day: 8th June
- Autistic Pride Day: 18th June
- Doctor's Day: 1st July
- World Rabies Day: 28th September
- Children's Day: 14th November
- National Neonatology Week: 15–21 November
- World AIDS Day: 1st December

Image-based Learning

Supplementary suckling technique

Foremilk	Hindmilk
Beginning part of breast milk	End part of breast milk
Rich in protein, vitamins, minerals	Rich in fat
Helps in thirst	Helps in satiety value

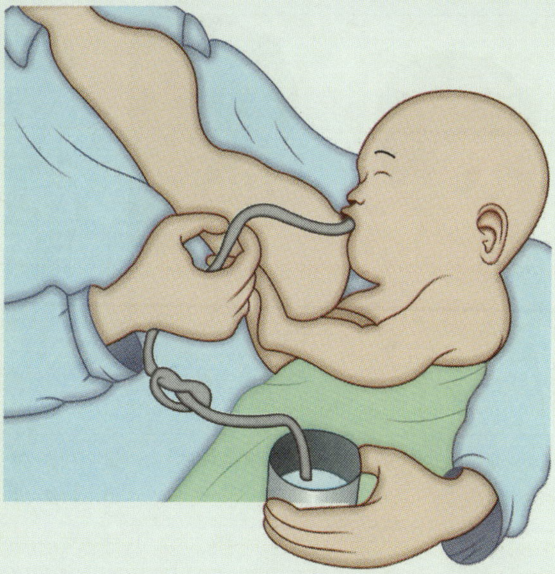

RECOMMENDED DAILY ENERGY REQUIREMENT/MAINTENANCE FLUID FORMULA NAME: HOLLIDAY SEGAR AND SEGAR FORMULA

- **0–10 kg:** 100 kcal/kg
- **10–20 kg:** 50 kcal/kg
- **>20 kg:** 20 kcal/kg
- **For example:** Baby is 9 kg—total fluid requirement of 24 hours will be 900 mL
- Or we can say 900 kilocalories
- **2nd example:** Baby is 12 kg—total fluid requirement will be 1100 mL or 1100 kilocalories

IMPORTANT FULL FORMS

- **IYCF:** Infant and Young Child Feeding
- **BFHI:** Baby-Friendly Hospital Initiative launched in 1991
- **BPNI:** Breastfeeding Promotion Network of India
- **WABA:** World Alliance for Breastfeeding Action
- **IMS Act:** Infant Milk Substitute Act

DO YOU KNOW?

First breast milk bank was started in which city in India: Mumbai.

"If you don't sacrifice for what you want. What you want becomes the sacrifice."

9. SEVERE ACUTE MALNUTRITION

"Discover who you are."

- WHO defines severe acute malnutrition (SAM) as:
  - Weight for height <-3 SD (standard deviation)
  - Mid-upper arm circumference (MUAC) <11.5 cm
  - Edema
- Kwashiorkor: Deficiency of proteins
- Marasmus: Deficiency of calories + proteins

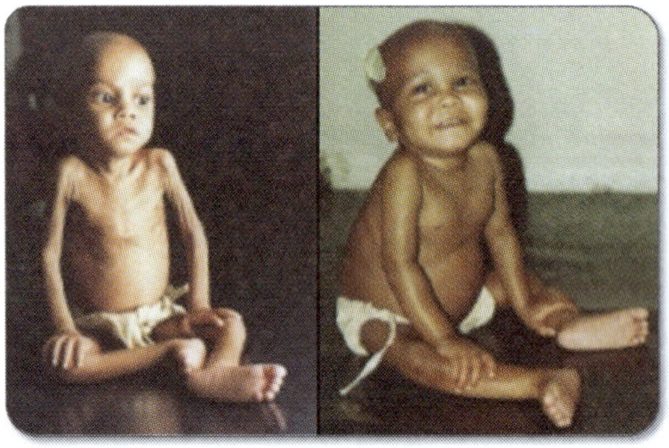

Marasmus Kwashiorkor

MEASURING MID UPPER ARM CIRCUMFERENCE

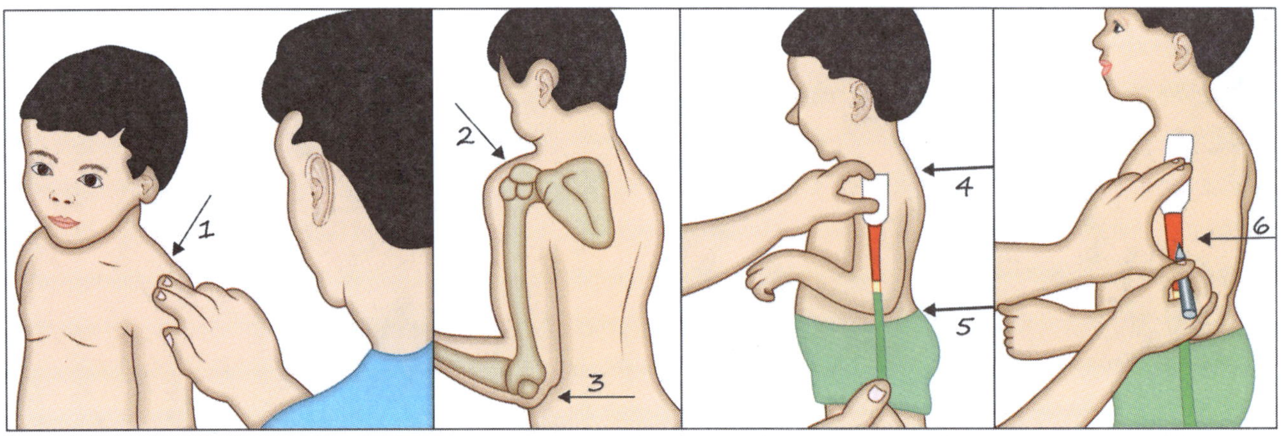

1. Locate tip of shoulder
2. Tip of shoulder
3. Tip of elbow
4. Place tape at tip of shoulder
5. Pull tape past tip of bent elbow
6. Mark midpoint

- Fatty baby/anasarca baby is kwashiorkor
- Skinny baby with baggy pant appearance is marasmus

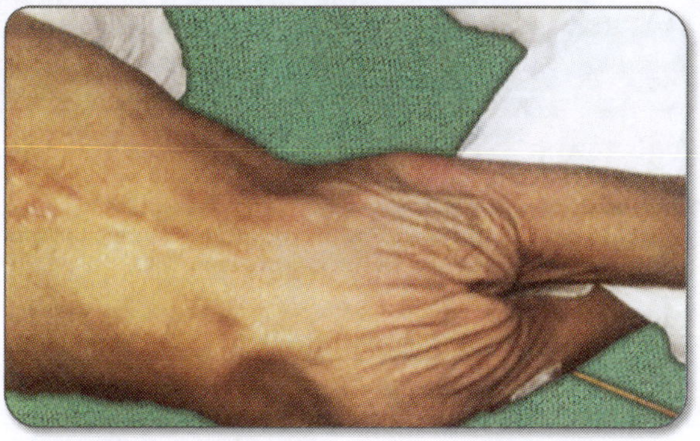

Baggy pant appearance—marasmus

SHAKIR TAPE

- Used by health worker
- To measure mid-upper arm circumference (MUAC)
  - **<11.5 cm:** Severe malnutrition (red color)
  - **<12.5 cm:** Borderline malnutrition (yellow)
  - **>12.5 cm:** Normal (green)

INDICATORS OF MALNUTRITION

- **Acute malnutrition/wasting:** Decrease weight for height <–2 SD (standard deviation)
- **Severe wasting:** Decrease weight for height <–3 standard deviation
- **Chronic malnutrition/stunting:** Decrease height for age <-2 SD
- **Severe stunting:** Decrease height for age <–3 SD
- Parameter changes in acute on chronic malnutrition is weight for age
  - Theory of adaptation is seen in: Marasmus
  - Theory of dysadaptation is seen in: Kwashiorkor
  - Liver findings
  - Kwashiorkor: fatty liver (kwashiorkor baby is fatty therefore we will see fatty liver)
  - Marasmus: atrophic changes (marasmus baby is skinny therefore, we see atrophic changes in liver)
- When do we give iron: Rehabilitation
- Triad of kwashiorkor: Mental changes, edema, apathy
- Triad of complication of SAM: Hypoglycemia, hypothermia, infection

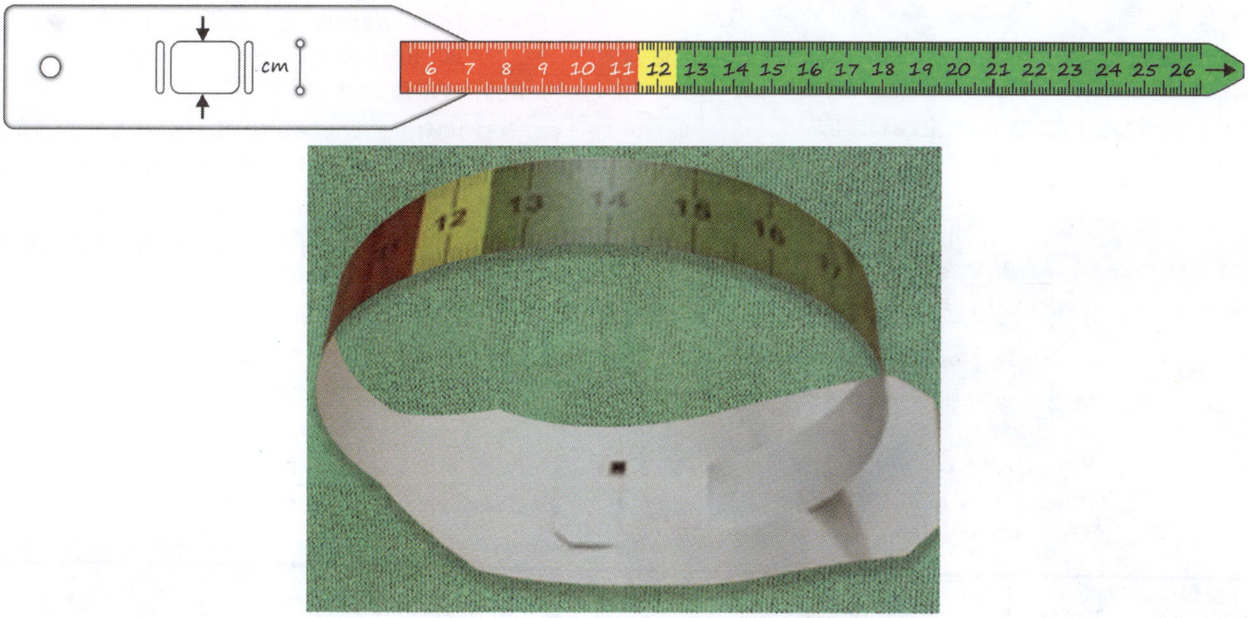

Shakir tape

- Flaky paint dermatosis also known as crazy pavement dermatosis
- Hyperpigmented patches which may peel easily seen in kwashiorkor

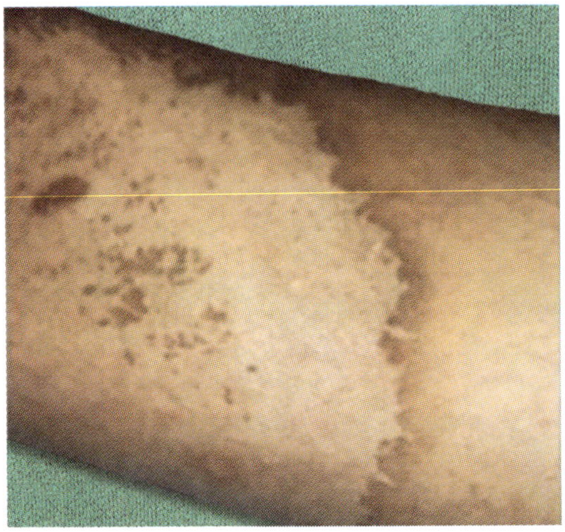

Flaky pant dermatosis

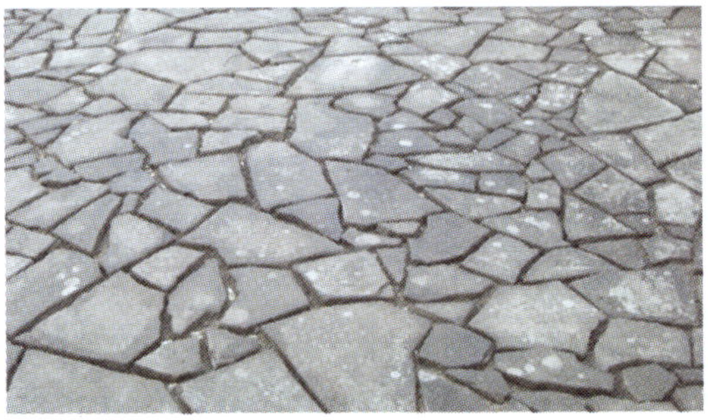

Crazy pavement dermatosis

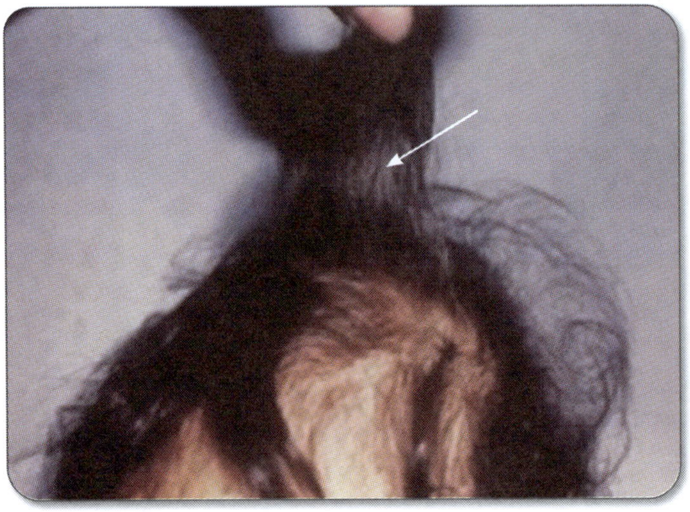

Flag sign

- Flag sign: Alternate band of shiny and dull areas in a hair follicle seen in kwashiorkor.

COMPLICATIONS OF SEVERE ACUTE MALNUTRITION (SAM)

	Stabilization		Rehabilitation
	Days 1–2	Days 3–7	Weeks 2–6
Hypoglycemia	------→		
Hypothermia	------→		
Dehydration	------→		
Electrolytes	------	------	------→
Infection	------	------→	
Micronutrients	no iron		with iron →
Cautious feeding	------	------→	
Catch-up growth		------	------→
Sensory stimulation	------	------	------→
Prepare for follow-up		------	------→

- Hypoglycemia cut off: <54 mg/dL
    - Treatment:
        - Asymptomatic hypoglycemia: Give 50 mL 10% dextrose/sucrose solution
        - Symptomatic hypoglycemia: 5 mL/kg 10% dextrose, follow with 50 mL of 10 and dextrose
- Hypothermia cut off
    - Remember three numbers – 36.5/35.5/35
    - <36.5°C is neonatal hypothermia cut off
    - <35.5°C is rectal hypothermia cut off in SAM
    - <35°C is axillary hypothermia cut off in SAM
    - **Treatment:**
        - Place the child in draught free area
        - Ensure head is covered
        - Skin to skin contact
        - Feeding 2 hourly
- Dehydration without shock
  Best answer will be ORS.

How often to give ORS	Amount to give
Every 30 minutes for first 2 hours	5 mL/kg weight
Alternate hours for up to 10 hours	5–10 mL/kg**

- Dehydration with shock
  15 mL/kg RL (ringer lactate) with 5% dextrose or half normal saline with 5% dextrose

Dose of Micronutrients

- Vitamin A dose:
  - **<6 months: 50,000 IU**
  - **6-12 months: 1 lakh IU**
  - **>1 year: 2 lakh IU**
  - If the age is >1 year <8 kg the dose will be 1 lakh IU
  - Vitamin k dose: 2.5 mg intramuscular
  - Potassium: 3-4 mEq/kg/day
  - Folic acid: 5 mg to be given on day 1 followed by 1 mg/day till day 14
  - Zinc: 2 mg/kg/day
  - Iron: Iron is never started in the beginning (rehabilitation phase) as it causes free radical generation and it will be flare-up the infection. It is started in the stabilization phase at the dose of 3 mg/kg/day
- **Treat infections:**
  - Without complication: Start oral amoxicillin for 5 days
  - Infections with complications: Inj. ampicillin and inj. gentamicin

FEEDING IN SEVERE ACUTE MALNUTRITION (SAM)

WHO recommended starter diet in SAM	F 75 diet	F 100 diet
Calories	75	100
Protein	0.9 g	2.9 g
Lactose	1.3 g	4.2 g

Imp PYQs

Q. When to discharge SAM baby?

Ans:

- 15% weight gain from the date of admission.
- >5 g/kg/day weight gain for 3 consecutive days.
- Mother is confident enough to take care of the baby.
- All the micronutrients are given for 14 days.
- Child is free from infection.
- Antibiotic course has been finished.
- Child appetite has returned.
- Immunization is complete.

Imp PYQs

Q. What is failure to respond in SAM?

Ans:

- Failure to regain appetite by day 4
- Failure to start to lose edema by day four
- Edema still present by day 10

"If you are not happy somewhere, walk away, you are not a tree."

10. MICRONUTRIENTS

"Realise your strength in life."

VITAMIN K

- **Exists in two forms:**
  1. **Vitamin K_1:** Phylloquinone
  2. **Vitamin K_2:** Menaquinone
- **Sources:** Green leafy vegetables
- **Absorption:** Jejunum
- **Primary site of storage:** Liver
- **Vitamin K dependent clotting factors:** Factor 2, 7, 9, 10
- **Deficiency causes:** Hemorrhagic disease of newborn (HDN)
- **Symptoms:** Bleeding from umbilical cord, ecchymosis

Classification of Hemorrhagic Disease of Newborn

- **Early onset:** Within 24 hours of life
- **Classical:** 1st week of life (normal breastfed babies who have not received vitamin K at birth)
- **Late:** 1–12 weeks—seen in liver disease
- **Treatment:** Vitamin K 0.5–1 mg

VITAMIN A

Xerophthalmia is a disease which is caused by the deficiency of vitamin A, results dry eyes.

Classification of Xerophthalmia by WHO

X1A	Conjunctival xerosis (earliest sign)
X1B	Bitot spots 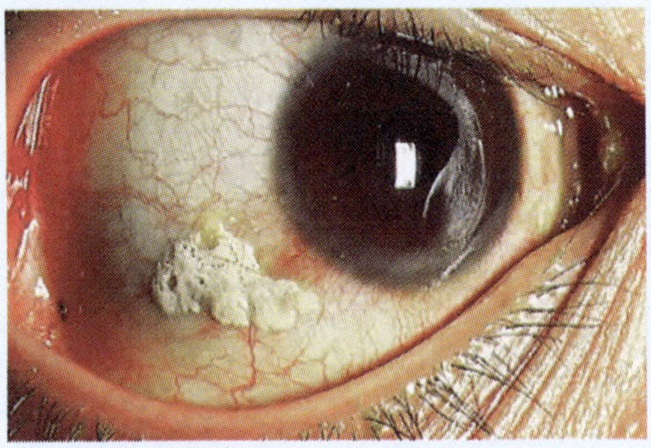
X2	Corneal xerosis*
X3A	Corneal ulceration in <1/3rd of cornea
X3B	Corneal ulceration in >1/3rd of cornea
XN	Night blindness (earliest symptom**)
XS	Scarring
XF	Fundal changes

Toad-like Skin: Phrynoderma is due to Deficiency of Vitamin A

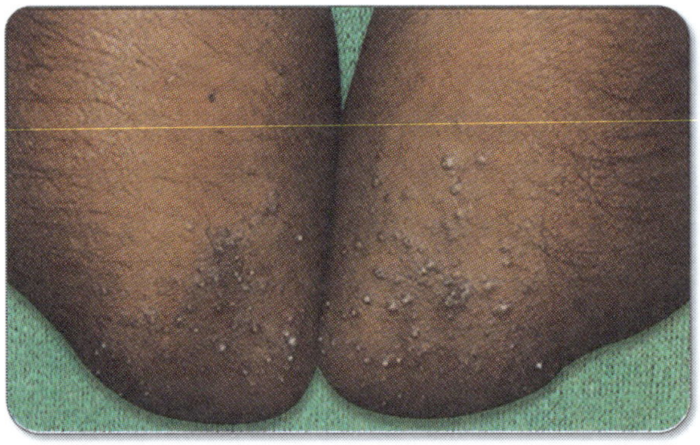

Phrynoderma

VITAMIN B_1—THIAMINE

- **Dietary source:** Human and cow milk, unpolished grains, eggs.
- **Deficiency:** Beriberi is caused by the deficiency of vitamin B_1 and also caused by consuming exclusive polished rice.
- **Types of beriberi:**
  - **Dry:** Affects the CNS causing—peripheral neuritis.
  - **Wet:** Heart failure and peripheral edema.
- **Severe thiamine deficiency causes: Wernicke-Korsakoff syndrome—triad:** Mental confusion, ataxia and ocular abnormalities.

VITAMIN B_2—RIBOFLAVIN

- **Dietary sources:** Meat, milk, eggs, cereals.
- **Deficiency:** Photophobia, corneal vascularization, glossitis, angular stomatitis.

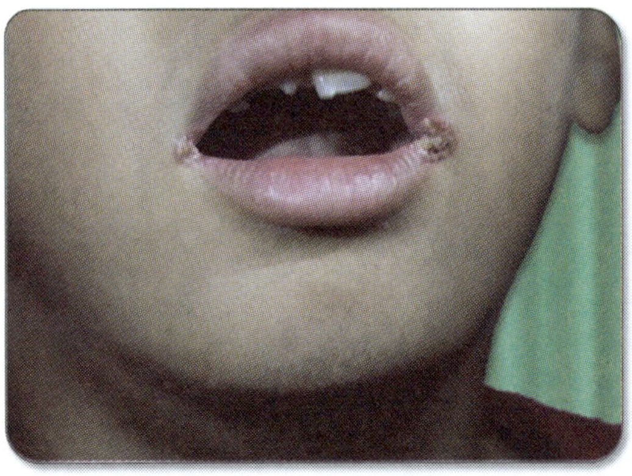

Angular stomatitis

VITAMIN B_3—NIACIN

- **Dietary source**: Milk, egg, meat, legumes, peanuts.
- **Deficiency** is seen in where the staple diet is maize.

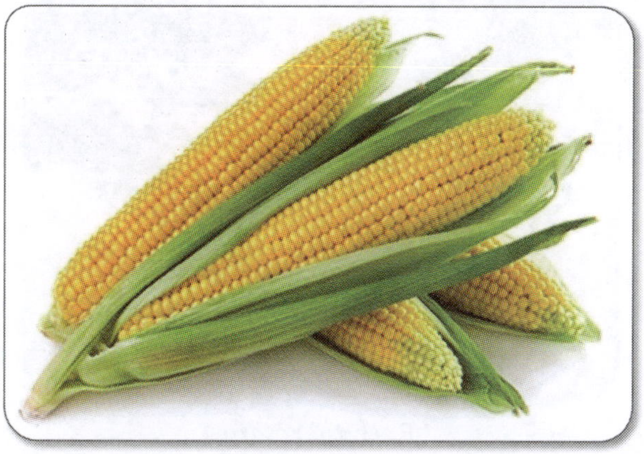

Corn

- Niacin is present in maize but in bound form and not easily absorbed.
- Niacin can be made in body by tryptophan, however, the conversion ratio is 60:1.
- 1 mg of niacin = 60 mg of tryptophan.
- Deficiency causes: "4 Ds"
    - D: Diarrhea
    - D: Dementia
    - D: Dermatitis
    - D: Death
- Symmetrical pigmented rashes seen in areas exposed to sunlight, give an appearance like a necklace known as "Casals necklace".

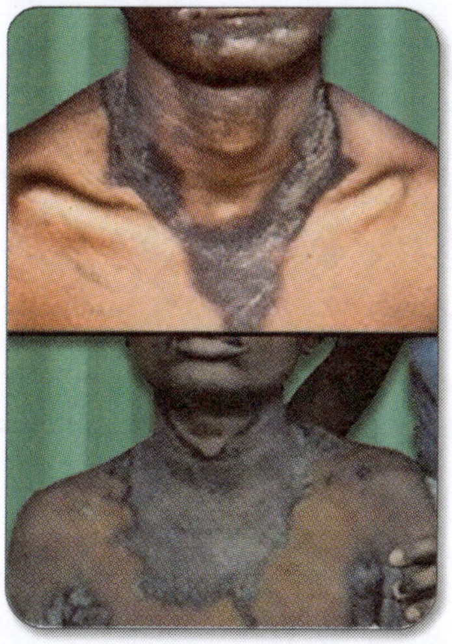

Casals necklace

- Disease which mimic Casals necklace like rash is Hartnup disease.
- Most children are symptomatic.
- Defect in the transport of amino acids including tryptophan*.

VITAMIN C

- Water soluble vitamin
- Active form of vitamin C
- L-ascorbic acid
- Dehydroascorbic acid
- **Functions:**
    - Collagen formation
    - Wound healing
    - Conversion of folic acid from one form to another. Therefore, vitamin C deficiency can lead to megaloblastic anemia*
    - Antioxidant
- **Sources:**
    - Citrus fruits
    - Coriander
    - Tomato + capsicum
- **RDA of vitamin C**
    - Older children: 40 mg/day
    - Pregnancy + lactation: 60–80
- Deficiency of vitamin C causes scurvy

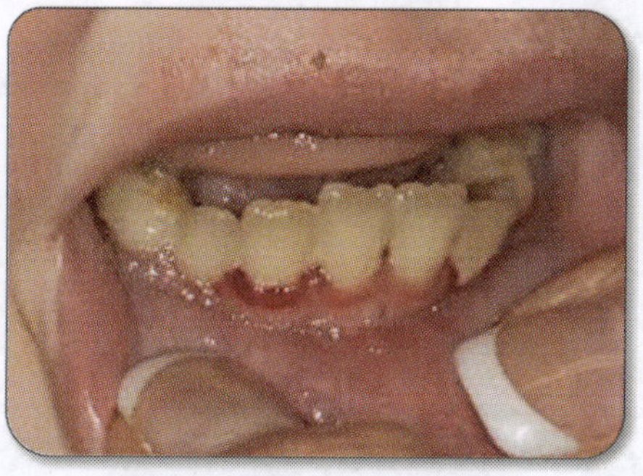

- Most common age group 6 months – 2 years
- **Clinical features**
    - Increased capillary permeability causing petechiae, purpura, ecchymosis
    - Subperiosteal hemorrhage
    - Swelling of the joint

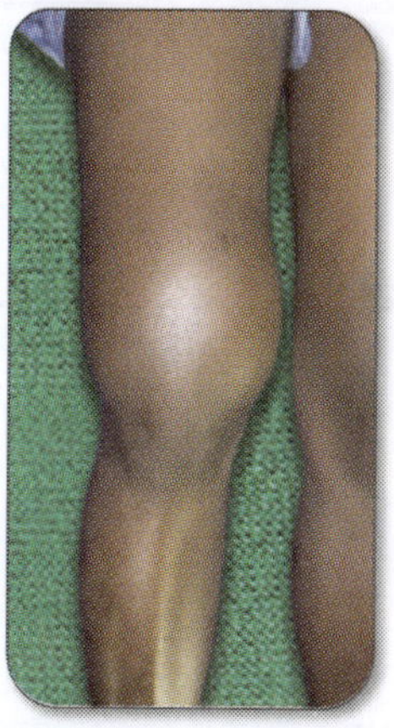

Swelling of joints

- Extreme restriction of movements
- Pseudo paralysis

- Baby screams while changing diaper and bathing
- Ground glass appearance of bone

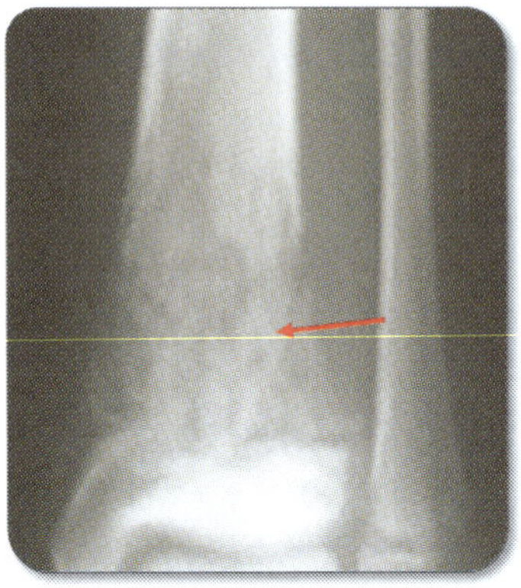

Ground glass appearance

- Wimberger's sign

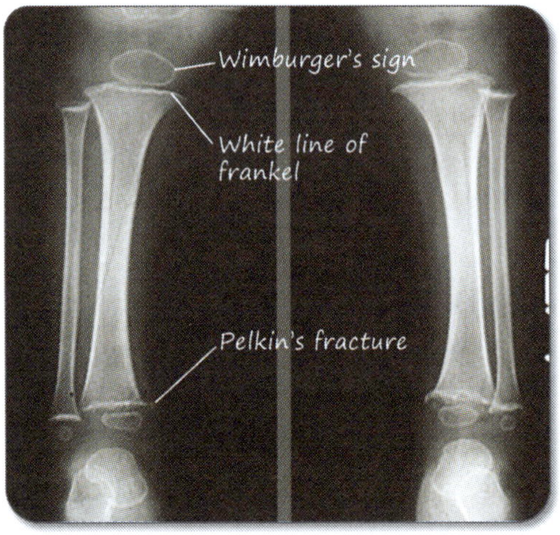

- White line of frankel
- Pelkin's fracture
- **Scorbutic rosary:** Beaded appearance at the cost chondral junction

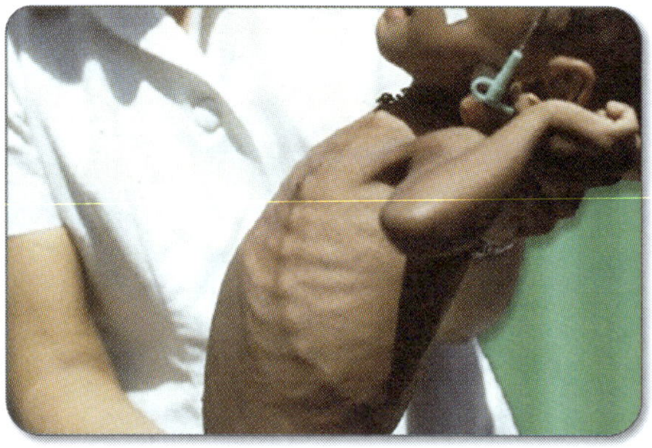

Rachitic rosary

- **Normal vitamin C levels in blood:**
  - 0.4–1.4 mg/dL
  - <0.1 mg/dL—scurvy
- **Rx:** Vitamin C 100–200 mg/day* 3 months

VITAMIN D/RICKETS

- **Vitamin D produced:** In the skin on exposure to sunlight—ultraviolet b radiation of wavelength 290–315 nm.
- **Sources of vitamin D:** Fatty fish, fish oil
- **Two forms of vitamin D:**
  1. Vitamin D_3, made in animals
  2. Vitamin D_2, ergocalciferol made in plants

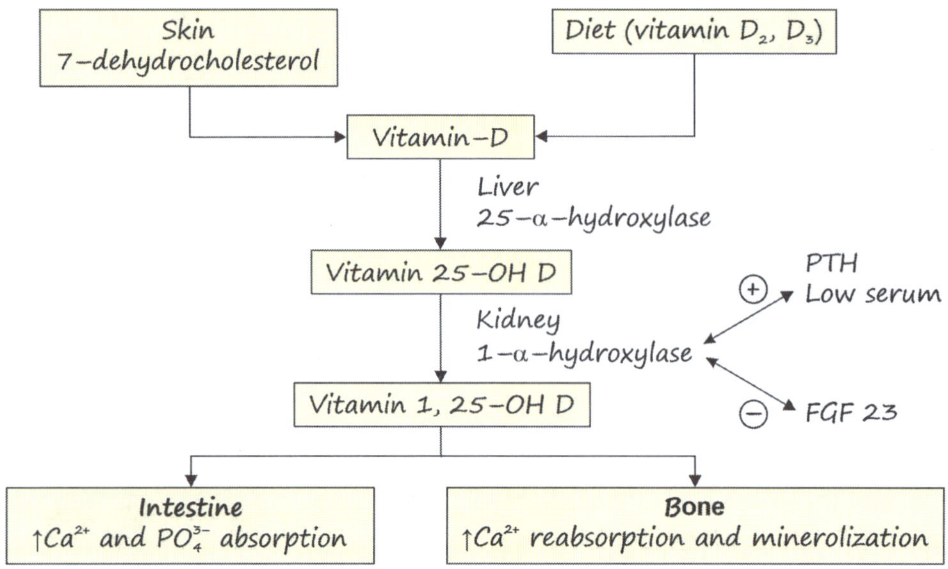

Vitamin D metabolizm

Rickets

- Most common cause of rickets is deficiency of vitamin D and/or calcium.
- It is a disease of growing bone.
- There is defective mineralization of the bone. (osteomalacia is defective mineralization of nongrowing bones)
- Mother's milk is deficient in vitamin D. Therefore breastfeed infant should be given vitamin D 400 IU for terms and 800 IU for preterms for the duration of one year.
- **X-ray findings:**
    - Cupping
    - Fraying
    - Splaying appearance

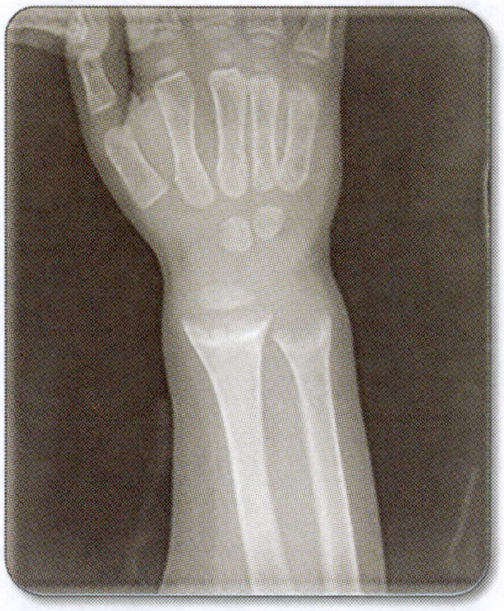

Rickets

Treatment

Age	Daily dose of vitamins for 12 weeks	Daily calcium supplementation
<6 months	2000 IU	30–75 mg/kg/day
6–12 months	3000 IU	30–75 mg/kg/day
<12 months	6000 IU	30–75 mg/kg/day

Vitamin D-Dependent Rickets (VDDR) Type I

- Autosomal recessive
- Deficiency of enzyme 1-α-hydroxylase.
- Leading to decrease in levels of 1, 25-Dihydroxyvitamin D

Levels of 25-OH vitamin D will be normal.

- Clinical features are similar to vitamin D deficiency:
    - Hypotonia
    - Growth failure
    - Delayed standing and walking
    - Convulsions due to hypocalcemia

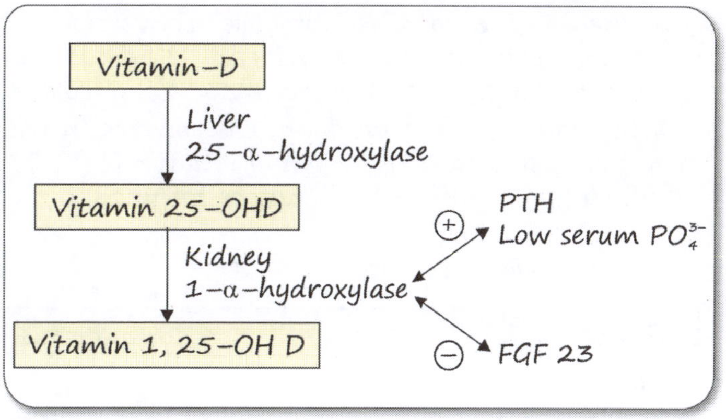

Treatment

Supplementation of 1, 25-Dihydroxyvitamin D with calcium supplementation.

Vitamin D-Dependent Rickets (VDDR) Type II

- Autosomal recessive
- Mutation in the gene encoding vitamin D receptor
- There will be raised levels of 1, 25-OH D
- It does not respond to vitamin D treatment
- ***Clinical features:***
    - Alopecia
    - Ectodermal defects (oligodontia—congenital absence of >6 teeth, milia)

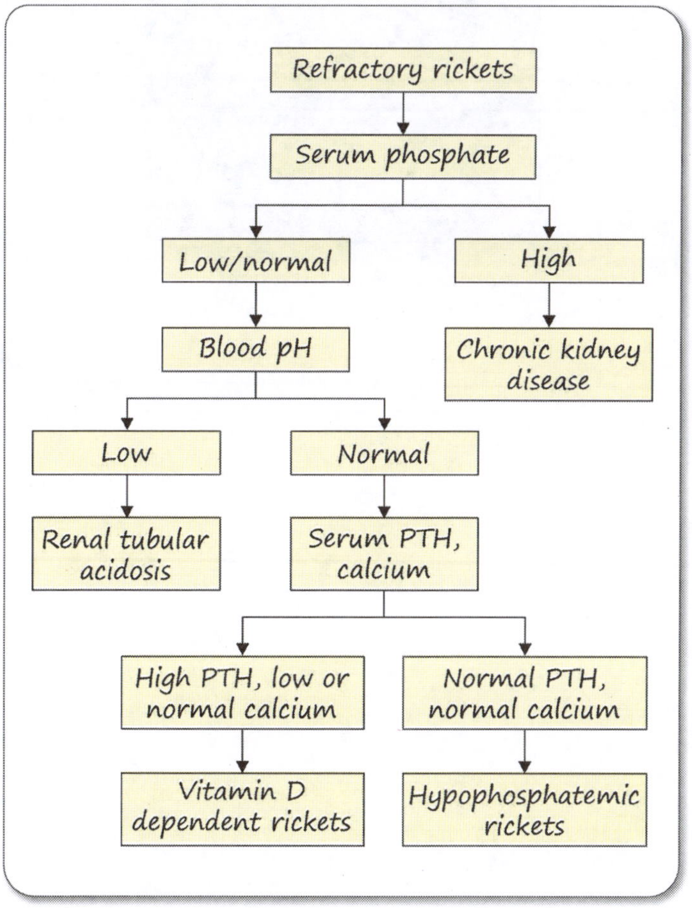

Refractory rickets

- Kidney is responsible for the conversion of 25 hydroxy vitamin D into 1, 25 dihydroxy vitamin D with the help of enzyme 1-α-hydroxide.
- When kidney is not working, the conversion will not happen and active form of vitamin D (1, 25 dihydroxy vitamin D) will not be formed.
- Normal function of 1, 25 dihydroxy vitamin D is phosphate reabsorption.
- Therefore, in chronic kidney disease, there is increase phosphate levels.

Serum Vitamin D Levels

Deficient	<12 nanogram/mL	<25 nanomoles/L
Insufficient	12–20 nanogram/mL	25–50 nanomoles/L
Sufficient	>20 nanogram/mL	>50 nanomoles/L
Toxic	>100 nanogram/mL	>250 nanomoles/L

ZINC

- **Deficiency**: Acrodermatitis enteropathica

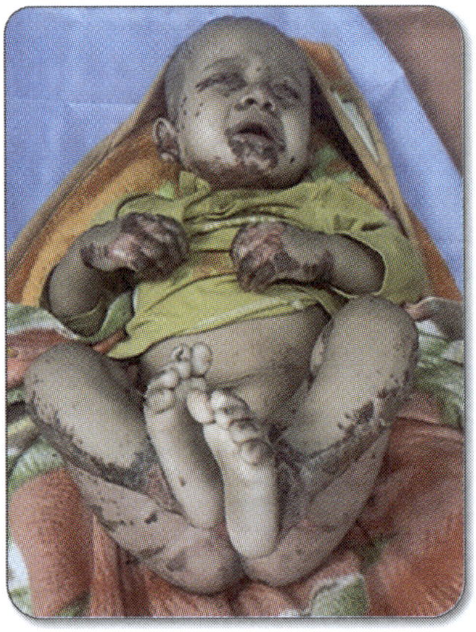

Acrodermatitis enteropathica

- **Inheritance:** Autosomal recessive
- **Clinical features:**
    - Perioral and perivaginal rash
    - Diarrhea
    - Failure to thrive
    - Impotence
    - Seen in the weaning period
- **Gene mutation**: SLC39A4

Extra Points

- Goat's milk is poor source of folate.
- Therefore, children who are on goat milk can lead to megaloblastic anemia.

11. VACCINES

"People say motivation doesn't last long well neither does the bathing, that's why we recommend it everyday."

INTRODUCTION

Vaccine is a substance used to stimulate the production of antibodies and provide immunity against the disease.

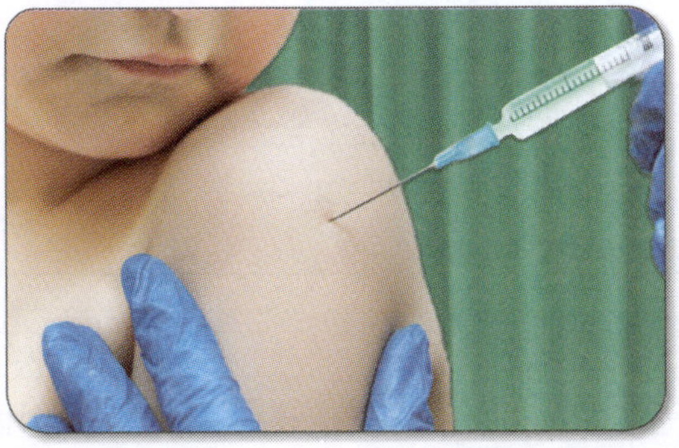

TYPES OF VACCINE

- S: Subunit vaccine
- T: Toxoid vaccine
- A: Attenuated live vaccine
- R: Recombinant vaccine
- K: Killed vaccine
- P: Polysaccharide vaccine

ROUTES OF VACCINE

- **Intranasal:**
  - H1N1
  - COVID vaccine
- **Oral:**
  - Rotavirus
  - OPV
  - Typhi oral
  - Vitamin A
- **Subcutaneous:**
  - Measles
  - MMR
  - Varicella
  - Meningococcal polysaccharide
  - JE
  - Yellow fever
  - Typhoid (s/c or IM)
- **Intradermal:**
  - IPV
  - Rabies
  - BCG
- **Intramuscular:**
  - Pentavalent
  - Hepatitis B
  - Tetanus
  - Hepatitis A
  - Hib
  - PCV (pneumococcal)
  - HPV
  - DPT
  - TT

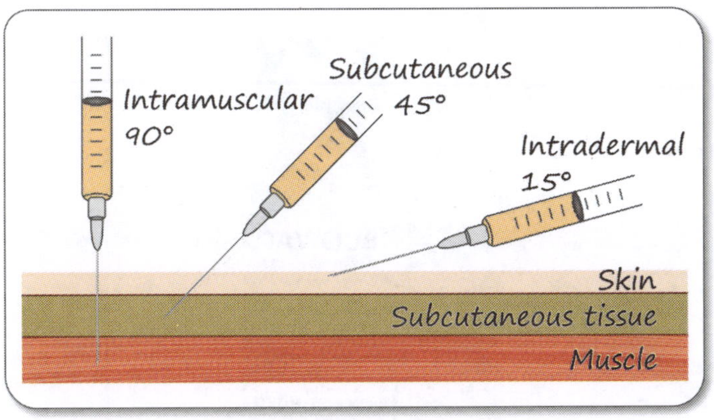

Routes of vaccine

Golden Points

- Which route we do not use for vaccination: intravenous
- All the vaccines are stored under 2°–8°C except OPV which is stored under –20°C

LIGHT-SENSITIVE VACCINES

- BCG
- DPT
- MMR
- HPV
- Rotavirus

WHERE TO KEEP THE VACCINES

- Freezing compartment: OPV
- Top compartment: BCG, measles
- Lower: Diluent
- Middle: DPT, TT, Pentavac, Hep A, B, Typhoid, varicella

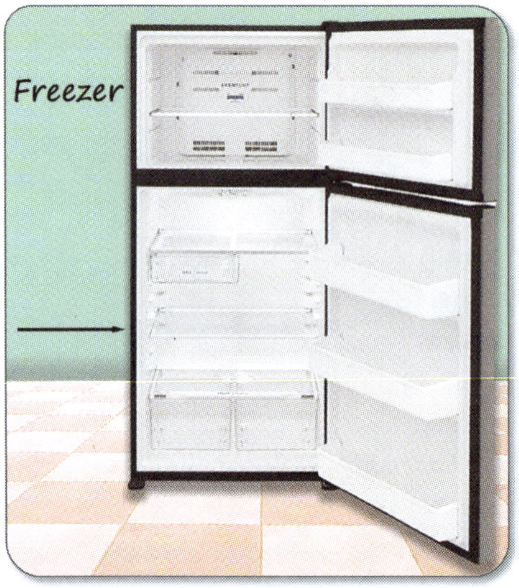

Vaccine	Substrate
DPT	Thiomersal (preservative) Aluminum hydroxide (adjuvant)
Measles	No preservative
BCG	No preservative
OPV	Magnesium chloride (thermostabilizer)

VACCINE VIAL MONITOR (VVM)

- *If the inner square is white and the outer circle is blue—vaccine is good to use.*
- *If the inner square matches the outer circle—vaccine is not good to use.*
- *Inner square is darker than outer circle—vaccine is beyond discard point.*

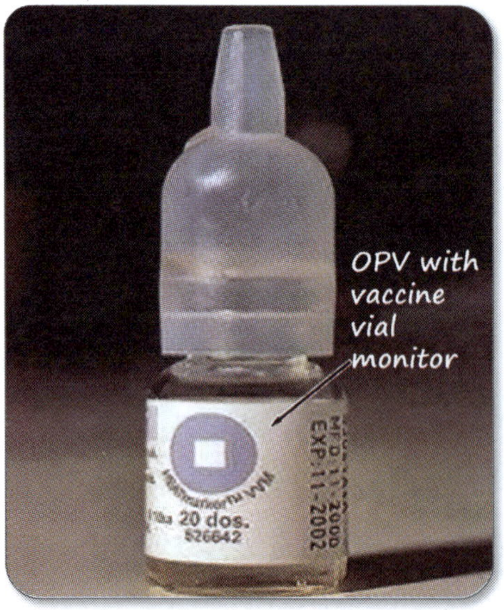

Extra Points

If anyone is allergic to eggs, then he/she should be careful of yellow fever and influenza vaccine.

LATEST NATIONAL IMMUNIZATION SCHEDULE

Age	Vaccine
At birth	BCG, bOPV-0, Hep B-0
6 weeks	bOPV-1, Pentavalent-1, Rotavirus-1*, fIPV-1, PCV-1*
10 weeks	bOPV-2, Pentavalent-2, Rotavirus-2*
14 weeks	bOPV-3, Pentavalent-3, Rotavirus-3, fIPV-2, PCV-2*
9 months	MR-1*, JE-1*, PCV-3*
16–24 months	DPT-B1, bOPV-B, JE-2*, MR-2*
5–6 years	DPT-B2
11–13 years	HPV-1*, HPV-2*

Important Points

- ***Vaccine which causes maximum cry***—DPT
- ***Vaccine which can cause seizures***—pertussis
- ***Vaccine which is contraindicated if the patient had intussusception***—rotavirus
- *Rotavirus vaccine is given to prevent diarrhea and the most common side effect of rotavirus vaccine is diarrhea.*

BCG VACCINE

- **Full form:** *Bacillus Calmette-Guerin vaccine*
- *Live vaccine*
- *BCG vaccine contains 0.1–0.4 million live bacilli per dose*
- **Strain:** *Danish 1331*
- **Diluent:** *Normal saline*
- **Form:** *Freeze-dried form*

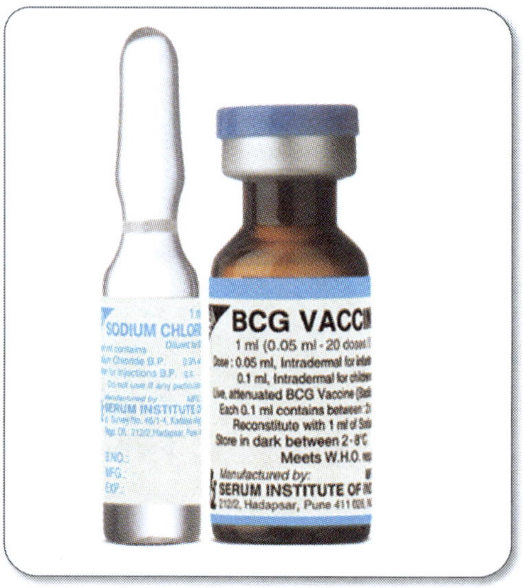

- **Protects from:** Extra pulmonary tuberculosis.
- **Route:** Intradermal.
- **Store:** 2°–8°C.
- **Catch up:** Till 1 year.
- BCG scar develops by 3 months of life.

BCG-Scar

- BCG prevents mainly from extrapulmonary TB.
- **Side effects:**
  - BCG adenitis* if given subcutaneous BCG
  - Osteitis* ulceration, infection

IAP LATEST VACCINATION GUIDELINES

Age	Vaccine
At birth	BCG, bOPV-0, Hep B1
6 weeks	DPT-1, **IPV-1**, Hep-B2, HiB-1, PCV 1, Rotavirus 1
10 weeks	DPT-2, **IPV-2**, Hib-2, PCV-2, Rotavirus-2
14 weeks	DPT-3, **IPV-3**, Hib-3, PCV-3, Rotavirus-3
6 months	**bOPV-1, Hep B3**
9 months	bOPV2, **MMR-1, Typhoid conjugate**, JE-1
12 months	**IPV-B1, Hib-B1, PCV-B1, Hep A1**
15 months	DTP-B1, MMR-2, **Varicella 1**, JE-2
18 months	**Hep A 2**
2 years	**Typhoid conjugate-B**
4–6 years	DPT B2, bOPV-3, MMR-3, Varicella-2
11–12 years	Tdap, HPV-1, HPV-2

Golden Points (Strain Used in Vaccine)

- **Edmonston Zagreb strain, Schwarz strain, Moraten strain:** Measles
- **Jeryl Lynn:** Mumps
- **Polio:** Lansing, Leon, Brunhilde
- **Oka strain:** Varicella
- **Danish 1331:** BCG
- **RA 27/3:** Rubella
- **Typhoid Oral:** Ty21
- **Cholera:** Dukoral, Shanchol*
- **Rabies:** Pitts More Strain*
- **Yellow fever:** 17D*
- **Hepatitis A:** HM175
- **Diphtheria:** Park Williams 8
- **JE vaccine:** Nakayama Strain, Beijing Strain, SA 14-14-2 (Used In India)
- **Swine Flu vaccine:** A7/California/2009*

Extra Points

Drugs given intranasal:

- COVID vaccine
- H1N1
- Febrile seizure
- Desmopressin in hemophilia
- Diabetes insipidus
- Coryza

POLIO VACCINE

- **Two types of polio vaccine:**
  1. Oral polio vaccine live (Sabin).
  2. Inactivated* polio vaccine: killed (Salk).
- On 25th April there was a switch from trivalent OPV to bivalent OPV.

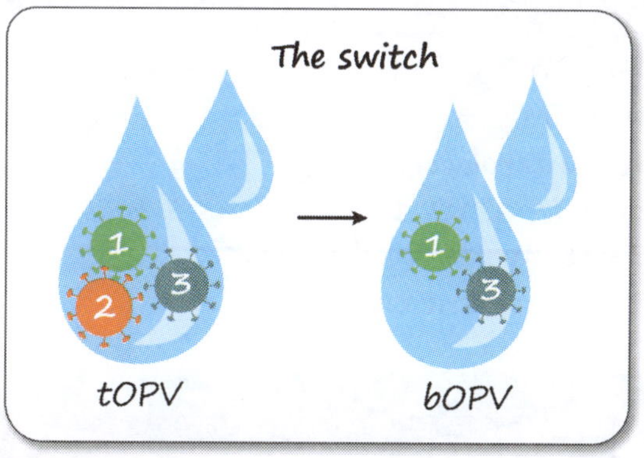

- Removing the type 2 component as interferes with the immune response.
- Birth dose of polio cannot cause vaccine associated paralytic polio (VAPP).
- Last case of polio reported was in Jan 2011.

- India was certified polio free on 27th march 2014.
- **Dose:** 2 drops
- **Route:** Oral
- **Schedule:** Birth—zero dose, 6, 10, 14 then booster at 15–18 months and 5 years.
- **IPV (inactivated polio vaccine)**
    - **Dose:** 0.5 mL
    - **Route:** IM/SC (0.5 mL) ID (0.1 mL) (ID right upper arm)
    - **Schedule:** 6 weeks, 14 weeks
    - ID - 2 doses

    Or
    - IM – 1 dose – 14 weeks

HEPATITIS B VACCINE

- **Schedule:** Birth, 6 week, 6 months
- **Route:** Intramuscular
- **Dose:** 0.5 mL
- **Site:** Anterolateral aspect of thigh

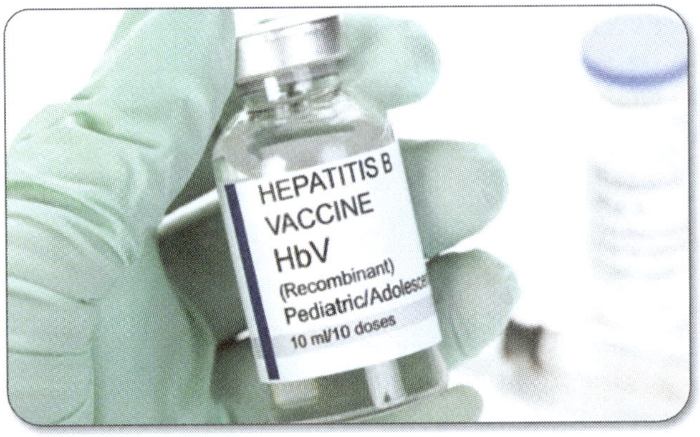

Diphtheria, Pertussis, Tetanus Vaccine (DTP)

- **Dose:** 0.5 mL.
- **Route:** IM.
- **Site:** Anterolateral thigh.
- **Schedule:** 6, 10, 14 weeks and 2 booster doses at 15–18 months and 5 years.
- **ADV:** Persistent cry.

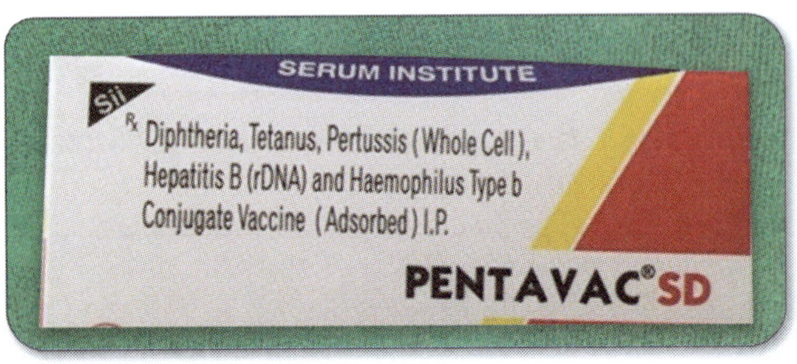

MEASLES VACCINE

- Live vaccine.
- **Strain:** Edmonston-Zagreb
- **Diluent:** Distilled water
- **Adv:** May cause Thrombocytopenic purpura*
- **Measles minimum age:** 9 months or 270 completed days
- **Side effect:** Toxic shock syndrome
- **Route:** S/C
- **Site:** Right upper arm
- **Dose:** 0.5 mL
- Unused measles vaccines should be discarded within 4–6 hours.

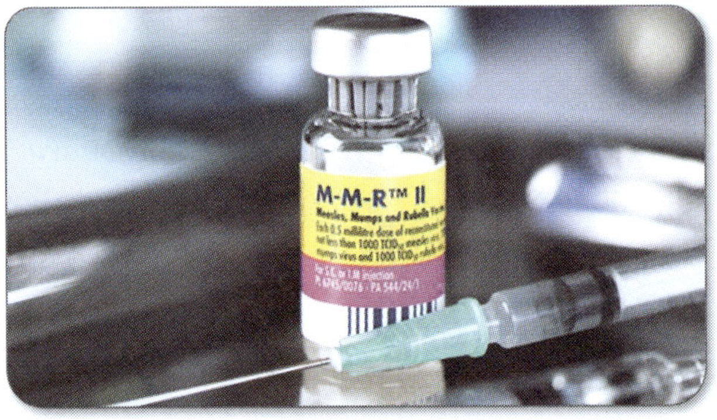

ROTAVIRUS VACCINE

- Oral live.
- **RotaTeq (3):** 2 mL - 6, 10, 14 weeks pentavalent.
- **Rotarix (2):** 1.5 mL 10, 14 weeks monovalent.
- **ROTAVAC:** 5 drops – 3 dose 6, 10, 14 weeks.
- **Side effect:**
    - Diarrhea
    - Vomiting
    - Intussusception

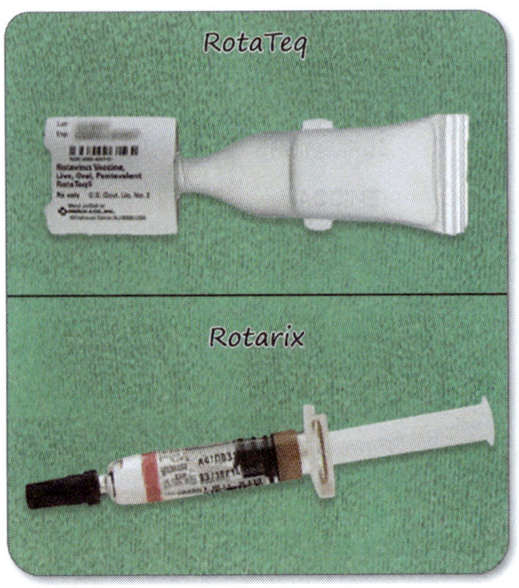

CHICKEN POX VACCINE

- **Dose:** 0.5 mL.
- **Route:** SC.
- **Schedule:** 15 months and 4–6 years.

RABIES

- **World rabies day:** 28th September.
- Approach to dog bite.
- First clean the wound with soap and running water for 10 minutes.
- Then categorize the wound:
    - Category 1: Only reassurance, no treatment
    - Category 2: Inj TT (tetanus toxoid) + ARV (antirabies vaccine)
    - Category 3: Inj TT + ARV + ARS (antirabies serum)

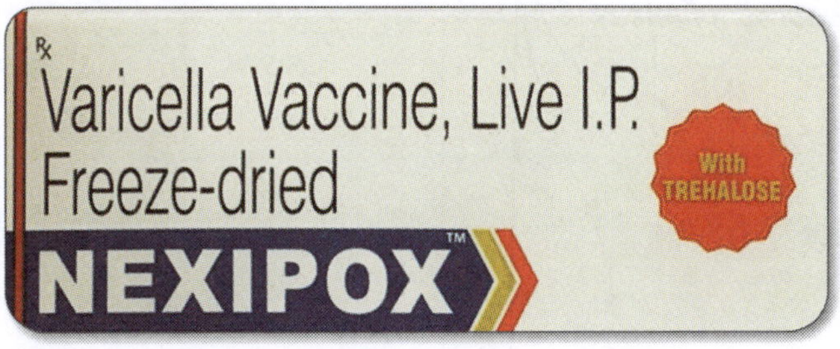

Golden Points

- Anti rabies serum (ARS) is given once in lifetime
- **Schedule of ARS:** Day 0, 3, 7, 30
- **In ARS we have two options:**
    1. Human rabies immunoglobulin: 20 IU/kg: (max. 1500).
    2. Equine rabies immunoglobulin: 40 IU/kg: (max. 3000).

HPV VACCINE (HUMAN PAPILLOMA VIRUS VACCINE)

- **Cervarix:** Protects from strain 16 and 18
    - **Schedule:** 0, 1 month
- **Gardasil:** 6, 11, 16, 18
    - **Schedule:** 0, 1, 6 months

"If the world was blind, how many people you would have impressed."

12. HEMATOLOGY AND INFECTIOUS DISEASE

LYMES DISEASE

- Most common vector-borne disease is caused by spirochete Borrelia burgdorferi.
- Bite of the infected tick: Blacklegged tick/Deer tick.

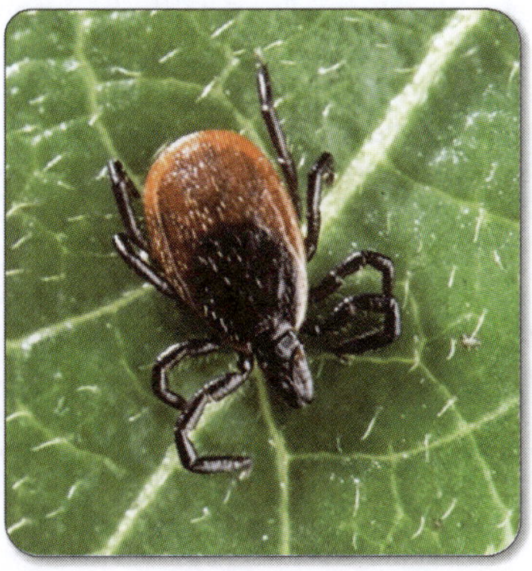

Blacklegged tick

- Erythema migrans

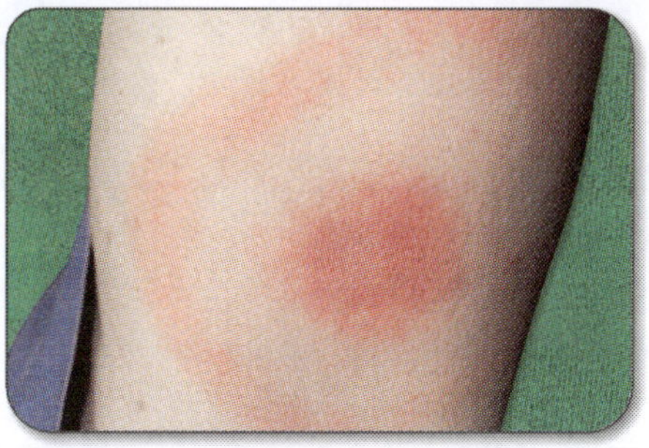

- It's typically a circular red area that is sometimes clear in the middle forming a bull's-eye pattern.

Treatment: Doxycycline/amoxicillin

MALARIA

- Caused by: Four species of genus plasmodium
    1. Plasmodium vivax—occurs in India
    2. Plasmodium falciparum—occurs in India
    3. Plasmodium ovale
    4. Plasmodium malariae

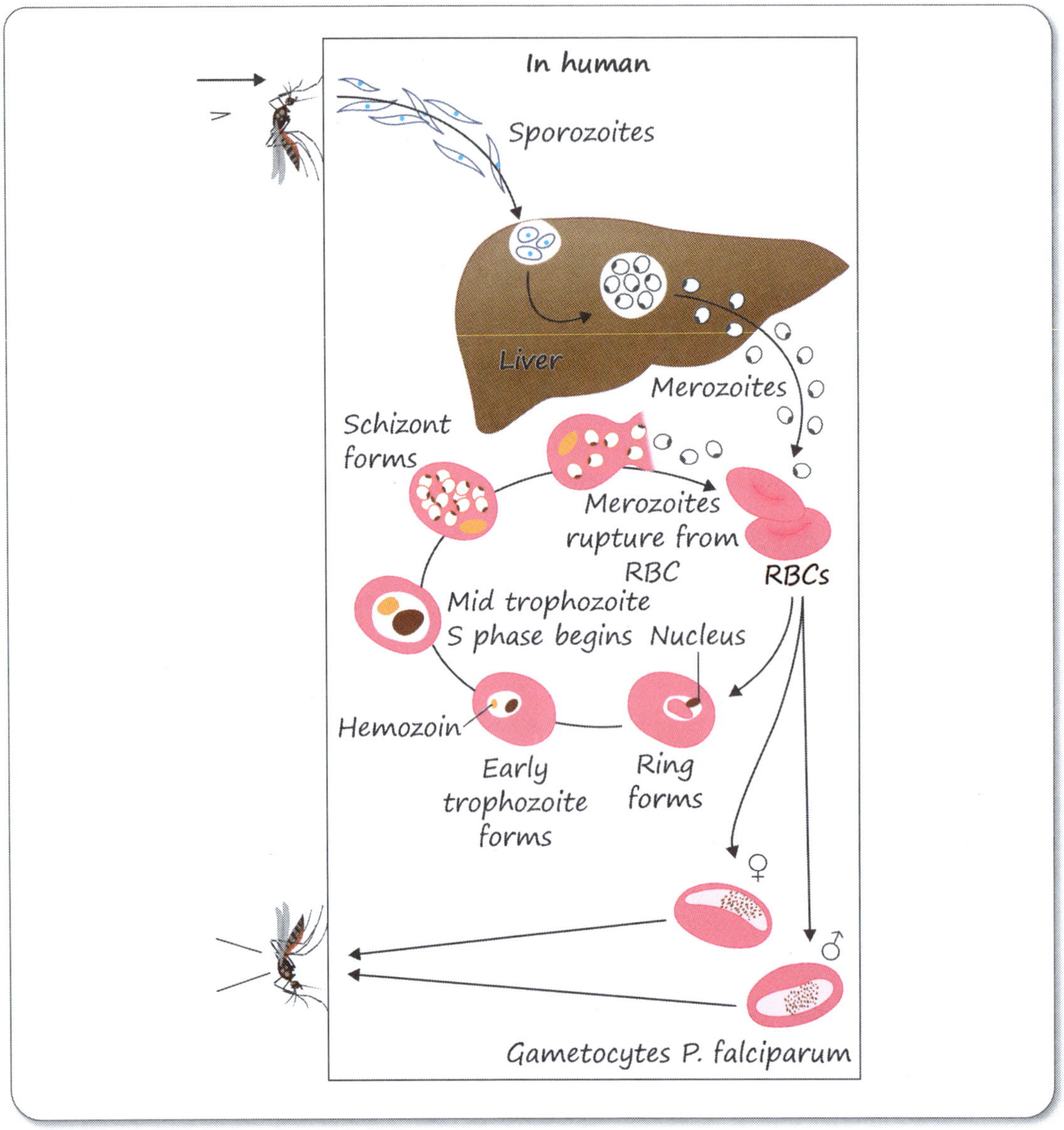

Lifecycle—Malaria

- **Life cycle:**
    - Hepatic phase
    - Erythrocytic phase
    - Gametocytes phase
- **Clinical features:**
    - Fever
    - Muscle pain
    - Lethargy
    - Abdominal pain
    - Hepatosplenomegaly with developing anemia

Severe Complication of Malaria

- Symptomatic malaria with signs and evidence of vital organ dysfunction is known as severe or complicated malaria.
- Features:
    - Cerebral malaria: Unarousable coma
    - Severe anemia: Hb <5 g/dL, hematocrit <15%
    - Hypoglycemia <40 mg/dL
    - Respiratory distress (acidosis) pH <7.35, bicarbonate <15 mmol/L
    - Circulatory collapse/shock (algid malaria): Defined as systolic BP <50 mm Hg in children
    - Pulmonary edema
    - Renal failure: Serum creatinine >3 mg/dL or urine output <0.5 mL/kg/hr
    - Jaundice: Serum bilirubin >3 mg/dL
- Gold standard investigation of choice:* Light microscopy of well stained thick and thin films

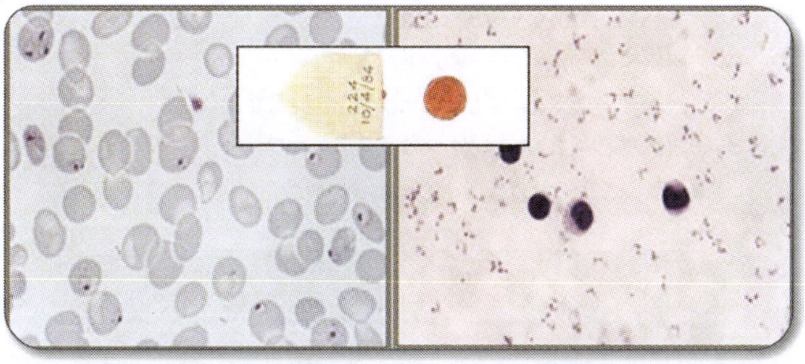

Thick smear	Thin smear
10 times more sensitive than thin smear	Identification of plasmodium species
Detects even at low levels of parasitaemia	Response to therapy
Skilled staff required	

Rapid Diagnostic Test for Malaria (RDT)

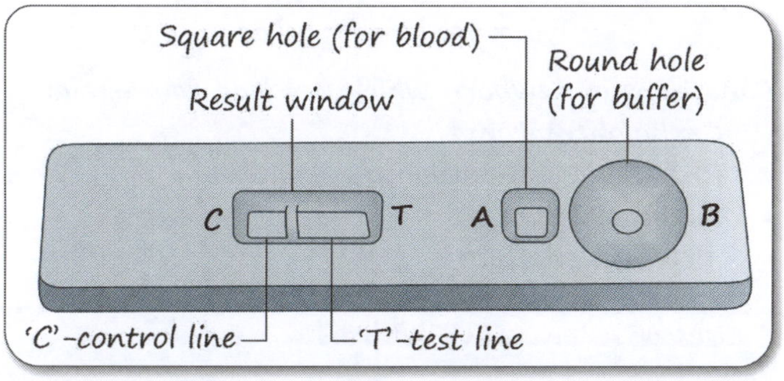

pfHRP2 (histidine rich protein)	pLDH/Vivax specific	pAldolase/ pLDH
Falciparum specific	Vivax specific	Detects malaria, not species
Sensitivity 95% and specificity 95.2%	Sensitivity 95% and specificity 98.5%.	
Cannot differentiate between new infection and recent infection. pfHRP2 + in blood for 1–5 weeks.	Rapidly negative after treatment, however can be positive due to the presence of gametocytes.	

- **Rx for uncomplicated P. vivax malaria**
  - Chloroquine: At 0, 6, 24, 48 hours
  - 10 mg/kg/day followed by 5 mg/kg/day
  - Total dose 25 mg/kg
  - To prevent relapse—what to add?
    Primaquine 0.25 mg/kg once daily for 14 days
  - Before starting primaquine: Get G6PD done as primaquine causes hemolytic anemia in G6PD deficiency patients
- **Rx for uncomplicated P. falciparum**
  - Artesunate 4 mg/kg od for 3 days and single dose of Sp
    S: Sulfadoxine
    p: Pyrimethamine

ITP–IDIOPATHIC THROMBOCYTOPENIC PURPURA/WERLHOF DISEASE

- ITP is the most common bleeding disorder present in children between 1 and 7 years of age.
- ITP is an immune mediated disorder against the platelet glycoprotein IIb/IIIa complex.
- Hallmark: Increase in megakaryocyte.
- Clinical features:
  - Bruising
  - Ecchymosis
  - Fall in platelet

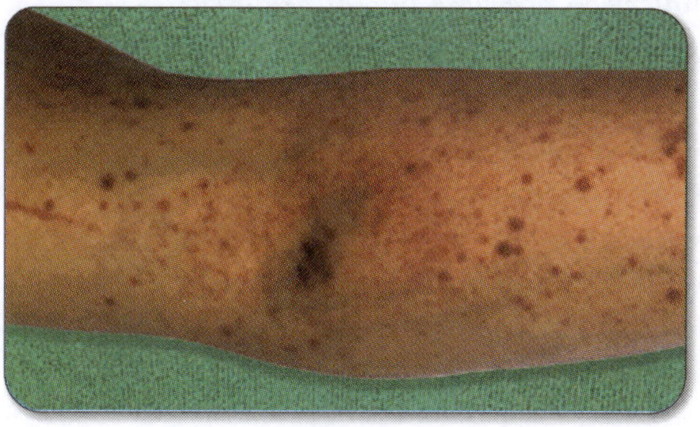

Purpura

Treatment

- Platelet count >20 thousand: Wait and watch
- Platelet count >20 thousand with bleeding:
  - IVIg: 1 g/kg/day
  - Dexamethasone: 20 mg/m^2 4 days
  - Prednisolone: 1-2 mg/kg/day for 2-3 weeks

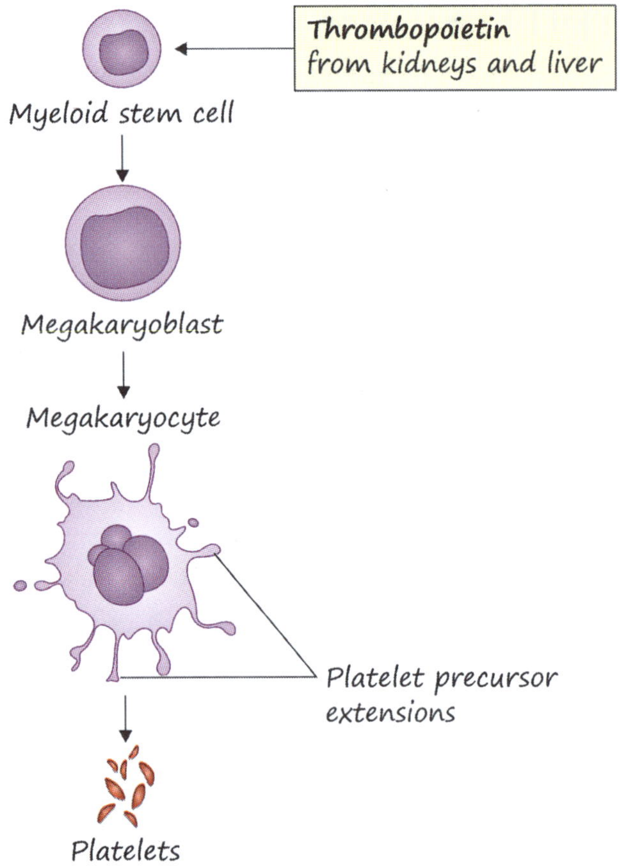

> **Golden Points**
>
> **Indication of giving IVIg in pediatrics**
> - ITP: Idiopathic thrombocytopenic purpura
> - GBS: Guillain-Barré syndrome
> - KD: Kawasaki disease
> - MMN: Multifocal motor neuropathy
> - CLL: Chronic lymphocytic leukemia
> - CIDP: Chronic inflammatory demyelinating polyneuropathy
> - Neonatal jaundice

ANEMIA

- To heal a wound, you need to stop touching it!
- Anemia is a sign, not a symptom.
- Definition: Hb level in the blood has two standard deviation below the mean for the age and sex.
- For 6 months – 5 years
  - Hb <7 g/dL—severe anemia
  - Hb 7-10 g/dL—moderate anemia
  - Hb 10-11 g/dL—mild anemia
  - Hb >11 g/dL—nonanemic

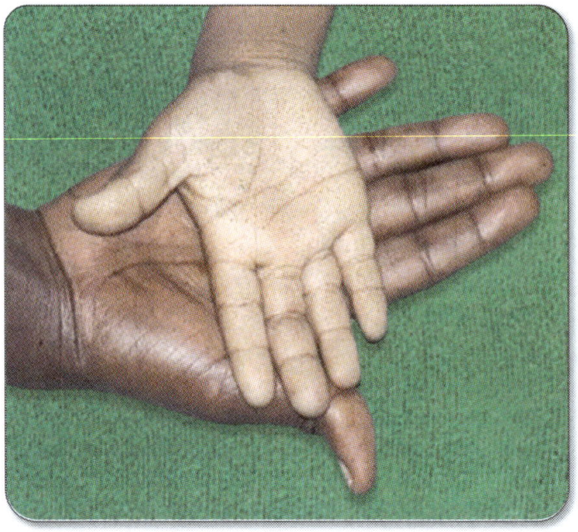

How to look for pallor

Conditions in newborn which can lead to anemia:
- Cephalohematoma
- Rh/ABO incompatibility
- Enzymopathies
- Membranopathies

Causes of Anemia in Children

- **During weaning time:** Iron deficiency anemia (6 months – 2 years)
- **CMPA:** Cow milk protein allergy (bloody diarrhea)
- **A child on pure veg diet and goat milk:** Megaloblastic anemia

Differential Diagnosis of Microcytic Hypochromic Anemia

> **Mnemonic—SHITAL**
>
> S – Sideroblastic anemia
> H – —x—
> I – Iron deficiency anemia
> T – Thalassemia
> A – Anemia of chronic disease
> L – Lead poisoning

	RDW	Serum iron	TIBC	Serum ferritin	FEP
Iron deficiency	Inc	Dec	Inc	Dec	Inc
Alpha Thal	Norm	Norm	Norm	Norm	Norm
Beta Thal	Norm	Norm	Norm	Norm	Norm
Hgb E Disease	Norm	Norm	Norm	Norm	Norm
Anemia of chronic disease	Norm	Dec	Dec	Inc	Inc
Sideroblastic anemia	Inc	Inc	Norm	Inc	Dec
Lead poisoning	Norm	Norm	Norm	Norm	Inc

Golden Points

- What is reticulocyte count?
  - Precursor of RBC
  - Devoid of nucleus
  - Releases early in case of requirement
- High retic count is seen in:
  - Hemolysis: autoimmune hemolytic anemia, hereditary spherocytosis
  - Hemorrhage
  - Sepsis
- Low retic count is seen in:
  - Congenital or acquired aplastic anemia
  - Pure red cell aplasia
  - Parvovirus B19 infection
  - Bone marrow failure/storage disorder
  - Transient erythroblastopenia of infancy
- Low retic count + low serum iron + low ferritin + increased TIBC = iron deficiency anemia
- Low serum iron + high ferritin + low TIBC = anemia of chronic disease
- Low serum iron + normal or high ferritin + normal or low TIBC+ ESR, CRP elevated = acute inflammatory disease

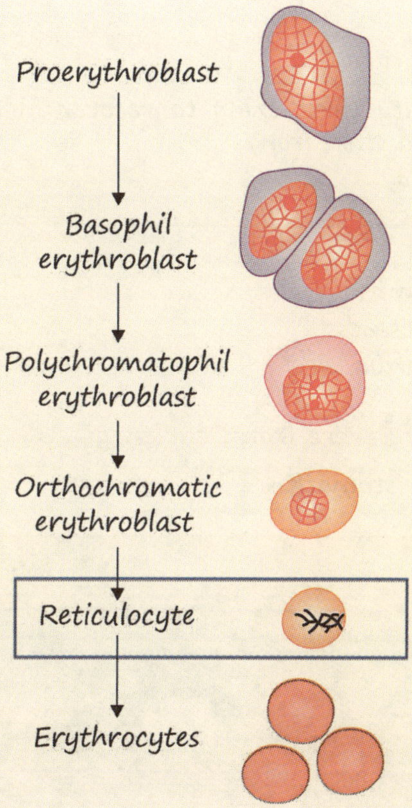

Iron Deficiency Anemia

- Factors that help in increasing iron absorption:
  - Ascorbic acid
  - Acidic pH
  - Sugar
  - Jaggery
- Breast milk contains small amount of iron
- But every baby is not given iron after birth because the bioavailability of this iron is 70–80% hence it is adequate for first 6 months of life
- Factors that help in decreasing iron absorption:
  - Calcium
  - Milk
  - Cereals
  - Legumes
  - Nuts
  - Tea, coffee, wine

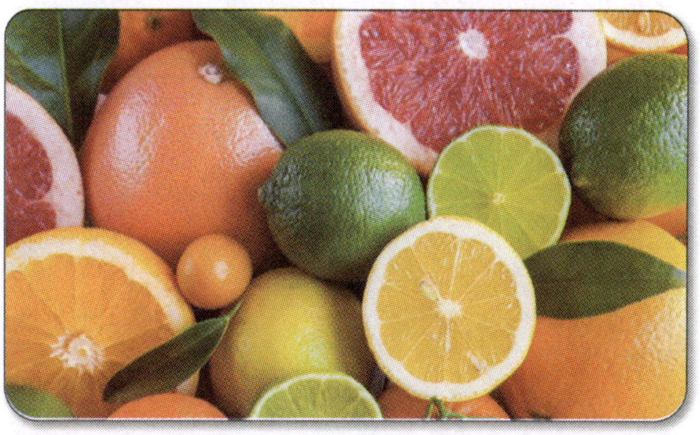

Absorption

Mnemonic—IFB

I – Iron is absorbed in duodenum

F – Folic acid is absorbed in jejunum (vitamin K is also absorbed in jejunum)

B – B_{12} is absorbed in ileum

- The best noninvasive test (gold standard) for evaluating iron status in the body: serum ferritin.
- The cutoff for serum ferritin in IDA: <12 ng/dL

Clinical Features

- Irritability (first thing to recover in 24 hours once you start iron)*
- Anorexia
- Weakness
- Fatigue
- Leg cramps
- Breathlessness
- Tachycardia

Features of Severe Iron Deficiency

- Angular stomatitis

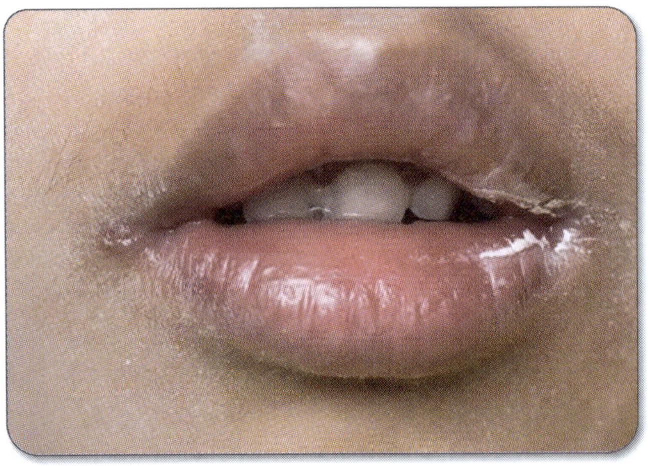

- Koilonychia: Spoon-shaped nail

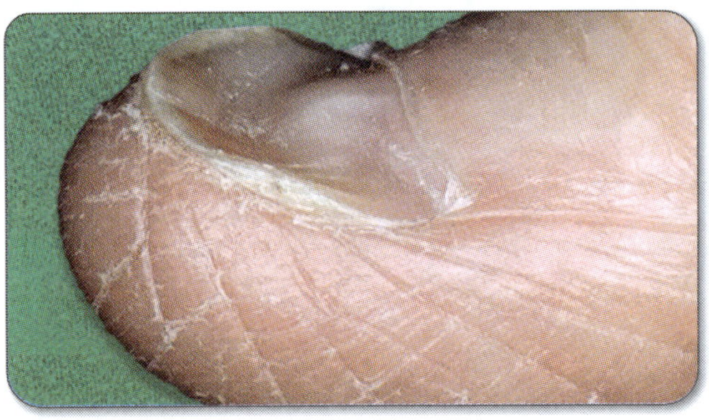

- Platynychia: Abnormally flat or broad nails
- Peripheral smear: Microcytic hypochromic anemia with pencil cells, target cells.
- Reticulocyte count will be raised
- Lab findings:
  - Low serum iron
  - High TIBC: >350 mg/dL
  - Most sensitive and specific marker in iron deficiency anemia: serum ferritin

Treatment

- Iron: 3–6 mg/kg/day
- Give empty stomach or in between meals

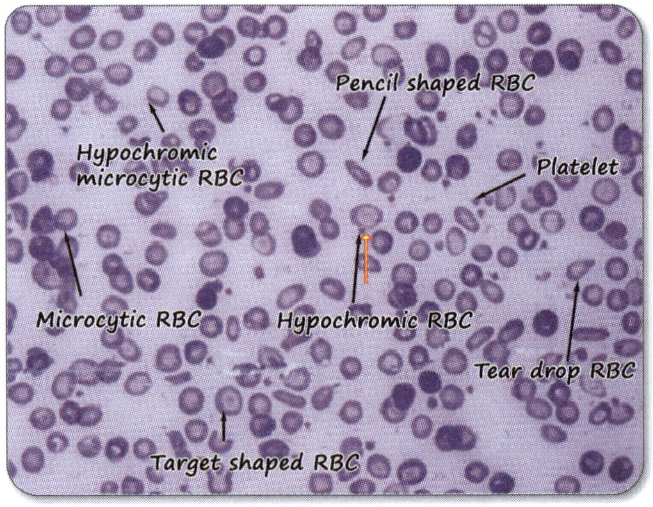

- It can cause gastritis, pain abdomen, constipation and diarrhea.
- Duration: 4–6 months.
- Irritability will decrease in 24 hours.
- Retic count will increase in 72–96 hours.
- Give vitamin C with iron therapy as it will improve the absorption.

Days of Appearance of Rash

- Very—varicella/chicken pox—fever with rash on day 1
- Sick—scarlet fever—fever with rash on day 2
- People—smallpox—fever with rash on day 3
- Must—measles—fever with rash on day 4
- Take—typhus—fever with rash on day 5
- Double—dengue—fever with rash on day 6
- Tablets—typhoid—fever with rash on day 7

MEASLES/RUBEOLA

- Cause: RNA virus—family Paramyxoviridae
- Incubation period: 8–12 days

Clinical Features

- Remember "3Cs"
  1. Cough
  2. Coryza
  3. Conjunctivitis (purulent)

Pathology

- Pathognomonic sign: Warthin-Finkeldey giant cells.

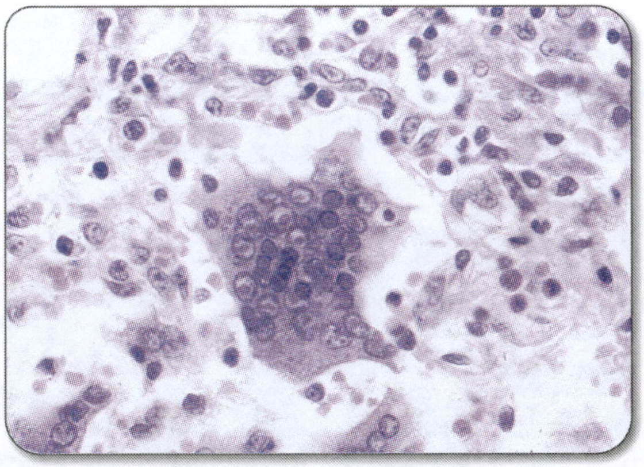

Warthin—Finkeldey giant cell

- Kolpkik spot: Discrete red lesions with bluish white spots in the center on the inner aspects of the cheek at the level of 1st and 2nd molar.

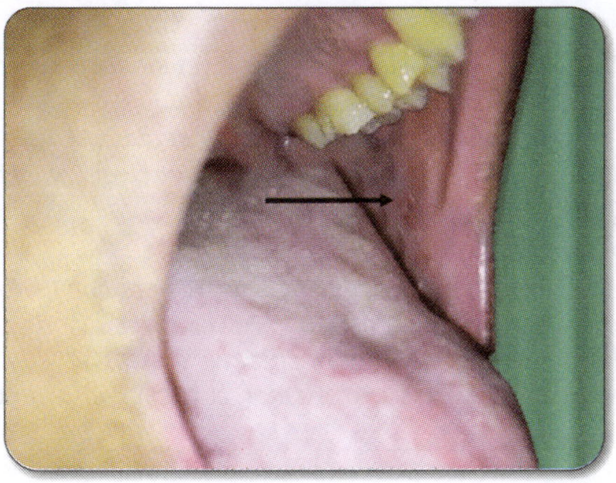

Koplik spots

- Most common complication: Otitis media.
- Most common cause of death: Pneumonia.
- Most common late complication: SSPE (subacute sclerosing panencephalitis).
- Management: Vitamin A.

SSPE: Subacute Sclerosing Panencephalitis

- Rare complication of measles begins at 7–13 years after primary infection*.
- 1st stage: Subtle change in school behavior, EEG normal
- 2nd stage: Massive myoclonus, consciousness is maintained.
- 3rd stage: Choreoathetosis, dystonia, lead pipe rigidity and altered sensorium.
- 4th stage: Loss of critical centers that support breathing, HR, BP.
- Diagnosis: Compatible clinical course and one of the following:
  - Measles antibody in CSF.
  - EEG findings.

Scarlet Fever

- White strawberry 1st day.
- Red strawberry 3rd day.

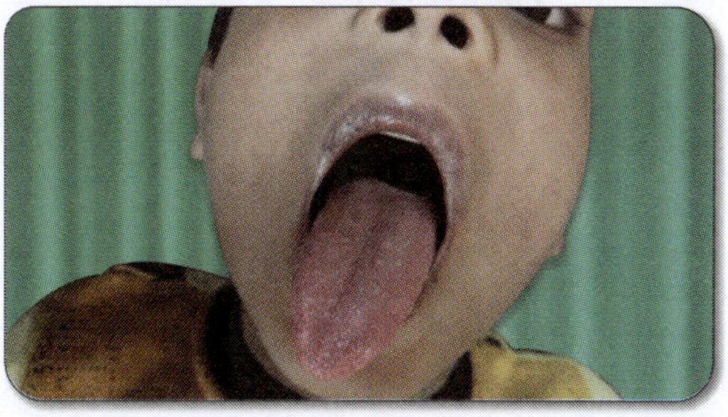

Strawberry tongue

- Sand paper like rash

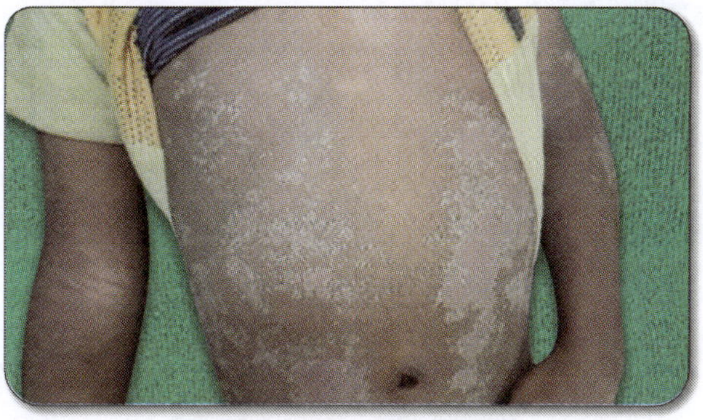

CHICKENPOX/VARICELLA

"It's ok if you don't like me, not everyone has a good taste."

- Cause: Varicella-zoster virus, DNA virus.
- Dew drop appearance.
- Period of infection: From 1–2 days before the rash until all vesicles are crusted.
- Pleomorphic rash.
- People with varicella should be isolated until lesions crust over.
- Centripetal rash (more toward the center).
- Maculopapular vesicular rash.

- Period of communicability: When all the vesicles get crusted
- Most common complication: Secondary bacterial infections

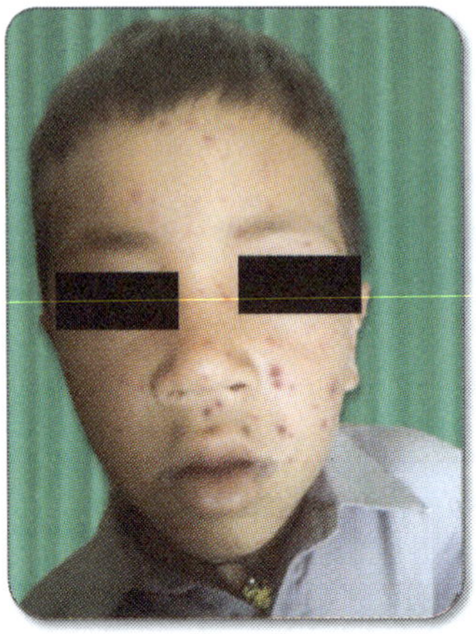

Varicella

Incubation Period

- Measles: 8–12 days
- Mumps: 2–4 weeks
- Chicken pox: 10–21 days
- Syphilis: 9–90 days
- Hepatitis A: 50 days

MUMPS

- Cause: RNA virus
- Clinical features:
  - Unilateral cheek swelling
  - Ear ache

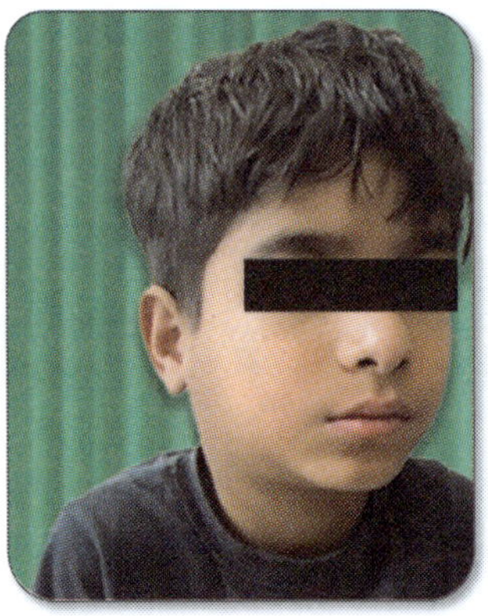

Mumps

Erythema infectiosum	Roseola infantum
5th disease	6th disease
Cause: Parvovirus B19	HHV-6 >7
Slapped cheek appearance	Nagayama spots
	Fever subsides then the rash appears

- Jaw tenderness while chewing
- Dryness of mouth
- Most commonly gland involved is parotid gland
- Most common age group: 5–15 years
- Infants are rarely affected due to the presence of transplacental maternal antibodies till nine months of life
- Reservoir of infection: man
- Most common complication: aseptic meningitis
- Mumps can cause infertility
- Symptomatic management: scrotal support/bed rest/steroids may help but it doesn't alter the course of disease

Slapped cheek appearance	Nagayama spots
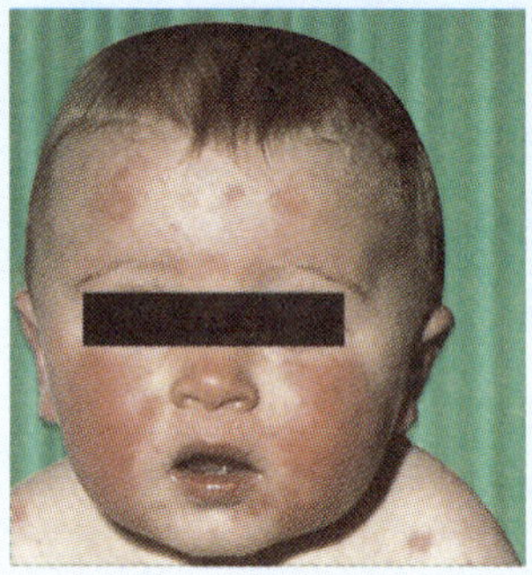	Fever subsides then the rash appears 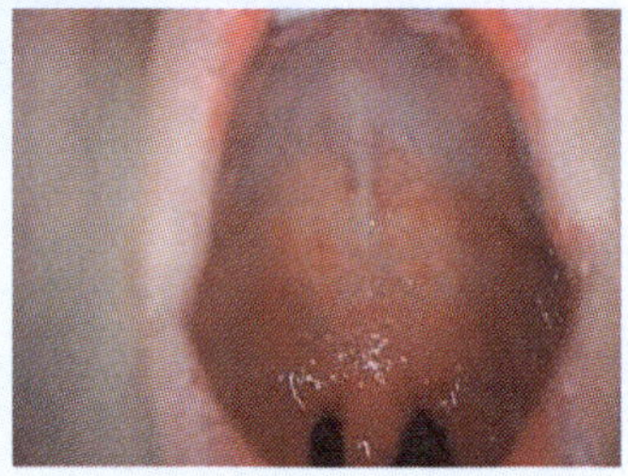

ENTERIC FEVER

"There is no elevator to success, we all have taken the stairs."

- The most common cause of fever lasting for >7 days in clinical practice in India.
- Cause: Salmonella enterica serovar typhi and Salmonella enterica serovar paratyphi A, B, C.
- Gram–negative bacteria.
- Incubation period: 7–14 days.
- It penetrates the mucosa and infects the lymphoid follicles and draining mesenteric nodes and disseminate into liver, spleen, bone marrow, gall bladder, Peyer's patches of the terminal ileum*.

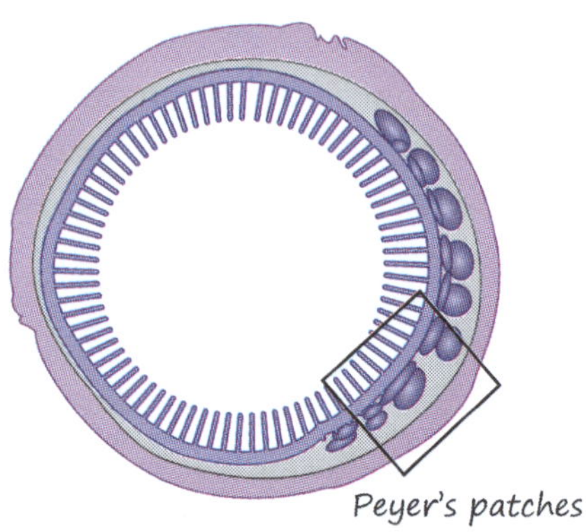

- The most common complication is intestinal bleeding/perforation in 2nd to 3rd week of illness
- Why there is bleeding? Due to the erosion of the necrotic Peyer's patches

What is complicated/severe enteric fever?

- Delirium
- Coma
- Shock
- Mortality is as high as 50%
- Mode of transmission: fecal-oral
- Gold standard—blood culture
- Drug of choice—ceftriaxone 100 mg/day
- Uncomplicated—oral—cefixime 20 mg/kg/day
- Duration: 14 days
- 2nd line—azithromycin 20 mg/kg/day
- Other 2nd line—chloramphenicol, amoxicillin, cotrimoxazole
- Dose: 0.5 mL
- Route: IM (intramuscular)
- Site: anterolateral aspect of thigh
- Schedule: 9–12 months, booster at 2 years
- Storage: 2°–8°C

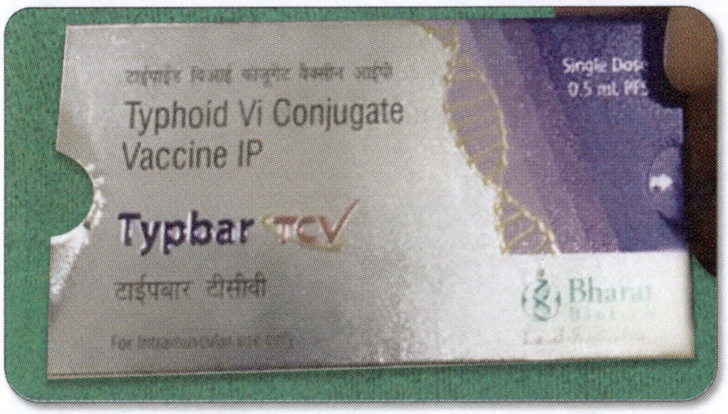

DENGUE FEVER

- It is a vector-borne disease
- Caused by: 4 dengue serotypes-denv 1, denv 2, denv 3, denv 4 - arboviruses
- Family—Flaviviridae
- It is an RNA virus
- Transmitted by: Bite of infected female aedes mosquitoes
- Amplifying host: Human
- Second episode of dengue is more severe than the first one.

Phases of Dengue Fever

- Febrile phase
- Critical phase
- Recovery phase

Febrile Phase

- High grade fever + facial flushing
- Body ache
- Myalgia
- Arthralgia
- Positive tourniquet test/Hess test
- Presence of 10 or more petechiae per square inch indicates a positive finding

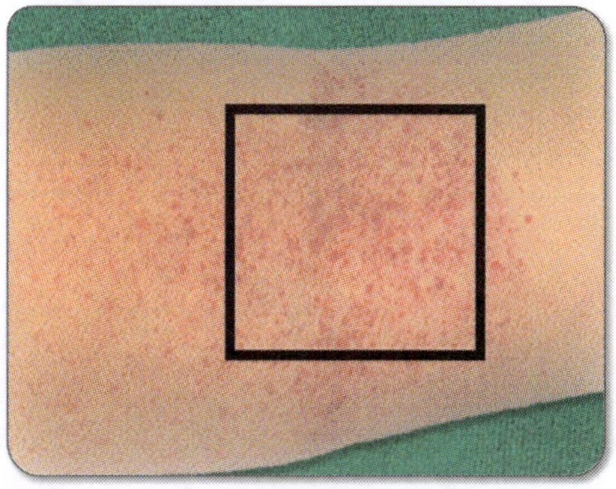

Hess test

Critical Phase

- No fever
- Fall in platelets
- Increase In PCV/hematocrit

Recovery Phase

- Appetite returns
- Isles of white in the sea of red

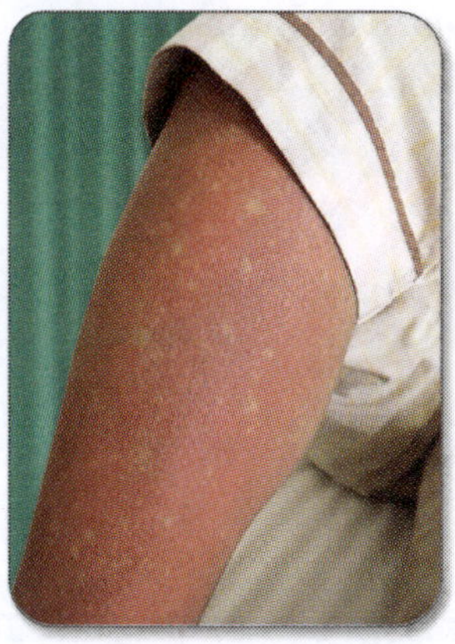

Recovery phase of dengue fever

Investigation

- NS1 will be detectable from onset of fever till on day 5.
- Following a dengue infection, 80% patients show detectable IgM antibodies by day 5, 99% by day 10 that peaks to day 14 and are undetectable by 2–3 months.

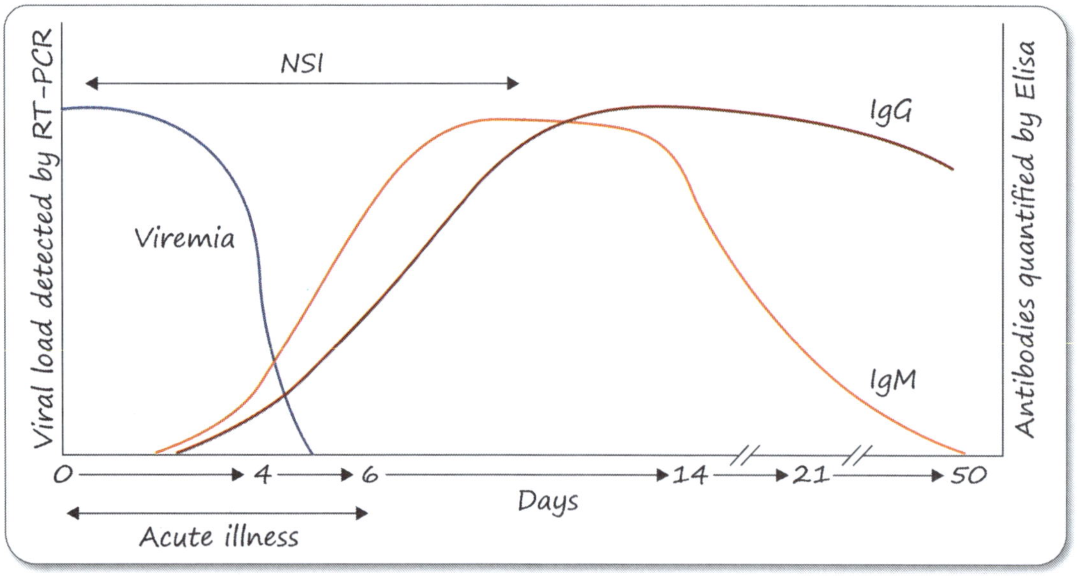

- IgG rises later, declines slowly and remains detectable at low levels for life.

Treatment

- Paracetamol
- Vitals monitoring
- Contraindication: Aspirin/NSAIDs should not be given as it will lead to mucosal bleeds.

Important Points

Dengue Fever with Warning Signs are:

1. Pain Abdomen
2. Persistent vomiting
3. Clinical fluid accumulation
4. Mucosal bleed
5. Liver >2 cm

Dengue fever with risk factors
Hospitalize
NS/RL at 7 mL/kg/hr
Assess after 1 hour

No improvement	Improvement
10 mL/kg/hr	5 mL/kg/hr
Assess at 2 hours	Improved
No improvement	3 mL/kg/hr
15 mL/kg/hr	Continue IV fluids until stable for 24 hours
Assess at 3 hours	Discharge
No improvement Colloids at 10 mL/kg/hr	

Prevention

- Aerial sprays/fogging with malathion
- larvicides
- No stagnation of water in open places, bathroom, kitchen
- Mesocyclops: A shell fish a larvivorous micro-crustacean.

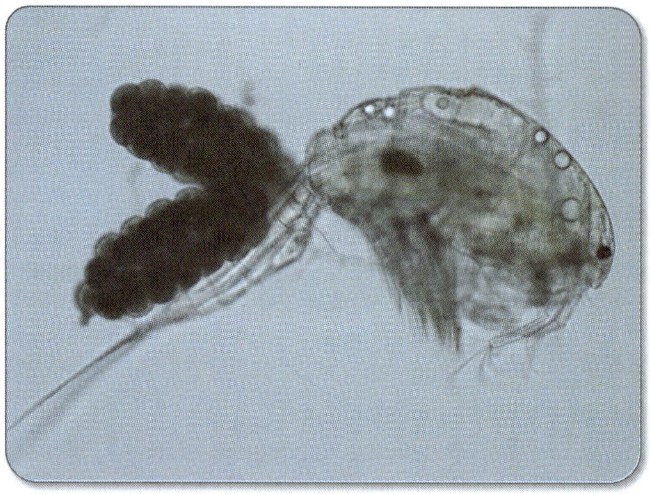

Mesocyclops

DIPHTHERIA

- Bacterial infection
- Gram-positive bacillus
- Cause: Corynebacterium diphtheriae
- Transmission: Droplets
- Portal of entry: Respiratory tract
- Incubation period: 2–5 days

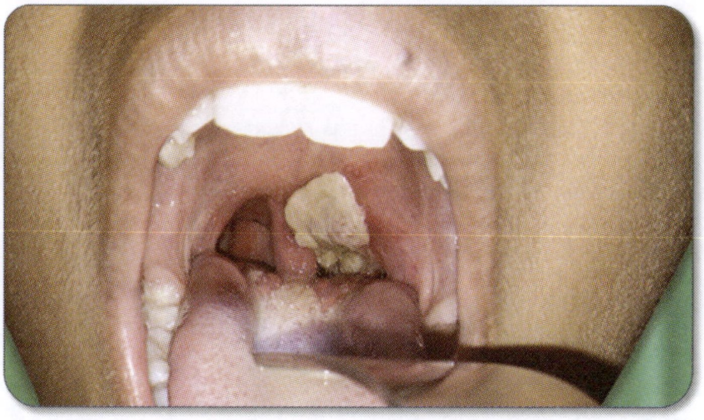

Pseudomembrane of diphtheria

Clinical Features

- Anterior nares are the most common sites of infection
- Fever
- Malaise
- Toxic look
- Nasal twang
- Nasal regurgitation
- Descending paralysis
- Sore throat
- Dysphagia
- Muffled voice
- Bull neck appearance due to cervical lymphadenopathy

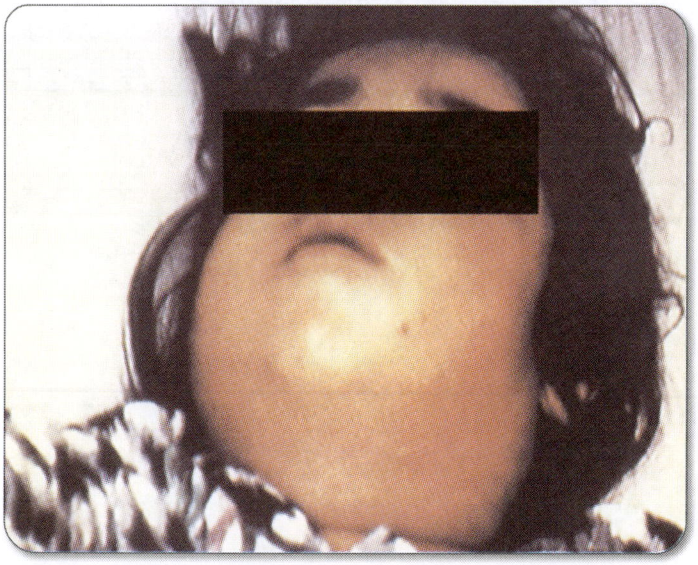

Bull neck appearance

Common Forms

- Nasal diphtheria
- Pharyngeal diphtheria

What happens in laryngeal diphtheria?

- Brassy cough
- Stridor, respiratory distress

Most Common Complications

- 1st week complication: Respiratory failure
- 2nd week complication: Myocarditis
- 3rd week complications: Ocular palsy, loss of accommodation and visual blurring
- 3rd–6th week complications: Generalized polyneuritis and renal—oliguria, proteinuria
- Diagnosis: Albert stain of a swab from oropharynx

Treatment

Antitoxin: 20,000 units – 1,20,000 units depending on the site, extent, toxicity, size of membrane.

TUBERCULOSIS

"Grow through, what you go through."

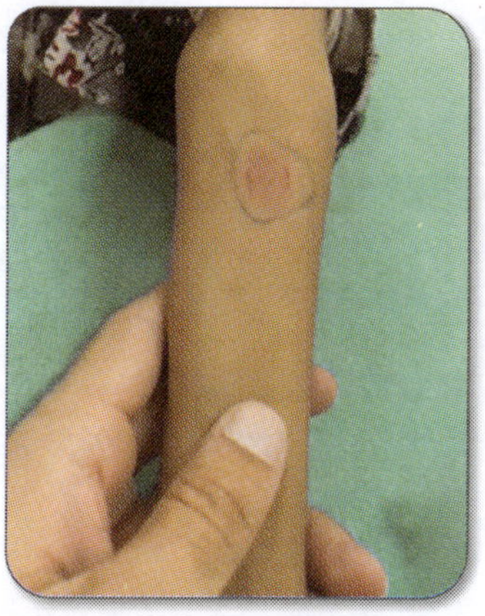

Positive mantoux

Approach

- Cough >2 weeks
- Fever >2 weeks
- Significant weight loss (>5% weight loss in 3 months)
- Peripheral painless lymph node swelling

Mantoux Test/Tuberculin Skin Test

- When to check?
  - 48–72 hours
  - Measured transversely
- False positive Mantoux is seen in
  - BCG vaccination
  - Infections due to atypical mycobacteria

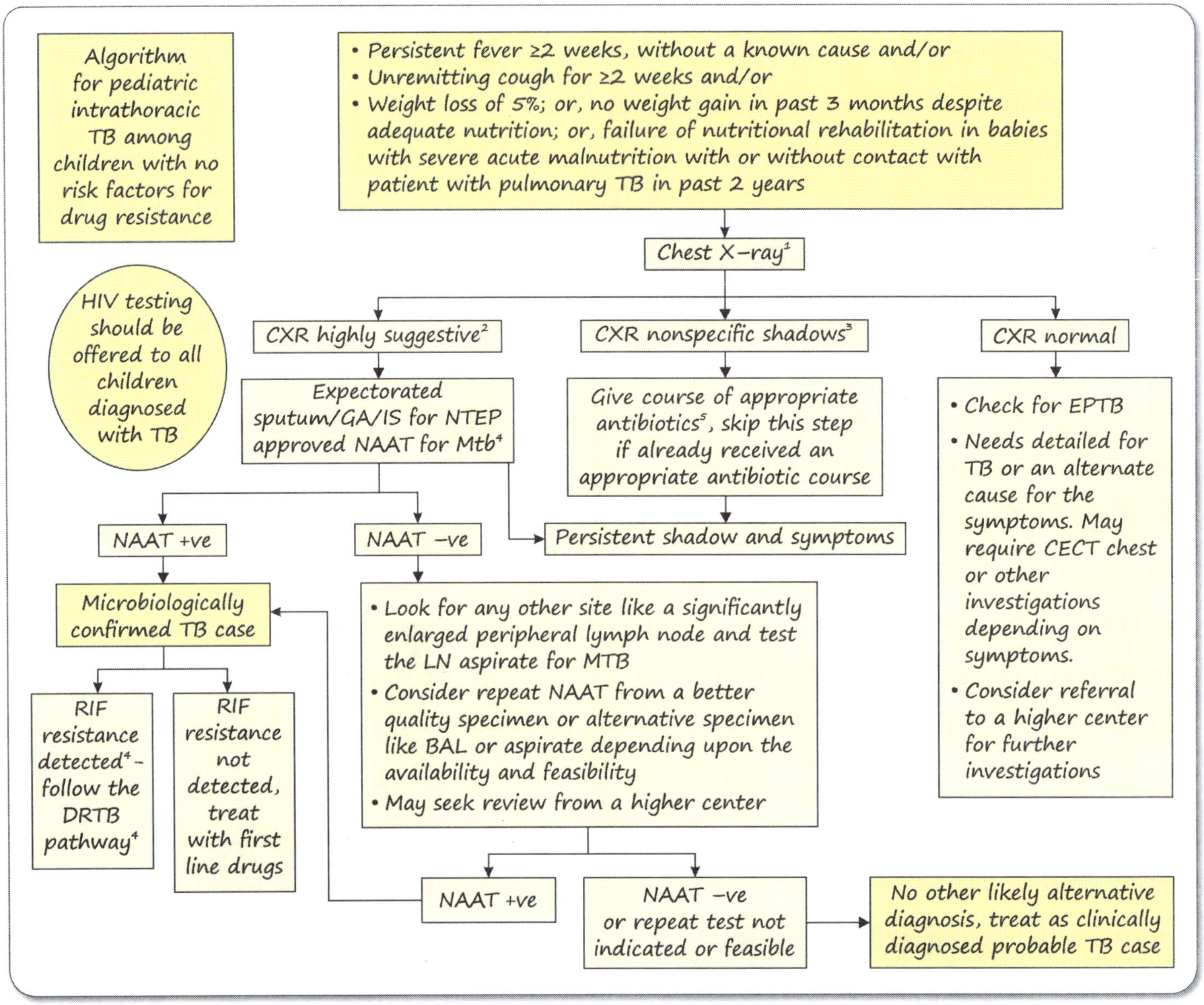

Golden Point
Most common organ involved by congenital TB: liver

Where all we give steroids in TB?

- **TBM:** It will reduce the inflammation
- Endobronchial TB
- Tuberculous massive pleural effusion
- Miliary TB
- Tuberculous pericardial effusion

"People who hate me, motivate me."

13. RENAL SYSTEM

"You are your only hope."
"Be hopeful with life."
"Change of your life is just around the corner."

FACTS

- The fetal bladder is visualized by 10–14 weeks of gestation.
- Beyond 16 weeks, amniotic fluid is principally dependent on urine production during gestation.
- Kidneys can be visualized on ultrasound by 12–13 weeks.
- Oliguria is defined as urine volume <0.5 mL/kg/hr.
- Polyuria is defined as urine output >4 mL/kg/hr.

Serum creatinine	Normal value
<6 years	0.2–0.5 mg/dL
>6 years	0.4–0.7 mg/dL
Urea	20–30 mg/dL

- GFR = K × height (cm)/serum creatinine (mg/dL)
- K = Constant (0.45)

ALPORT SYNDROME/HEREDITARY NEPHRITIS

- Genetic disorder of glomerular basement membrane.
- X-linked recessive 85%, autosomal recessive 10%.
- Autosomal dominant 5%.
- Type 4 collagen mutation (mutation in the gene encoding the alpha subunit of collagen 4 (col4a).

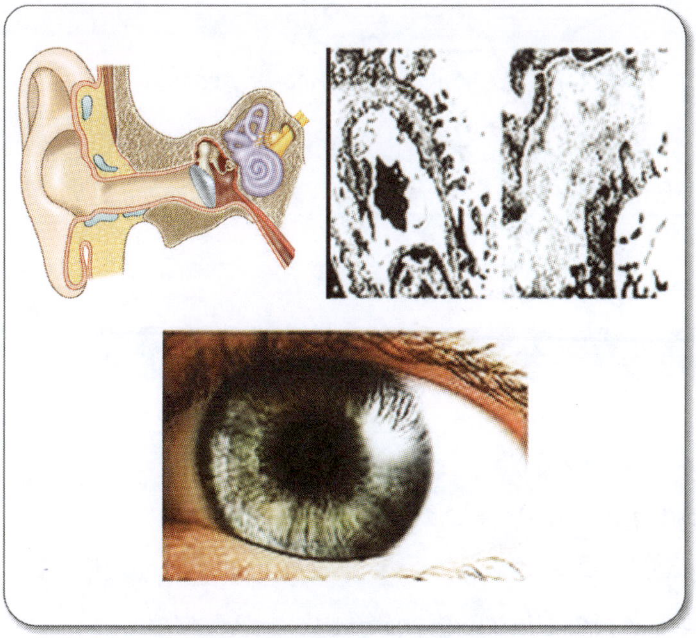

Triad of Alport syndrome

Triad

- Sensorineural hearing loss (SNHL).
- Anterior lenticonus: Cone-shaped deformation of the anterior or posterior lens surface.
- Hematuria/proteinuria (ACE inhibitors are used as therapeutic).

PRUNE-BELLY SYNDROME/EAGLE-BARRETT SYNDROME/TRIAD SYNDROME

- Deficient abdominal muscles/laxity.
- Undescended testicle.
- Urinary tract abnormalities.
- Prognosis depends on the degree of pulmonary hypoplasia and renal dysplasia.

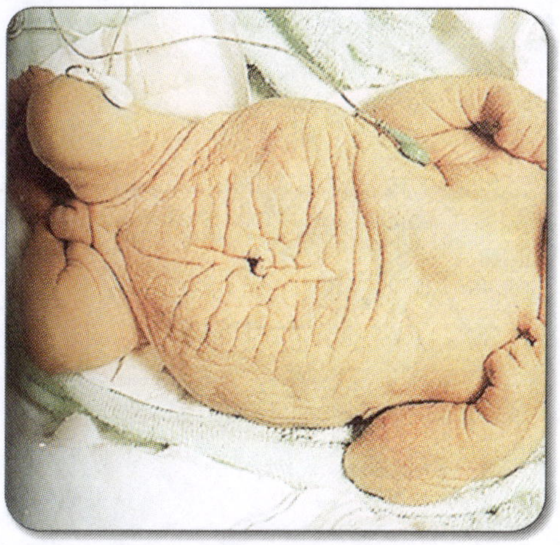

Prune-Belly syndrome

NEPHROTIC SYNDROME

- Characteristics:
  - Hypoalbuminemia <3 g/dL
  - Hyperlipidemia >200 mg/dL
  - Massive proteinuria >1 g/m²/day

Normal proteinuria	<4 mg/m²/hr
Non-nephrotic range proteinuria	4–40 mg/m²/hr
Nephrotic range proteinuria	>40 mg/m²/hr

- Most common cause: Primary (Idiopathic)
- Secondary causes:
  - SLE
  - Hepatitis B
  - Amyloidosis
  - Vasculitis

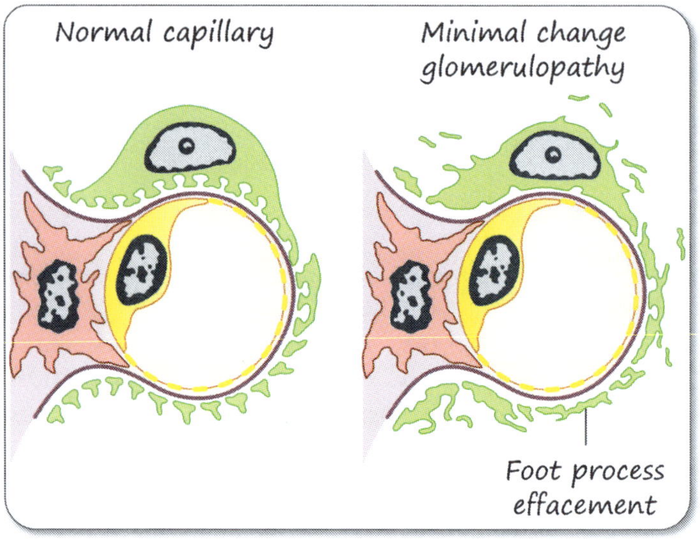

Types

- Minimal change nephrotic syndrome (MCNS)/ steroid-sensitive nephrotic syndrome.
- Nephrotic syndrome with significant lesion.
- Electron microscopy findings in MCNS—Foot process effacement.

Investigations

- Urine routine
- Full blood workup
- CBC, LFT, KFT, urine culture
- Chest X-ray
- We must rule out tuberculosis before starting steroids.
- Heat coagulation test.

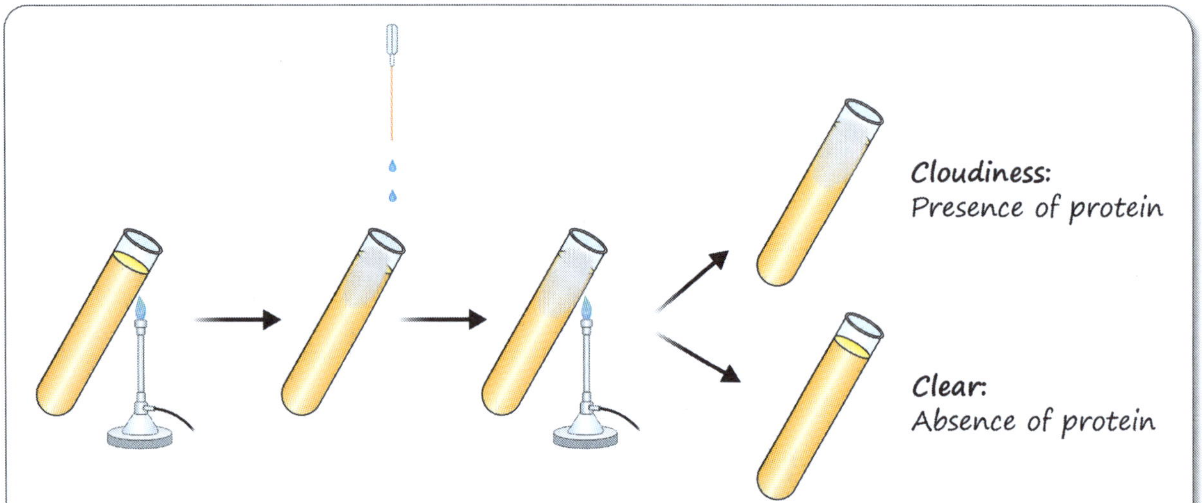

Heat coagulation test

- Qualitative test

Interpretation of heat coagulation test

Sample	Observation
Nil	No cloudiness
Trace	Faint cloudiness—(<0.1 g/dL)
+	Cloudiness without granularity + 0.1 g/dL
++	Granular cloudiness ++ 0.1–0.2 g/dL
+++	Precipitation with clumps (flocculation) +++ 0.2–0.4 g/dL
++++	Thick solid ppt ++++ > equal to 0.5 g/dL

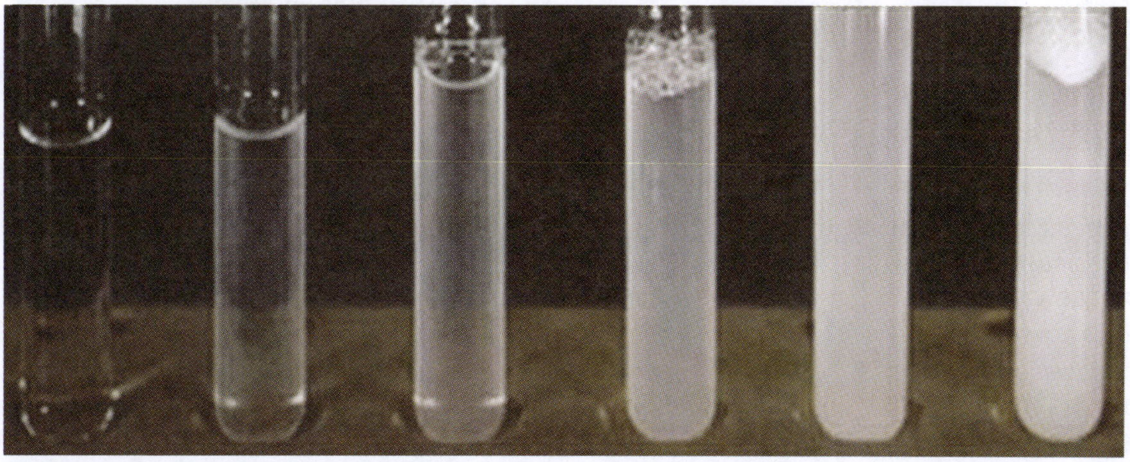

WHAT IS INFREQUENT RELAPSE

- 3 or <3 episodes in 1 year: Infrequent.
- Frequent: 4 or more in 1 year.

Important Definitions

- **Remission:** Early morning 3 consecutive days urine protein nil/trace or proteinuria <4 mg/m^2/hr.
- **Relapse**: Early morning 3 consecutive days urine protein 3+ 4+ in a patient who has remission previously or proteinuria >40 mg/m^2/hr.
- **Steroid-dependence:** Within 14 days of discontinuation of steroids, patient comes with a relapse.
- **Steroid-resistant nephrotic syndrome:** Absence of remission despite daily prednisolone @ 2 mg/kg/day for 6 weeks.

First Episode How to Treat

Start prednisolone 2 mg/kg/day (60 mg/m^2/day) for 6 weeks followed by 1.5 mg/kg/day (40) on alternate day for next 6 weeks.

Frequent Relapse Approach

- Start prednisolone 2 mg/kg/day (60 mg/m^2/day) till the patient goes into remission.
- Followed by alternate day 1.5 mg/kg/day (40 mg/m^2) for 4 weeks.
- Total duration 5–6 weeks
- Followed by long-term alternate day dose of prednisolone should be 0.3–0.7 mg/kg/day.

Steroid Sparing Agents

- Levamisole 2–2.5 mg/kg/day (side effect: leukopenia).
- Cyclophosphamide 2–2.5 mg/kg/day (side effect: leukopenia/hemorrhagic cystitis/gonadal toxicity).
- Mycophenolate mofetil: 20–25 mg/kg/day.
- Cyclosporine/tacrolimus (causes hirsutism/gum hyperplasia).
- Rituximab.

Indications of Renal Biopsy

- Age <1 or >10 years
- Gross or persistent microscopic hematuria
- Low blood C3
- **Hypertension**
- Secondary nephrotic syndrome.
- Before starting with cyclosporine or tacrolimus.
- Failure to remission despite 4 weeks of therapy.

Complications of Nephrotic Syndrome

- Electrolyte imbalance
- SBP—Caused by **Streptococcus pneumoniae**
- RVT—Renal vein thrombosis

Drug of choice of steroid-dependent nephrotic syndrome: (mnemonic—cycle)

- Cyclophosphamide
- Levamisole (first choice)

Drug of choice of steroid-resistant nephrotic syndrome (mnemonic – CT scan)

- Cyclosporine (first choice)
- Tacrolimus

CONGENITAL NEPHROTIC SYNDROME

- NPHS 1 gene mutation
- Present at birth or within 3 months of life
- **Clinical features:** Anasarca, hypoalbuminemia, oliguria followed by:
  - Failure to thrive
  - Recurrent infections
  - Progressive renal failure by 2–3 years
- **Antenatal screening:** Elevated levels of alpha-fetoprotein in maternal serum and amniotic fluid.

Extra Points

- NPHS 2 gene mutation: Focal segmental glomerulosclerosis/steroid-resistant nephrotic syndrome
- WT1 gene—Denys-Drash syndrome
- Lmx1b—Nail-Patella syndrome

URINARY TRACT INFECTION (UTI)

- Most common cause: E. coli
- During infancy incidence of UTI boys > girls
- Beyond infancy—girls > boys
- **Clinical features**
  - **In neonates:**
    - Fever
    - Diarrhea
    - Poor weight gain
    - Vomiting
    - Jaundice
    - Lethargy
  - **In children:**
    - Pain/crying while passing urine
    - Straining during passing urine/dribbling
    - Urgency/hesitancy/frequency

Predisposing Factors of UTI

- Female sex
- Age <6 months
- Voiding dysfunction
- Vesicoureteral reflux (VUR)
- Constipation
- Repeated catheterization

Investigation

- Urine routine and culture-growth of significant number of organisms of a single species in the urine.
- <2 years: suprapubic aspiration or catheter

- **How many colonies count in suprapubic aspiration is significant?**
  Any colonies on suprapubic aspiration and >50,000/mL on urethral catheterization are considered significant.
- **What is Asymptomatic Bacteriuria**
  The occurrence of significant bacteriuria in the absence of symptoms is termed Asymptomatic bacteriuria.
  >5 leukocytes per high-power field in centrifuged sample are useful for screening.
- **What is Significant Bacteriuria**
  Significant bacteriuria is a colony count of >105/mL of a single species in a clean catch sample.
  Oral—cefixime – 10 mg/kg/day.
  IV—ceftriaxone—75–100 mg/kg/day.

Duration

- **Simple UTI—7 days**
- **Complicated UTI—14 days**

Features of Complicated UTI

- Fever >39°C
- Systemic toxicity
- Vomiting + dehydration
- Renal angle tenderness
- Creatinine high

Features of Simple UTI

- Low-grade fever
- Dysuria
- Frequency
- Urgency + without symptoms of complicated UTI

Evaluation Following the First Episode of UTI

- <1 year: USG (ultrasound)/MCU (micturating cystourethrogram)/DMSA renal scan
- 1–5 year: USG/DMSA (dimercaptosuccinic acid)/MCU (if DMSA or USG is abnormal)
- >5 year: USG (if USG normal, then: DMSA/MCU)

- Circumcision reduces the risk of recurrent UTI in infant boys, and might have benefits in patients with high-grade VUR.

Patient, proteinuria with hypertension, RBC cast in urine with recent history of URTI: We will think of Nephritic syndrome.

"Be the change you wish to see in others."

14. MUSCULOSKELETAL SYSTEM

OSTEOGENESIS IMPERFECTA

"Thousands of candles can be lighted from a single candle, be the candle."

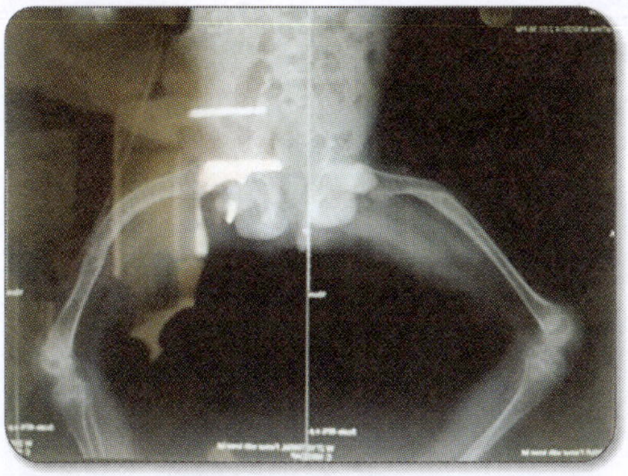

Multiple fractures

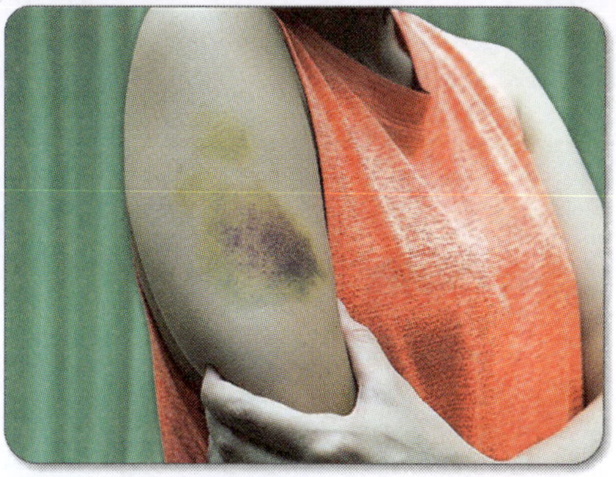

Easy bruisability

Osteogenesis imperfecta (OI) is also known as brittle bone disease.

Triad:

- History of blue sclera
- Recurrent fractures
- Early deafness

Classification

Silence Classification

Defect is in the collagen.

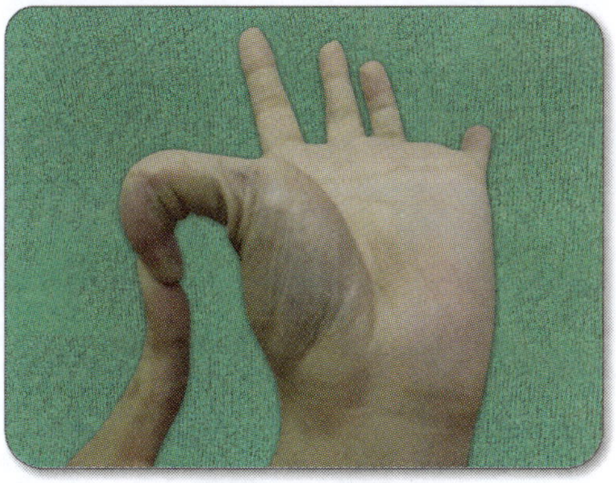

Hyperextensible joints

Clinical Features

- Hyperextensible joints
- Easy bruising
- Joint laxity
- Short stature
- **Type of OI which is lethal in prenatal period:** Type 2
- Baby will be stillborn/die in first year
- Intrauterine fracture/crumpled appearance
- Popcorn appearance of metaphysis

Diagnosis

As early as 16 weeks of gestation.

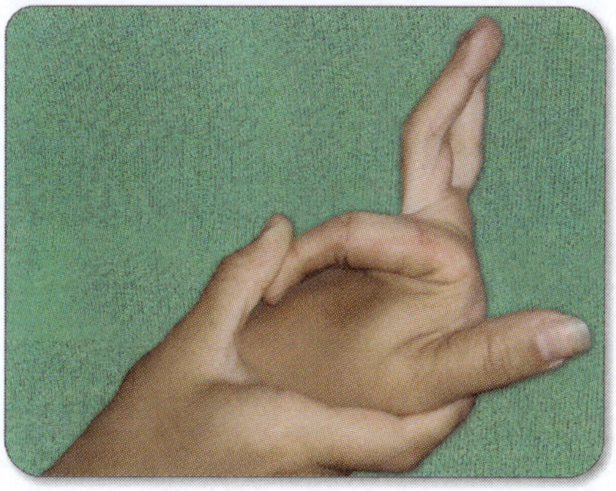

Hyperextensible joints

Complications

- Recurrent pneumonia
- Declining PFT
- Brain stem compression
- Hydrocephalus

Treatment

- Physical/psychological support
- Treat the fracture
- Bisphosphonates (IV pamidronate or oral olpadronate or risedronate).

Percentage of recurrence:

- For autosomal dominant OI, the risk of an affected individual passing the gene to the individual's offspring is 50%.
- For autosomal recessive OI, the recurrence risk is 25% per pregnancy.

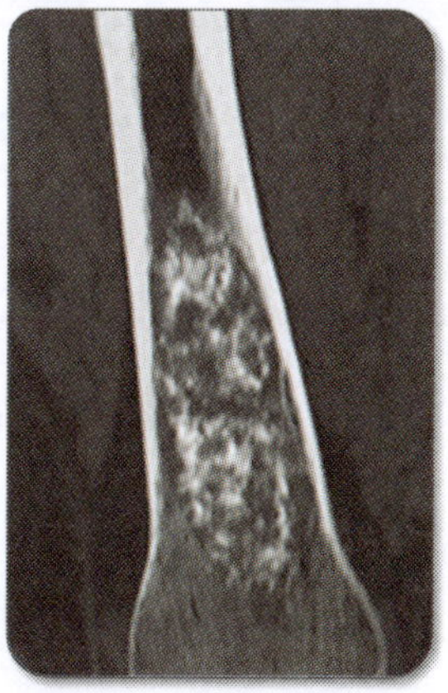

Popcorn appearance of metaphysis

MUSCULAR DYSTROPHY

Major types of muscular dystrophy are:

- Duchenne muscular dystrophy (DMD)
- Becker muscular dystrophy
- Myotonic muscular dystrophy
- Facioscapulohumeral muscular dystrophy/ Landouzy-Dejerine disease

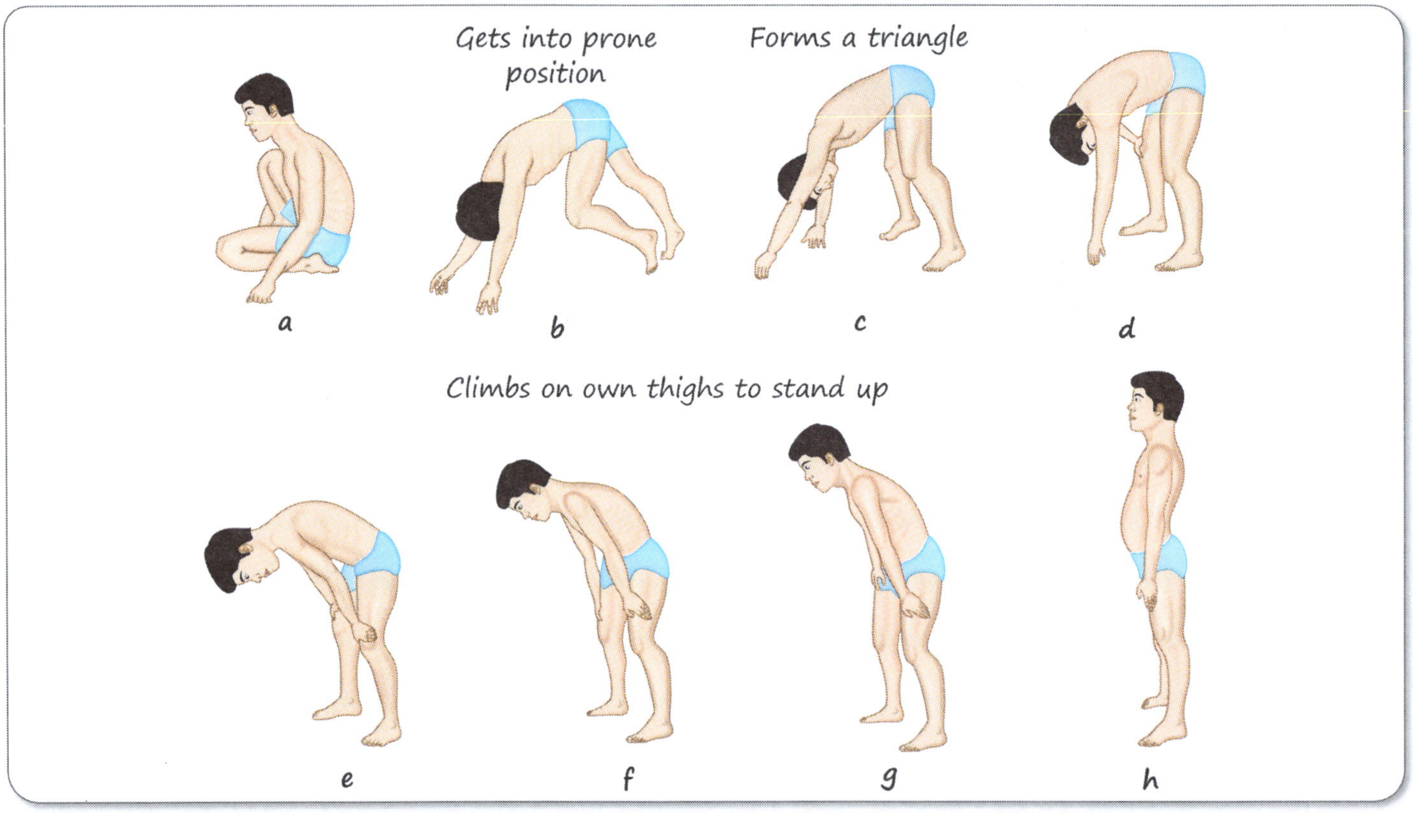
Gets into prone position
Forms a triangle
a
b
c
d
Climbs on own thighs to stand up
e
f
g
h

Gower sign

Duchenne Muscular Dystrophy (DMD)

- DMD is the most common hereditary neuromuscular disease.
- **Genetics:** X linked recessive: XP21 (dystrophin gene) is affected.
- **Clinical features are:**
  - Progressive weakness
  - Developmental delay
  - Pseudohypertrophy of calf muscles and wasting of thigh muscles
  - After calves, next common site is tongue
  - Gower sign **(Image)**
  - Evident by 3 years, fully expressed by 5–6 years
  - Indicates weakness of proximal muscles
  - Patient uses hands and arms to walk up from squatting position due to lack of hip and thigh muscles strength
- Glucocorticoids decrease the rate of apoptosis and decelerate myofiber necrosis.
- Death at 18–20 years of age

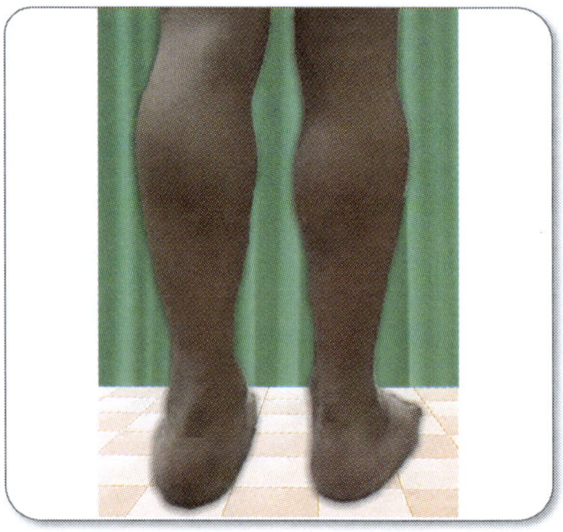

Pseudohypertrophy of calf muscles

- Other muscles having hypertrophy are:
  - Vastus lateralis
  - Infraspinatus
  - Gluteus maximus
  - Triceps
  - Masseter

- **Age of loss of independent ambulation:** 8.8–10.5 years
- **Most common cause of death in DMD:** Respiratory insufficiency and cardiomyopathy

Imp PYQs

Q. Which is more severe—Duchenne (DMD) or Becker?

- Duchenne
  - Early onset <6 years
  - More severe and fast progression
  - History of delayed walking
- **Diagnosis:** Serum creatine kinase (CK) is greatly elevated (N- <160 IU/L) 15-35,000 IU/L
- PCR of dystrophin gene confirms the diagnosis
- If PCR is normal, muscle biopsy with dystrophin immunocytochemistry is done.
- **Findings in muscle biopsy:**
  - Necrosis and attempted regeneration of attempted muscle fibers.
  - Later everything is replaced by fat
- **Complications are:**
  - Contractures
  - Cardiomyopathy
  - Malignant hyperthermia after anesthesia
- **Treatment:**
  - Physiotherapy
  - Steroids
  - Cardiac decompensation

Myotonic Muscular Dystrophy

- 2nd most common muscular dystrophy
- Facial weakness
- Invert V-shaped upper lip
- Loss of muscle mass in temporal fossa
- Autosomal dominant – Chromosome 19q (long arm) 13

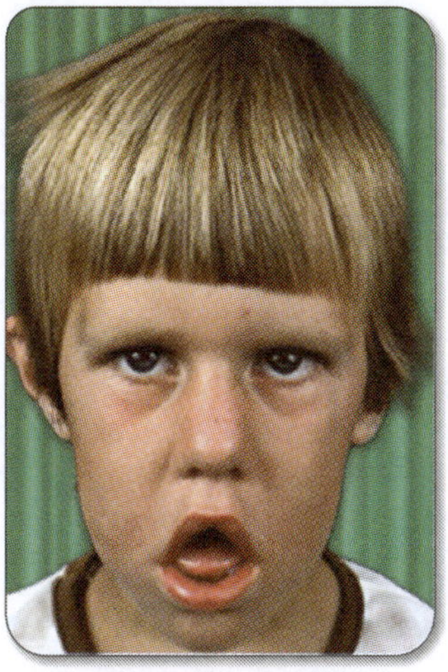

Inverted V shape upper lip

- **Dysfunction in multiple organs:** GIT uterus, endocrinopathies
- **Myotonia:** Very slow relaxation of muscles after contraction seen >5 years of age.

Facioscapulohumeral Muscular Dystrophy (Landouzy-Dejerine Disease)

- Autosomal dominant
- Scapular winging is the first sign
- Usually after a sports injury or breast surgeries
- Hearing loss and retinal vasculopathy
- Flattening of deltoid contour
- Gower sign is also seen
- Calf hypertrophy is not a feature, foot drop may be seen
- **Common complications:**
  - Lumbar lordosis
  - Kyphoscoliosis

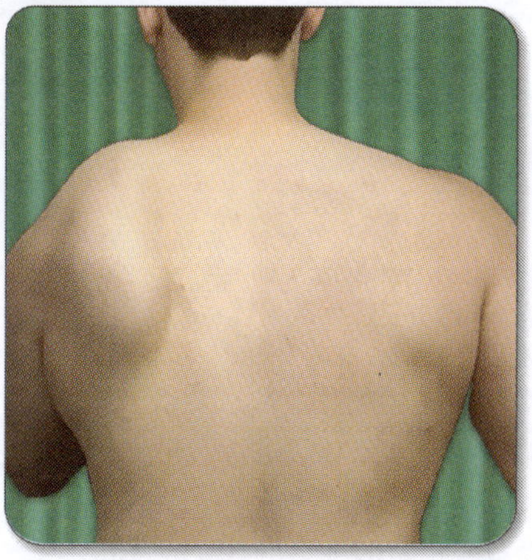

Winging of scapula

KLIPPEL-FEIL SYNDROME (KFS)

- Klippel-Feil syndrome is a congenital, musculoskeletal condition characterized by the fusion of at least two vertebrae of the neck.

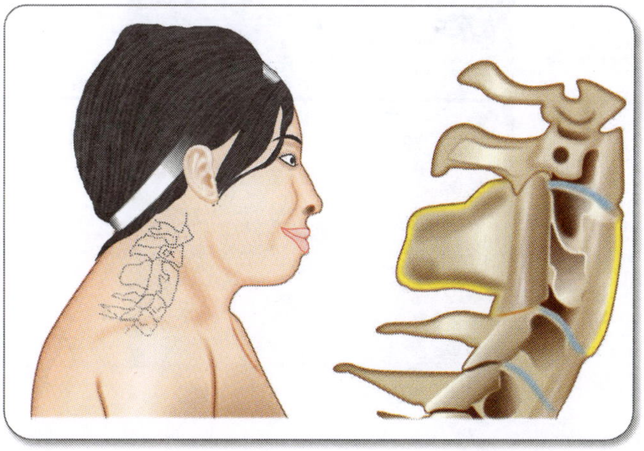

Webbed neck, fusion of vertebral

- ***Common symptoms:***
  - *Short neck*
  - *Low hairline at the back of the head*
  - *Restricted mobility of the upper spine*

TRACHEOESOPHAGEAL FISTULA (TEF)

"Everything will make sense at the end of journey."

- *The most common congenital anomaly of the esophagus is esophageal atresia.*

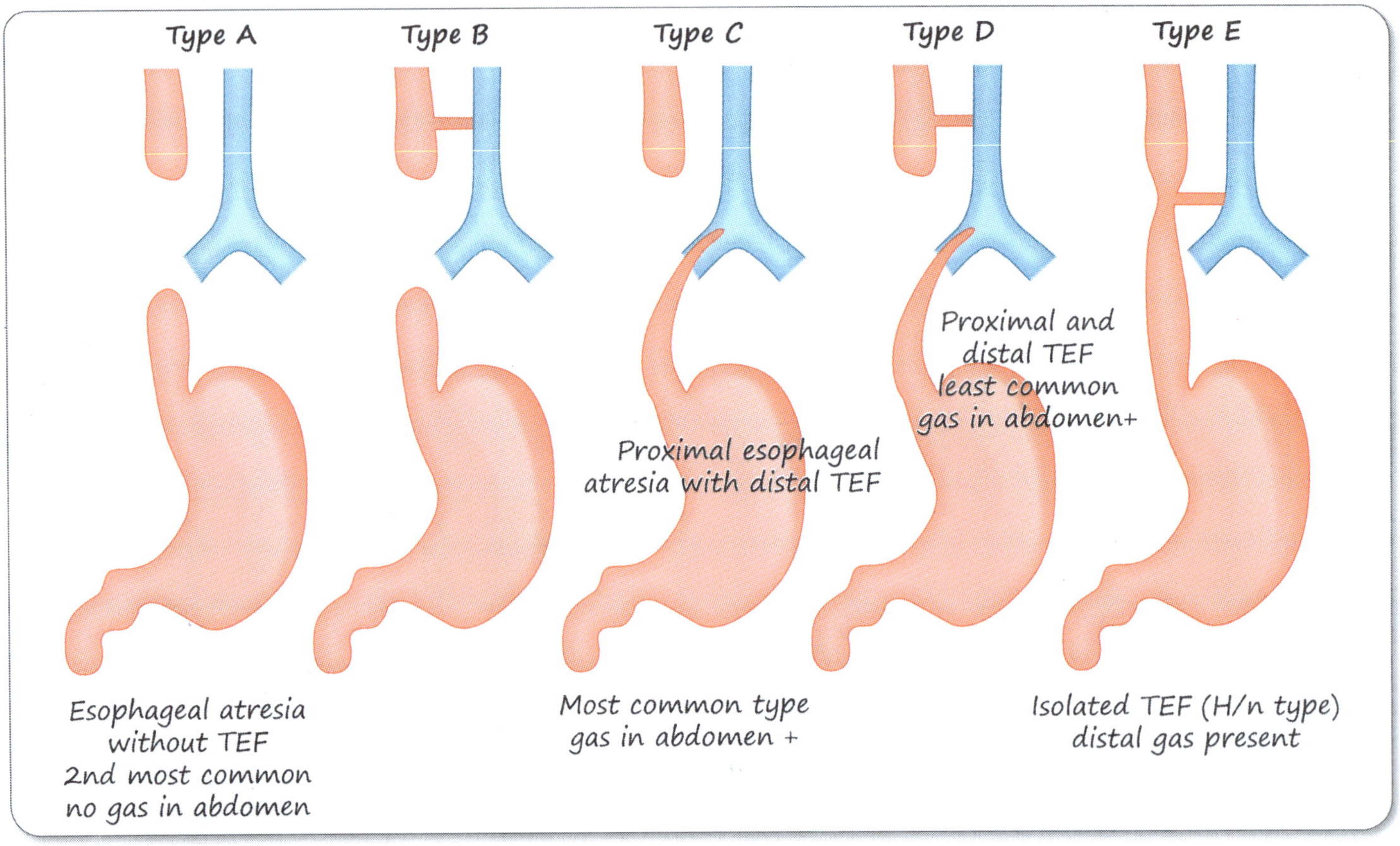

Types of TEF—Gross classification

- *Out of these >90% will have TEF.*
- *Gasless abdomen is seen in types A and B.*
- ***Gas in the abdomen:** Type C, D and E.*
- ***X-ray:** Coiling of the nasogastric tube.*

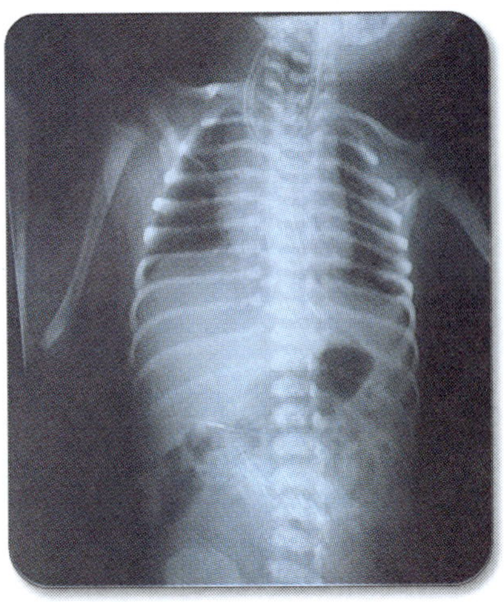

Coiling of the nasogastric tube

- *Associated with polyhydramnios due to inability of fetus to swallow amniotic fluid.*

- ***Clinical features:***
  - *Frothing*
  - *Excessive drooling and coughing with feeds*
  - *F/B → Cyanosis and respiratory distress*
- *Type H/N (TYPE E) presents later with recurrent pneumonia due to aspiration**
- ***Treatment:***
  - *Prone position*
  - *OG and put a slow suction device attached to it*
  - *IV fluids/antibiotics if infection +*
  - *Surgical repair*
  - ***Distance b/w both ends <3 cm:** Surgical repair and end-to-end anastomosis of esophagus*
  - *If the gap is more, then this is a bad prognostic criteria for surgery**. Gastrostomy is done and esophageal repair by conduits (stomach, jejunum).*
- ***Complications:***
  - ***Anastomosis leak:** Earliest complication***
  - ***Stricture formation:** Most common complication***
  - ***Other:** GERD, Barrett's esophagus*

CONGENITAL HYPERTROPHIC PYLORIC STENOSIS (CHPS)

"What we know is drop,
what we don't know is ocean."

- Most common surgical cause of nonbilious vomiting in infants.
- Forceful, projectile, postprandial nonbilious vomiting F/B voracious appetite.
- After vomiting, child is hungry with voracious appetite.

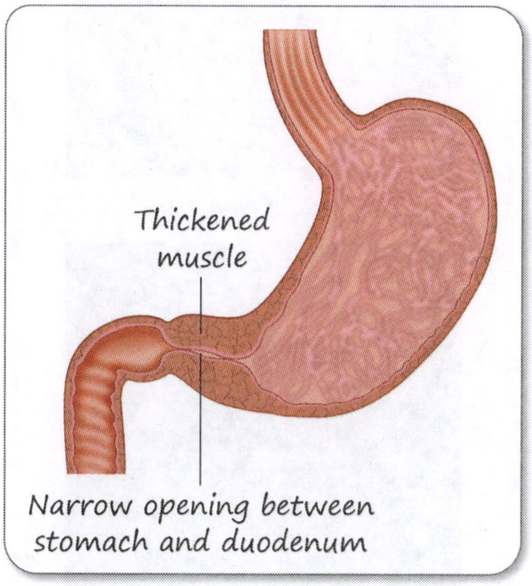

- Visible peristalsis from left to right
- Olive shape mass
- Males > females*
- **ABG:** hypokalemic hypochloremic metabolic alkalosis with paradoxical aciduria
- Maternal intake of erythromycin can lead to CHPS
- **AGE:** 2–6 weeks
- **Most specific and sensitive test:** USG
- **Most definitive test:** UGI contrast
- **Contrast findings:** String sign, double tract sign, shoulder sign
- **USG:** Target sign and antral nipple sign
- Pyloric thickness >4 mm and length >14 mm is diagnostic
- **Surgery:** Ramstedt's pyloromyotomy
- During feeding, place the infant in seated position after the surgery to limit the vomiting (don't keep the baby supine)

HIRSCHSPRUNG DISEASE (HD)

"Overthinking will kill your happiness."

- The most common congenital gut motility disorder.

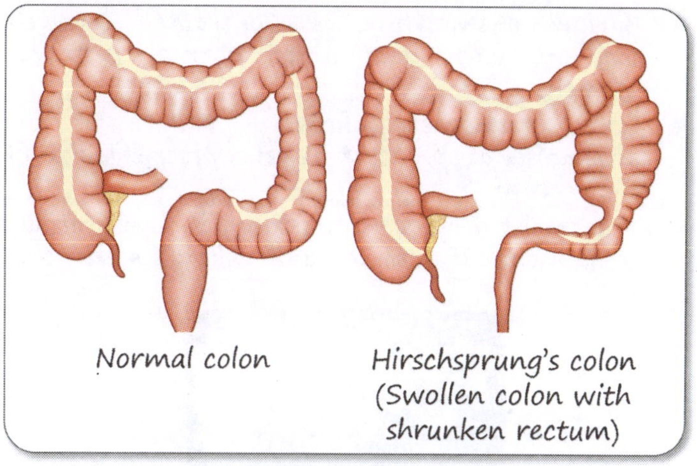

- Absence of ganglions in the submucosal and myenteric plexus of intestine
- Decreased peristalsis and contraction of the involved segment
- **Clinical features:**
  - Delayed passage of meconium
  - Bilious vomiting
  - Abdominal distension
  - Bilious vomiting
  - Rectum is empty but when finger is removed, there will be explosive discharge of foul-smelling stool**
  - Enterocolitis (fever, bloody stools) is usually seen b/w 2–4 weeks

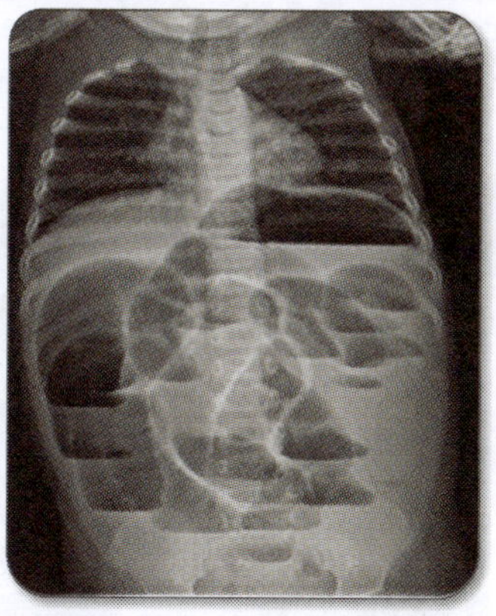

Multiple air fluid levels (intestinal obstruction)

- **Complications:**
  - Intestinal perforation
  - Constipation
  - Rectal bleeding
- **Diagnosis and treatment:**
  Intestinal (rectal) biopsy* findings:
  - Absence of ganglions
  - Nerve trunk hypertrophy
  - Increased acetylcholinesterase activity in involved segment

- Barium enema findings: Contracted involved segment with dilation of normal proximal segment.
- Rectal manometry findings: Failure of the internal anal sphincter to relax after dilation of the rectum.
- **Treatment:** Diversion colostomy is done initially to gain time if patient is not willing for surgery.

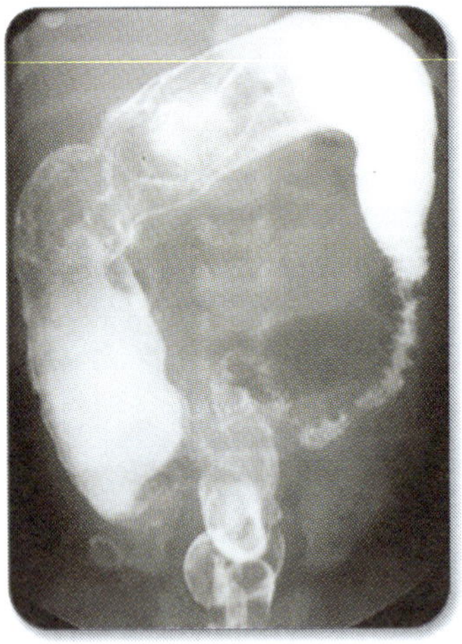

H.disease

INTUSSUSCEPTION

- Common cause of intestinal obstruction in 3 months–6 years.
- Telescoping of a proximal segment of intestine into a distal segment.
- Ileocolic intussusception is most common.

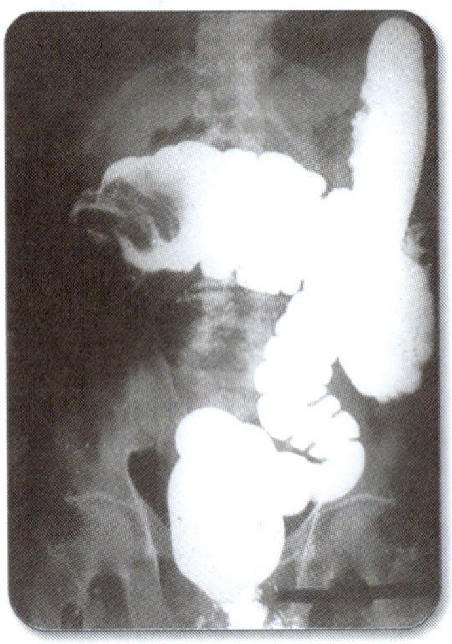

Claw sign: Intussusception

- **Triad:**
  - Pain abdomen
  - Palpable mass
  - Red currant jelly stool
- Barium enema—Claw sign
- Coiled spring sign
- Ultrasound—Doughnut sign

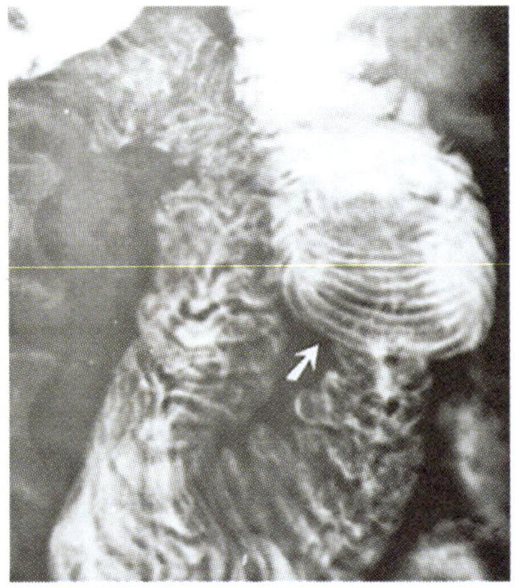

Coiled spring sign

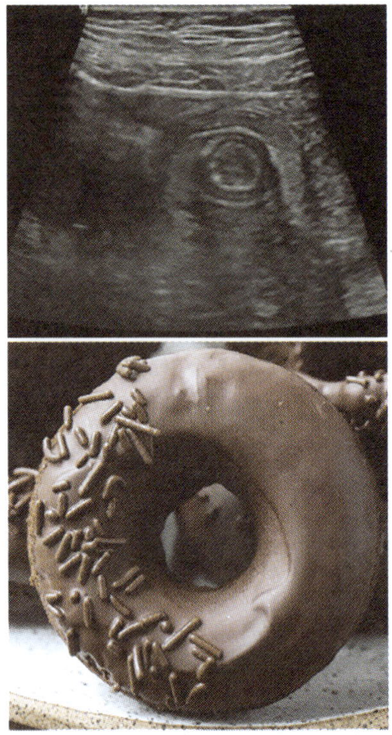

Doughnut sign

Golden Points

- Best diagnostic investigation for acute appendicitis in children is ultrasound.
- Children have thin abdominal wall—USG will be best for them.
- Even though USG does not have that much penetration power, appendix can be visualized.
- Best investigation for visualizing appendix would be CT abdomen, but that would expose the child to radiation; therefore, it is not the investigation of choice.

15. GIT/HEPATOLOGY

"If that's what you are
Then that's who you are
There's no use in fighting it
& If you are not gonna fight it
You might as well embrace it."

GASTROESOPHAGEAL REFLUX DISEASE (GERD)

- Most common esophageal disorder in children
- Passing the gastric contents of esophagus into the esophagus
- About 50% of healthy 3–4 months old infants regurgitate at least once per day.
- **Risk factors:**
  - Obesity
  - Esophageal atresia
  - Preterm babies
  - Cystic fibrosis
  - Cerebral palsy

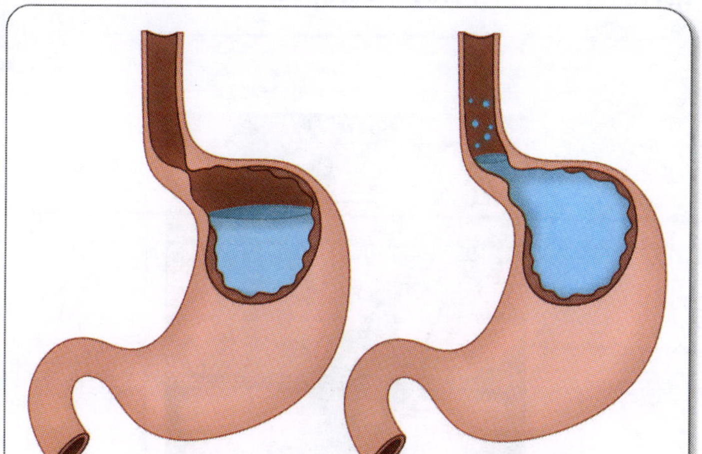

GERD

- **Clinical features:**
  - Regurgitation of feed
  - Not gaining weight
  - Heartburn
  - Hematemesis
  - Dysphagia
  - Odynophagia
- Stridor
- **Sandifer syndrome:** Arching of the back with spasmodic dystonia
- **Gold standard:** 24-hour pH recording
- **24-hour esophageal manometry:** Measurement of the esophageal acid exposure
- **UGI endoscopy:** Erosions/breaks in the distal esophageal mucosa
- **Complications:**
  - **Stricture esophagus**
  - **Barrett's esophagus**
- **Treatment:**
  - Lifestyle modifications/propped up 45°
  - Avoid tea/coffee
  - Trial of an extensively hydrolyzed protein formula.
  - H_2 receptor antagonist (ranitidine)
  - **PPI proton pump inhibitors:** Lansoprazole (treatment of choice)
  - **Surgery:** Nissen fundoplication

CELIAC DISEASE

- **Celiac disease is a disease of:**
  - Genes – HLA class 2 – HLA DQ2, HLA DQ8 (HLA – human leukocyte antigen)
  - Grains – gluten sensitivity
  - Hallmark lesions
  - Villus atrophy
  - Crypt hyperplasia
  - Increased intraepithelial lymphocytes (IELs)
- Patient is sensitive to gluten
- **Gluten is present in:**
  - Wheat
  - Chapati
  - Cake
  - Muffin
  - Burger
  - Pizza
  - Sandwich
  - Hot dog
  - Bread
- **Typical clinical features:**
  - **Vomiting**
  - **Diarrhea**

The celiac enteropathy

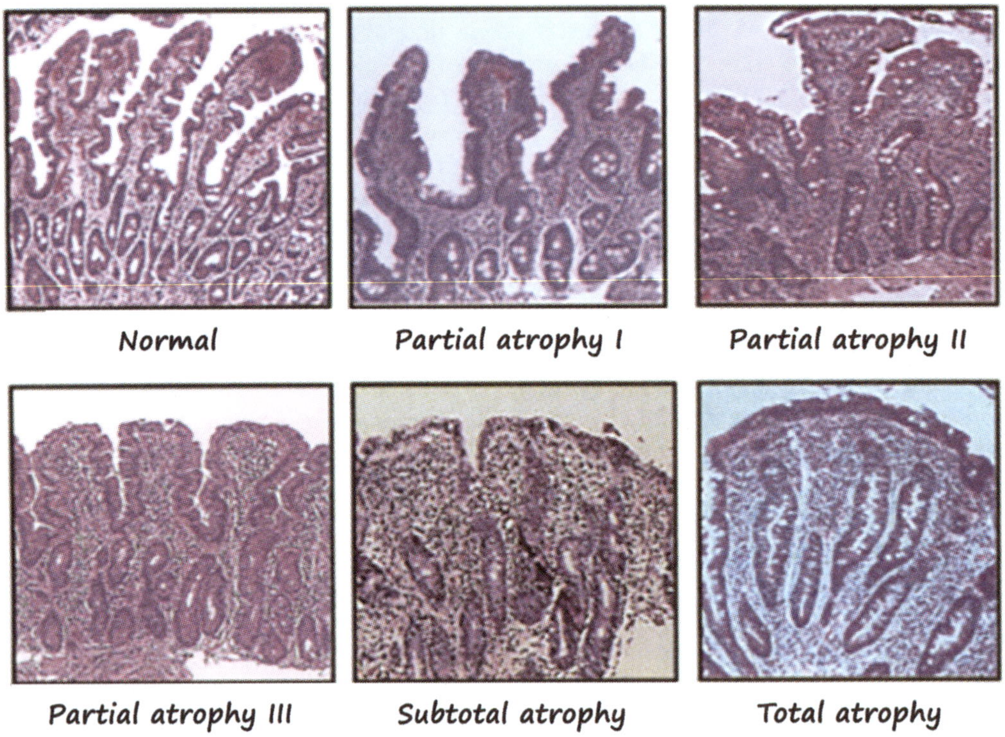

- Constipation
- Failure to thrive

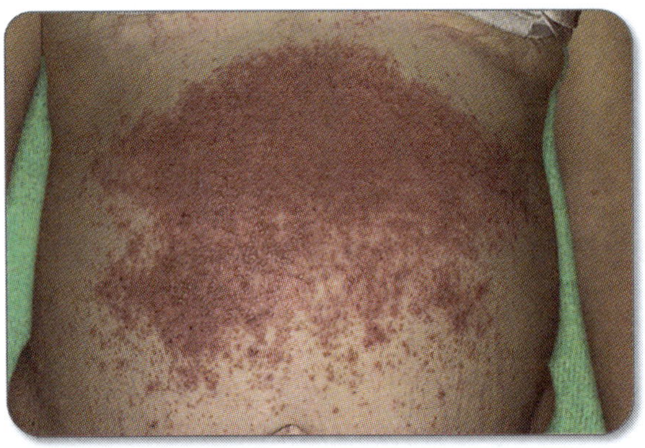

Dermatitis herpetiformis

- Extraintestinal manifestations are more common which are:
  - **Dermatitis herpetiformis:** Intense itchy blisters filled with water—elbows/knees/lower back
  - Failure to thrive
  - Short stature
  - Delayed puberty
  - Arthritis
  - Osteopenia
- **Most common extraintestinal manifestation of celiac disease:** Iron deficiency anemia.

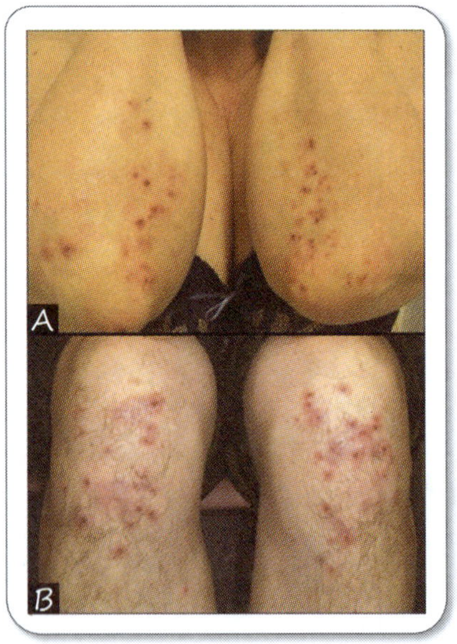

Dermatitis herpetiformis

- **MC cause of chronic diarrhea in children:** Celiac disease.
- Small bowel diarrhea is seen.
- **First serological testing:** tTg-IgA (Tissue transglutaminase IgA).
- **<2 years: EMA:** Endomysial antibodies.
- **Duodenal biopsy:** Scalloping.
- **The degree of villus atrophy and the number of IEL are based on:** Marsh Oberhuber classification.

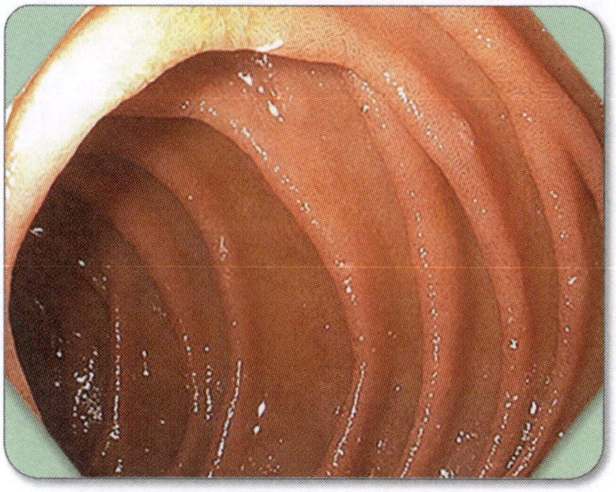

Duodenal biopsy—scalloping

- **Treatment:**
  - **What is not allowed?**
    - **B: Barley/bread**
    - **R: Rye**
    - **O: Oats**
    - **W: Wheat**
  - **What is allowed?**
    - **Maize**
    - **Sarso**
    - **Jowar**
    - **Pure oats (Jaee)**
    - **Rice**
    - **Corn**
    - **Potato**
    - **Soyabean**

CONSTIPATION

"Shine like a diamond."

- **Definition:** Difficulty in defecation sufficient to cause significant distress to the patient.
- Acute constipation less than four weeks.
- Chronic constipation more than four weeks.

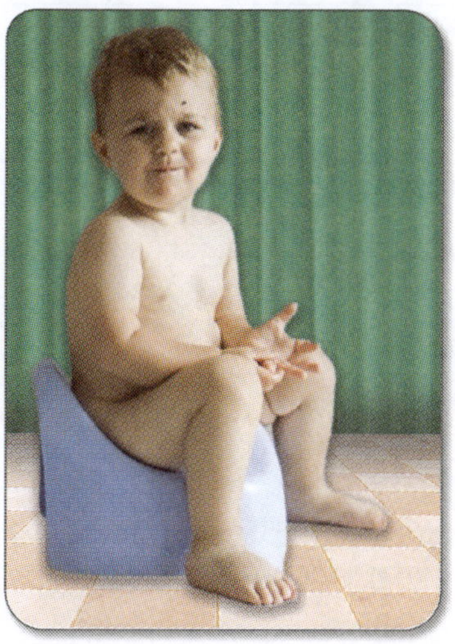

Golden Point

A stool frequency of less than or equal to two per week is considered abnormal for all ages.

- Functional constipation is defined by the presence of at least two or more of the following criteria for more than one month:
  - Two or few defecations per week
  - At least one episode of fecal incontinence per week
  - History of retentive posturing
  - History of painful or hard bowel movements
  - Presence of a large fecal mass in the rectum on per abdomen examination.

Clinical Features

- Abdominal pain
- Anorexia
- Urinary tract infection
- Psychological problems
- Screening in infant
- Tiptoe walking
- Tightening of buttocks in older children

Red flag signs:

- Failure to thrive
- Blood stool
- Recurrent fever, vomiting
- Lump in abdomen

Management

- **Disimpaction:** Polyethylene glycol (PEG) 1.5 g/kg/day for 3–4 days
- **Maintenance therapy:**
  - **Behavioral training:** Positive routine of sitting on toilet for passing stools after meal
  - **Dietary changes:** Fruits and vegetables
  - **Medications:** Lactulose 1–3 mL/kg/day

DIARRHEA

"Be humble – we all have a past."

- **Most common cause of diarrhea:** Rotavirus
- **Most common virus causing diarrhea:** Rotavirus
- **Most common bacteria causing diarrhea:** *E. coli*
- **Most common cause of dysentery:** Shigella
- **Definition:** Liquid/watery stool >3 times a day

Types of Diarrhea

- **Acute:** Usually <14 days.
- **Persistent:** Starts acutely/of presumed infectious etiology which lasts for >14 days.
- **Chronic:** Insidious onset of >2 weeks in children and >4 weeks in adults (noninfectious).
- **Antibiotic associated diarrhea:** Most commonly associated is amoxicillin.
- **Traveler's diarrhea:** Caused by enterotoxigenic strain of *E. coli.*

Clinical Assessment

Parameters	No dehydration	Some dehydration	Severe dehydration
Appearance	Well, alert	Restless, irritable	Lethargic, or unconscious, floppy
Eyes	Normal	Sunken	Very sunken
Thirst	Drinks normally, not thirsty	Thirsty, drinks eagerly	Drinks poorly or not able to drink
Skin pinch	Goes back quickly (<1 second)	Goes back slowly (1 second)	Goes back very slowly (2 seconds)

Treatment

No dehydration

- **ORS + Zinc**
- **Dose of zinc**
  - **<6 months** = 10 mg once a day
  - **>6 months** = 20 mg once a day
  - **Zinc is given for 14 days**

Oral rehydration solution (ORS) mOsm/L	Resomal rehydration solution for the malnourished
Glucose 75	125
NA 75	45 (less)
Citrate 10	7 (less)
K 20	40
Chloride 65	70

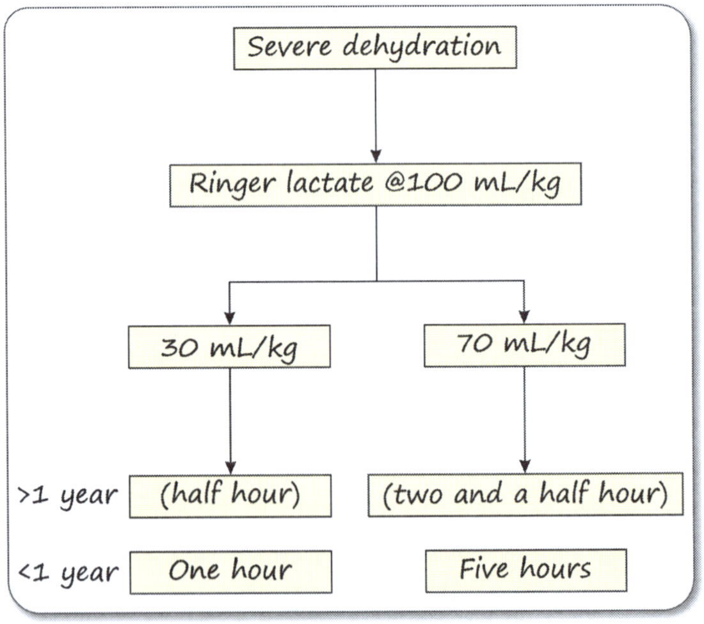

Management of severe dehydration

Some dehydration

- **Fluid of choice:** ORS
- **Dose:** 75 mL/kg over 4–6 hours

Severe dehydration

- **Fluid of choice:** RL
- To calculate the maintenance fluid, use the Holliday and Segar formula:
  - **1–10 kg:** 100 mL/kg
  - **10-20 kg:** 50 mL/kg
  - **>20 kg:** 20 mL/kg

> **Extra Point**
>
> If the child is thirsty or eagerly drinking the water that means the child is in some dehydration.

Conditions for Giving Antibiotics in Diarrhea

- Diarrhea with SAM
- Diarrhea with dysentery
- Diarrhea with rice watery stool

Important Terms

- **Tenesmus:** Sensation of incomplete evacuation of bowel.
- **Dysentery:** Blood while passing stool.
- **Hematochezia:** Fresh blood in the stool (Upper GI bleed).
- **Melena:** Black tarry stool (Lower GI bleed).
- Demarcation point of upper GI and lower GI bleed is ligament of Treitz located at the duodenojejunal flexure.
- Frothy diarrhea with perianal excoriation = lactose intolerance.

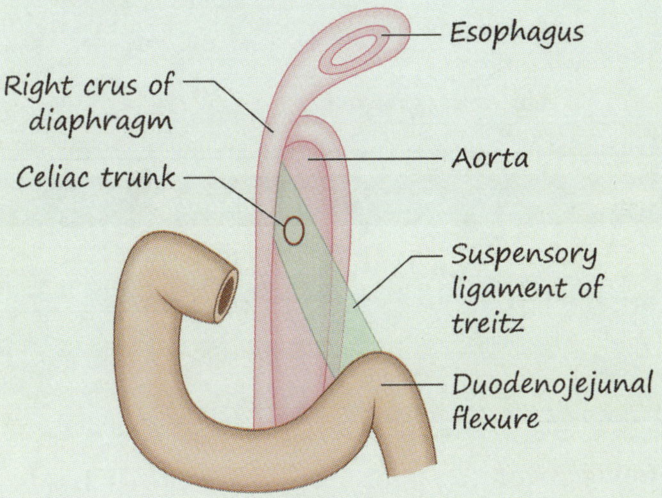

Extra Point

McBurney's point: It is the point between the lateral one third and medial two third of the line passing between the umbilicus and anterior superior iliac spine.

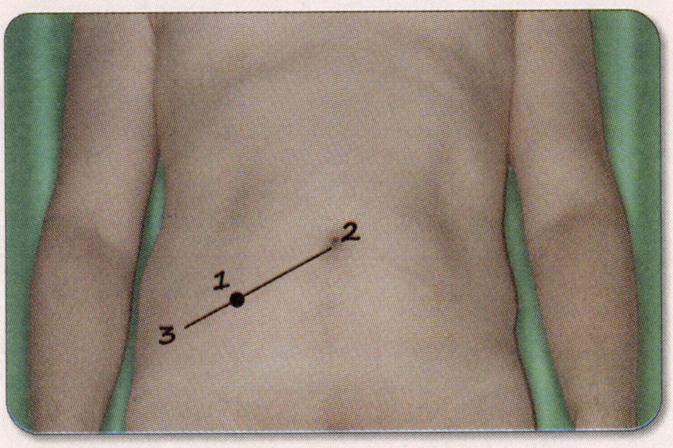

COW MILK PROTEIN ALLERGY (CMPA)

- CMPA is the most common food allergy in small children who are top fed.
- CMPA is of two types:
  1. **Immediate (IgE mediated)**
     - Occurs within minutes of milk intake
     - Vomiting, pallor, shock-like state, urticaria and swelling of lips.
  2. **Delayed (cell mediated):** Presents mainly with GI symptoms
- **Clinical features:**
  - **Diarrhea with blood and mucus**
  - **Respiratory symptoms:** Allergic rhinitis and asthma
  - **Atopic symptoms:** Eczema and Angioedema

Diagnosis

- **Gold standard:** Elimination and challenge test.
- Symptoms subside after withdrawal of milk and milk products.
- **Sigmoidoscopy:** We will see aphthous ulcers.
- **Rectal biopsy:** Plenty of eosinophils.

Treatment

- All animal milk products have to be removed.
- Soy or extensively hydrolyzed formula.
- A trial of continued breastfeeding till six months while the mother is placed on a milk product free diet.

ACUTE VIRAL HEPATITIS

- **The most common cause of acute viral hepatitis:** Hepatitis A followed by hepatitis E.
- **Fecal-oral route transmission:** Hepatitis A and E.
- **Clinical features:** Low grade fever, anorexia, vomit and jaundice.
- **On examination:** Hepatomegaly, splenomegaly, mild ascites.

Investigations

- Elevated lever function test
- Hyperbilirubinemia
- Marked elevated ALT/AST

Complications

- Acute liver failure
- Aplastic anemia
- Acute pancreatitis
- Hemolysis with renal failure in patients with G6PD deficiency
- Chronic liver disease

Management

- Oral intake is ensured.
- Intravenous fluids.
- Watch for complications like encephalopathy.

Prevention

- Sanitation
- Safe drinking water supply
- Hand wash
- Food hygiene
- Vaccination for hepatitis B

ACUTE LIVER FAILURE

Uncorrected coagulopathy (6–8 hours after giving vitamin K) with INR ≥ 1.5 with hepatic encephalopathy

Causes

Infections	Viral hepatitis A, B, E
Drugs	INH Rifampicin Pyrazinamide Acetaminophen Sodium valproate
Metabolic	Wilson disease Galactosemia Tyrosinemia Niemann-Pick disease
Autoimmune	Autoimmune liver disease
Vascular	Budd-Chiari syndrome

Stage: West Haven Staging*

Stage	Features	Reflexes
1	• Inconsolable cry • Inattention to task • Not acting like self • Disturbed sleep-wake cycle	Normal or hyper-reflexia, Asterixis absent
2	Same	Asterixis +ve
3	Somnolence/stupor/ combative	Asterixis +ve
4	**Comatose** 4a: responsive to pain 4b: nonresponsive to pain	Asterixis absent

Stage	EEG changes
1	Triphasic waves
2	Triphasic waves
3	Triphasic waves
4	Delta waves

Management

- Symptomatic management
  - Manage raised ICT (intracranial teusion) by:
    1. Mannitol
    2. Hypertonic saline
    3. Head end 30° elevation
  - Lactulose for constipation
  - N-acetyl cysteine—100 mg/kg/day

Management of a Child with Acute Liver Failure

Systems	Evaluation	Intervention, remarks
Airway and respiratory support	• SpO_2, pO_2, pCO_2 and pH • Pulse oximetry, pH, oxygen saturation	• Assisted ventilation in grade 111/1V encephalopathy or agitation with lower encephalopathy grades • Atracurium not dependent on hepatic elimination; useful when needing paralysis
Fluid, electrolyte and metabolic management	• Blood sodium, potassium, phosphate, urea creatinine; glucose, calcium, magnesium, lactate, pH • Central venous pressure • Urine ouput	• Start with 80% dextrose-based maintenance fluid for age and weight • Target euvolemia to ensure cerebral perfusion • Rapid fluid boluses can worsen cerebral edema • No evidence to support use of lactulose, L-ornithine, L-asparate and rifaximin • Consider kidney replacement therapy, if fluid overload, metabolic derangement

Contd...

Systems	Evaluation	Intervention, remarks
Cardiovascular support	• Heart rate, blood pressure, invasive arterial pressure, capillary refill time • Mixed venous oxygen saturation in patients on inotropes, trend in CVP, stroke volume variations, pulse pressure variations and response to fluid administration in hypotension	• Noradrenaline is the inotrope of choice to treat hypotension • Corticosteroids may alleviate adrenal insufficiency and treat refractory hypotension • Plasmapheresis, if high inotrope requirement • Consider emergency liver transplantation
Neurological monitoring and support	• Stage hepatic encephalopathy • Glasgow coma/AVPU score • Monitor for raised intracranial pressure, hypoglycemia, worsening of neurological signs, intracranial bleed	• Prevent raised intracranial pressure (ICP)/ neurological injury: Fever control, head end elevation to 30°, avoid fluid overload • Maintain serum sodium between 145 and 150 mEq/L. Nurse with minimal stimulation in a quiet environment • 3% saline, 20% mannitol (contraindicated in AKI) and transient hyperventilation may be used for increased ICP • Sedate, agitated or ventilated patient; avoid benzodiazepines. Morphine/fentanyl preferred • Early CRRT with renal impairment, HE grade III-IV with ammonia >150 ionol/L, or absolute ammonia l >200 µmol/L • Hepatectomy, if necrotic liver is believed to be causing raised intracranial hypertension, while awaiting emergency liver transplantation
Coagulation and hematological support	• Bleeding manifestations • Prothrombin time (INR), fibrinogen level, platelet count • INR does not predict bleeding risk	• Correction of INR by fresh frozen plasma, if bleeding manifestations and invasive procedures • Platelet count >50,000/mm³ reduces risk of bleeding • Consider plasma exchange for life-threatening bleeds or increased requirement for coagulation factor support (>30 mL/kg FFP in 24 hours) • Stress ulcer prevention using proton pump inhibitor
Secondary Infection	• Features of systemic inflammatory response syndrome are non-specific, and could be result of liver failure/necrosis • Daily surveillance cultures • Suspect infection, if sudden worsening/ hypotension/unexplained AKI/encephalopathy/SIRS	• Prophylactic broad-spectrum antibiotics and antifungals decrease frequency of infections. • Selective gut decontamination not recommended • CRP unreliable as a marker of sepsis
Nutrition		Enteral feed when possible; ensure 1 g/kg/clay of protein
Nonspecific supportive medications		• Role of N-acetylcysteine infusion in non-paracetamol-associated ALF is controversial

16. INBORN ERRORS OF METABOLISM

"Mistakes are proof that you are trying."
"Thought: Define your purpose
Identify your priorities
Stay focused on them
It's hard to be distracted when you know clearly what you want."

WHEN TO SUSPECT

- Sepsis like presentation with negative septic screen.
- Persistent vomiting, peculiar body/urine odor.
- Rapidly progressive encephalopathy with seizure.
- Parental consanguinity, significant family history.
- After initial normalcy there is acidosis, ketosis, and hypoglycemia.
- Unexplained acute illness in a previously well child.
- Recurrent coma/stroke/ataxia/cramps.
- Multisystem involvement with family history.

DISORDERS OF CARBOHYDRATE METABOLISM

- Glycogen storage disease
- Galactosemia
- Hereditary fructose intolerance

What are Carbohydrates

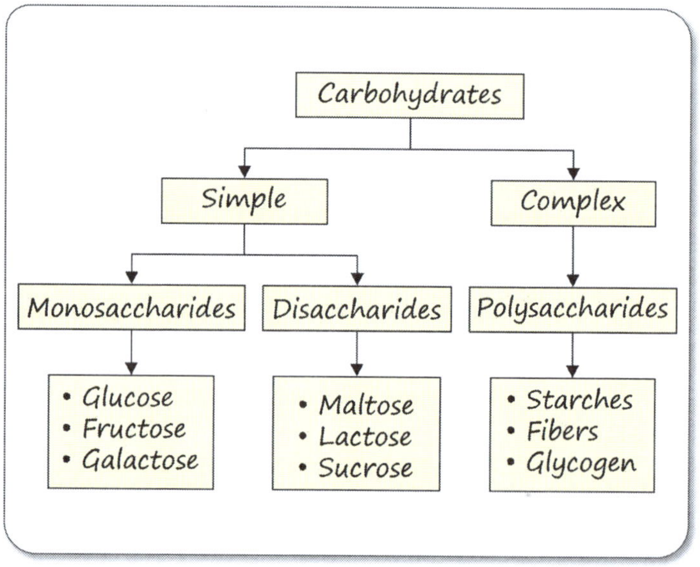

Glycogen Storage Disease

Type	Disease	Enzyme deficiency
2 – Mixed	Pompe disease* (INI-CET 2023)	Alpha 1,4 glucosidase/acid maltase
5 – Muscle	McArdle disease	Muscle phosphorylase
7 – Muscle	Tarui disease	Phosphofructokinase
1 – Liver	Von Gierke's disease	Glucose 6 phosphatase
3 – Mixed	Cori disease	Debranching enzyme
4 – Mixed	Anderson disease	Branching enzyme
6 – Liver	Hers disease	Liver phosphorylase

- Muscle Glycogen Storage Disease (GSD) (type 2, 5, 7 – mnemonic 2 + 5 = 7)
- Liver GSD type 1, 3, 4, 6 (mnemonic – violet color acha hai)
- Type 3 Cori disease—liver and muscle both are involved.
- Most common GSD in children is type 1: von Gierke's disease
- Most common GSD in adults is type 5: McArdle disease
- Best single answer for mixed is Pompe
- Best single answer for liver is von Gierke's
- Best single answer for muscle involvement is Mc Ardle disease

Von Gierke Disease

- Enzyme deficient: glucose 6 phosphatase
- Leads to glycogen accumulation in liver, kidney
- **Clinical features**:
  - Hypoglycemia, hepatomegaly
  - Jaundice is usually not seen
  - Hyperuricemia, hyperlipidemia, lactic acidosis

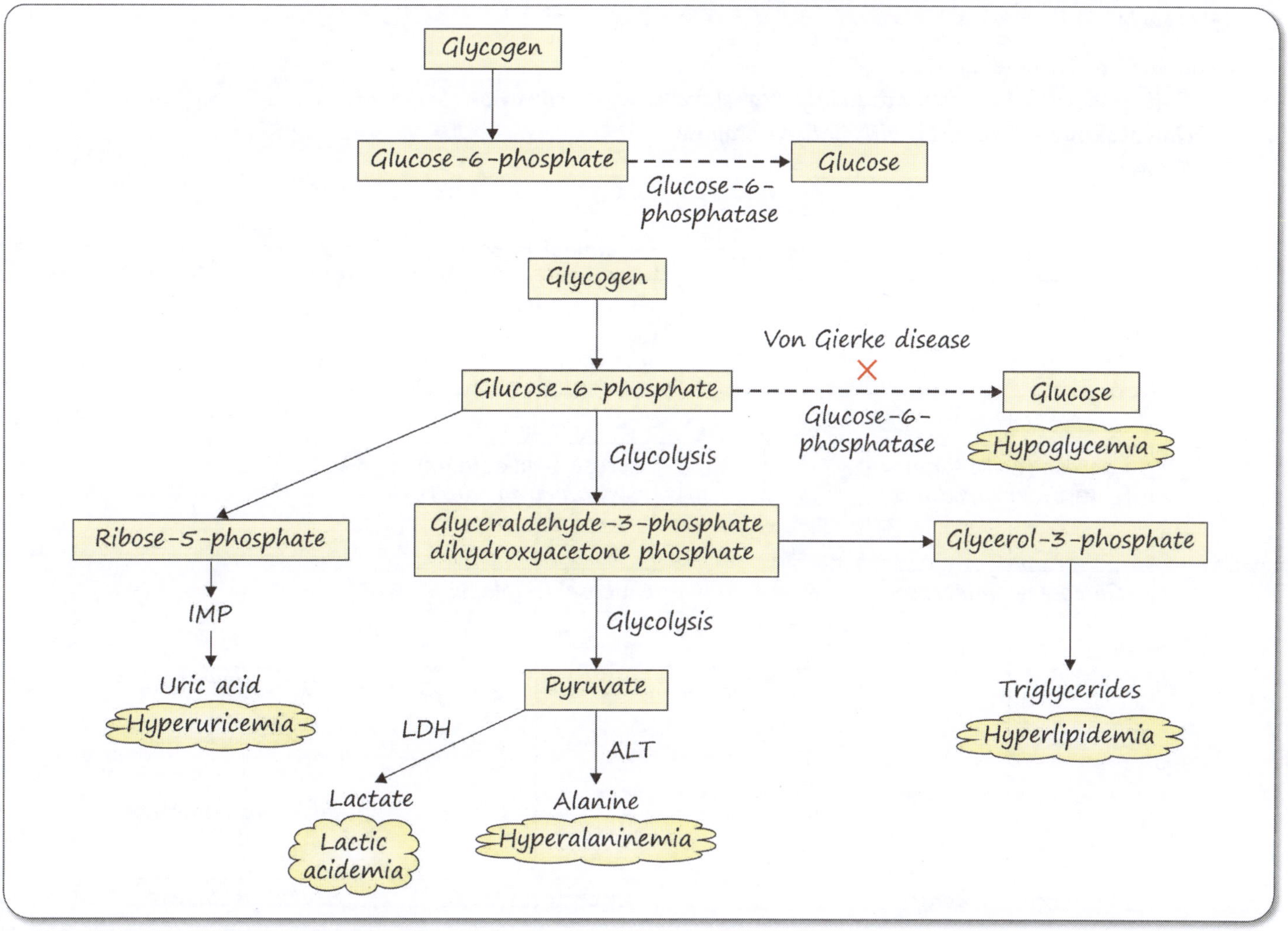

- Doll-like face

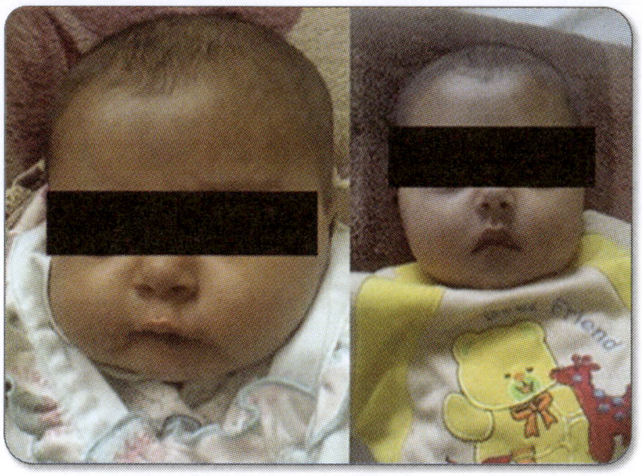

- Recurrent hypoglycemia
- Hepatomegaly (due to glucose 6 phosphate accumulates in liver)

- **Diagnosis**: liver biopsy
- **Rx**: (treatment)
  - High carbohydrate feeds—cornstarch and including nighttime feeds
  - Liver transplantation.

Pompe Disease (Type 2 GSD)

- **Enzyme deficiency**: Acid maltase/alpha 1,4 glucosidase
- Type 2 involves the muscle and heart.
- **Features**: Floppy child, coarse facies
- Hypotonia, hepatosplenomegaly
- **Chest X-ray**: Cardiomegaly**, heart failure
- **EEG**: Tall QRS with short PR interval
- **Treatment**: Enzyme replacement therapy
- **Prognosis**: Death before 2 years.

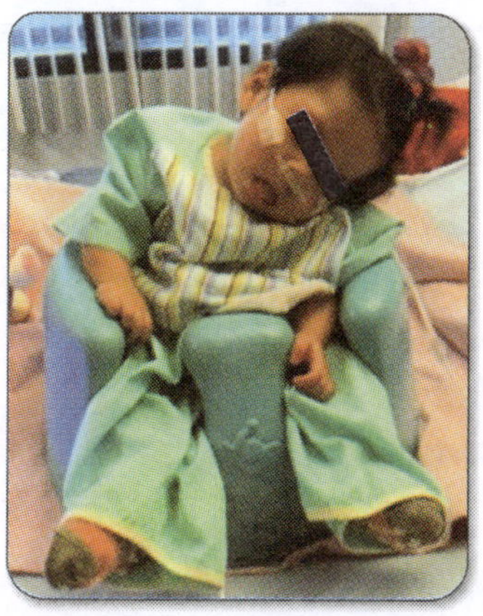

Galactosemia

- Deficiency of three enzymes:
  1. Galt galactose 1 phosphate uridyl transferase* most common
  2. **Galactokinase**: Presents with cataract alone
  3. Epimerase

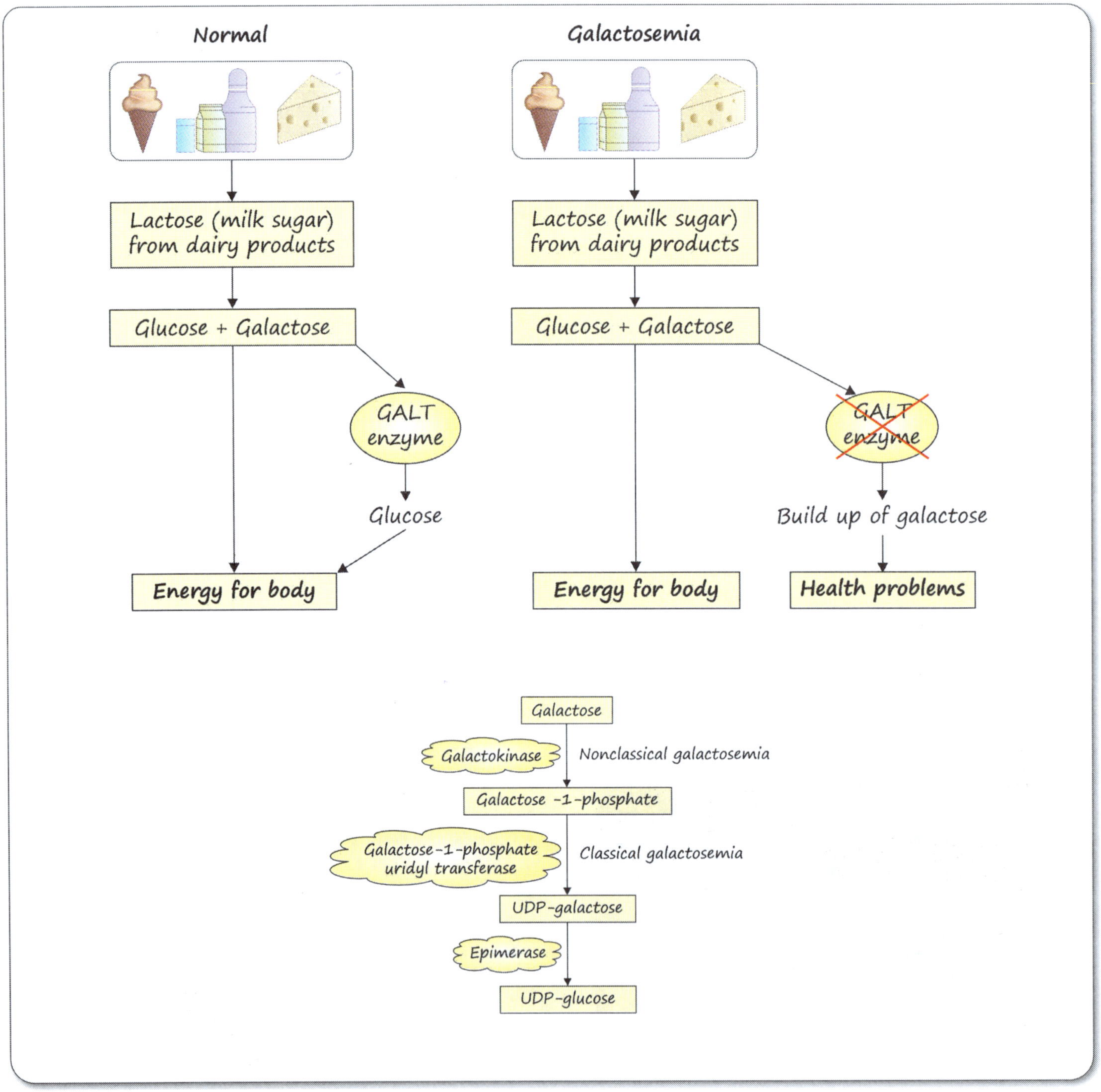

- **Clinical features:**
  - Jaundice
  - Hepatomegaly
  - Diarrhea
  - Vomiting
  - FTT
  - Seizures
  - Cataract
- **Diagnosis:**
  - Reducing substances in urine by benedicts test.

- Direct enzyme assay.
- Carrier testing and prenatal diagnosis

- **Rx:**
  - Eliminate milk and dairy products containing lactose
  - Soya-based diet

Key Points
- Breastfeeding is contraindicated.
- Cataract will be the only finding in galactokinase deficiency.
- Most common cause of sepsis in galactosemia is *E. coli*.

Hereditary Fructose Intolerance

- Accumulation of fructose 1 phosphate causes inhibition of glycolysis and gluconeogenesis.
- Causing hypoglycemia.
- Ingestion of fructose (sugar) leads to accumulation of fructose 1 phosphate.

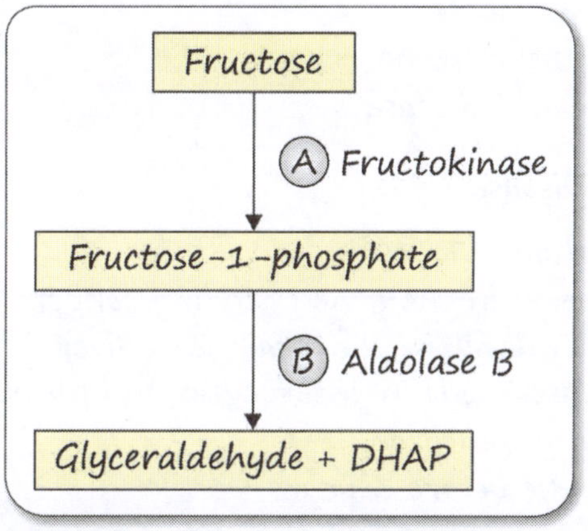

- **Clinical features:**
  - Hypoglycemia
  - Jaundice
  - Vomiting
  - Fructosuria
  - Failure to thrive (FTT)
  - Symptoms will come if we introduce fructose-rich food.
- **Diagnosis:**
  - Reducing substances in urine +ve by benedict's test
  - IV fructose tolerance test
  - Definitive diagnosis—aldolase B enzyme activity in liver
  - Gene-based diagnosis
- **Rx:**
  - Elimination of sources of fructose and sorbitol.
  - If the diet is restricted, intellectual impairment is reversed.

NEURODEGENERATIVE DISORDERS

The patient will present with loss of acquired milestones.

	Gray matter disease	White matter disease
Loss of social interaction	Early	Late
Seizures	Early	Late
Electroretinogram (ERG)	May be abnormal	Normal
Visual evoked response (VER)	May be abnormal	Normal

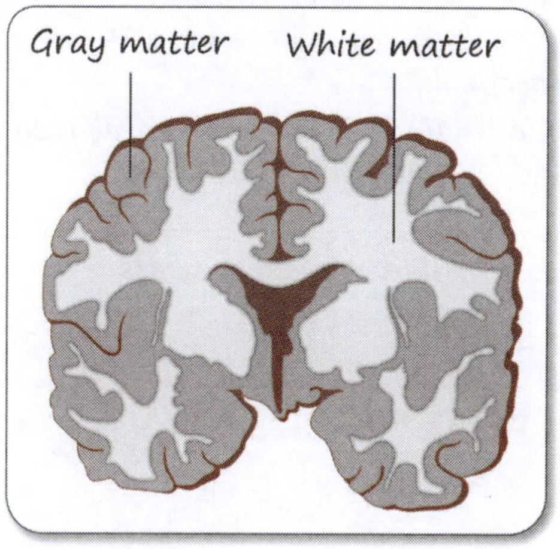

White Matter Disease

- Krabbe disease
- Alexander disease
- Canavan disease
- Metachromatic leukodystrophy

Krabbe Disease

- Neurodegenerative white matter disorder
- Myelin loss
- Globoid bodies in white matter
- Deficiency of enzyme galactocerebroside beta-galactosidase
- Autosomal recessive
- Chromosome 14q24
- Microcephaly
- **Clinical features:**
  - Vomiting
  - Feeding difficulties
  - Hypertonia
  - Blindness
  - Deafness
  - Absent DTR
  - B/L symmetrical basal ganglia hyperdensities

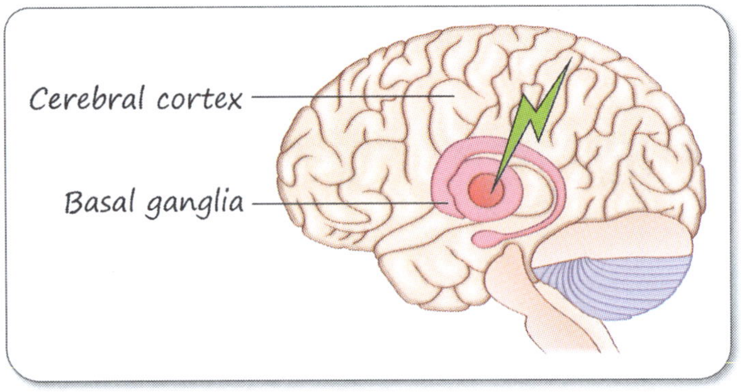

Alexander Disease

- Neurodegenerative disorder
- Mutation: GFAP gene—chromosome 17q21
- Glial fibrillary acidic protein (GFAP)
- Macrocephaly
- Specific finding: B/L symmetrical frontal white matter involving the U-fibers.

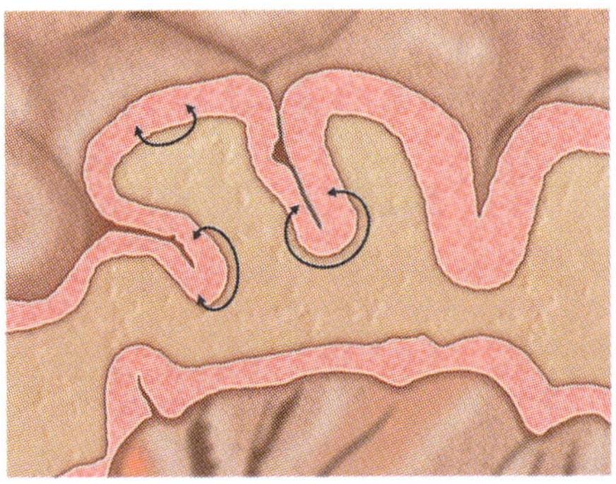
Subcortical U-fibers

Canavan Disease

- Deficiency of enzyme aspartoacylase.
- Accumulation of n-acetyl aspartic acid in brain.
- **Triad:**
  1. Hypotonia
  2. Head lag
  3. Macrocephaly
- **MR spectroscopy:**
  - Elevation of NAA peak and increase in NAA to choline ratio in white matter.
  - Both urinary and blood NAA levels are increased.

Metachromatic Leukodystrophy

- Autosomal recessive
- Deficiency of enzyme **Arylsulfatase A**.
- ARSA gene mutation chromosome 22q.
- Accumulation of cerebroside sulfate within myelin sheath.
- **Earliest sign**: Hypotonia
- **Diagnosis**: Urine examination
- Stripe sign/tigroid pattern

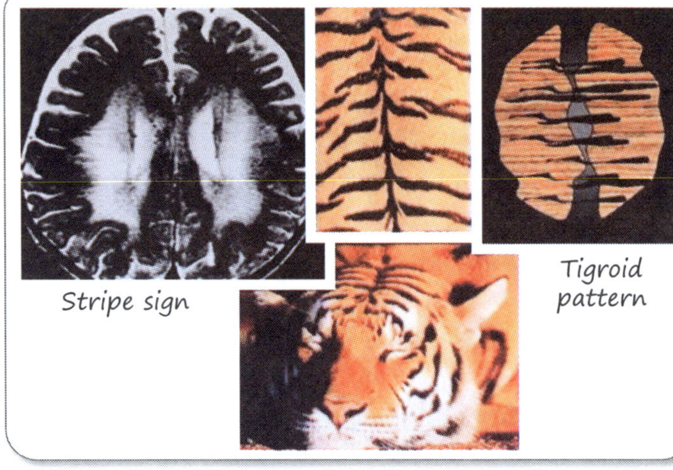

Gray Matter Disease

- Menkes disease
- Wilson disease
- Leigh's syndrome
- Tay-Sachs disease

Menkes Disease

- **Mutation**: ATP7A
- Mutation in the gene encoding copper
- Copper level in the brain and liver is low and increased level in enterocytes and fibroblasts
- Delayed dentition
- They die before 3 years
- Most common cause of death: Cardiac rupture
- Loss of previously attained developmental milestones
- Wormian bones
- Multiple fractures
- Flaring of ribs
- Kinky hair

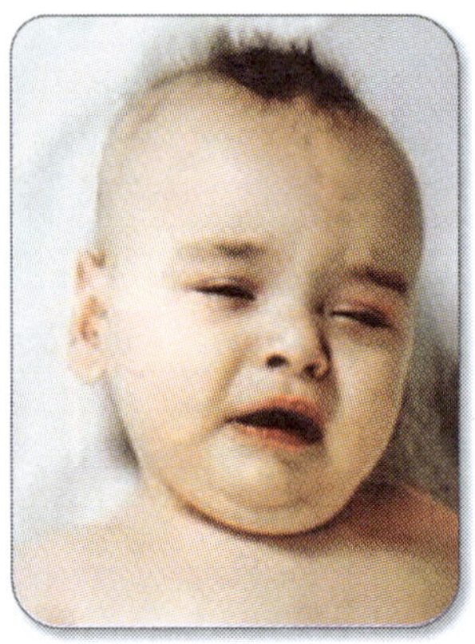
Kinky hair

- **Trichorrhexis nodosa**: Defect in the hair shaft characterized by thickening or weak points (nodes) that cause the hair to break off easily.

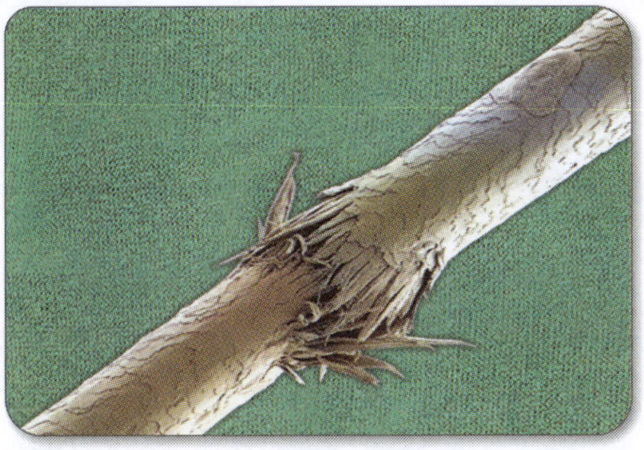

Trichorrhexis nodosa

- **Pathognomonic**: Pili torti is a rare hair condition characterized by fragile hair.
- 180° shifting of the hair shaft.

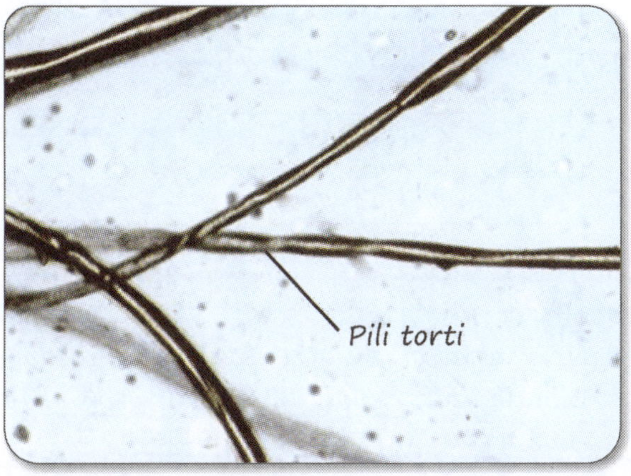

- **Cutis laxa**: In which the skin hangs loosely in folds. Patients develop a prematurely aged appearance.

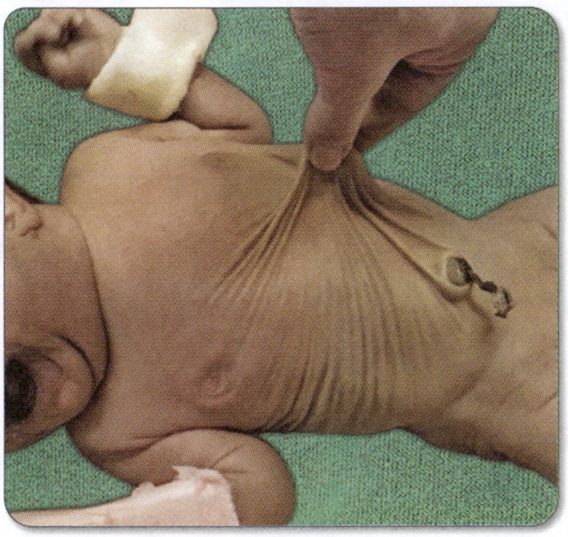

Cutis laxa

Wilson Disease (Hepatolenticular Degeneration)

- Autosomal recessive
- It is the major cause of chronic liver disease.
- **Discovered by**: Samuel Alexander Kinnier Wilson .
- Mutation in ATP7B gene mutation on chromosome 13q14.
- ATP7B gene helps in biliary copper excretion.
- Defective gene means decrease biliary copper excretion and copper accumulation.
- Inadequate incorporation of copper into apoceruloplasmin.
- Therefore, there will be decrease in serum ceruloplasmin levels.
- There will be free serum copper everywhere in the liver, eyes, and cornea.
- **Clinical features:**
  - Asymptomatic hepatomegaly (with or without splenomegaly)
  - Subacute or chronic hepatitis
  - Acute hepatic failure
  - Portal hypertension
  - Ascites
  - Variceal bleeding
  - Other symptoms (delayed puberty, amenorrhea)
- Type of tremor seen in Wilson disease: Wing beating tremor.

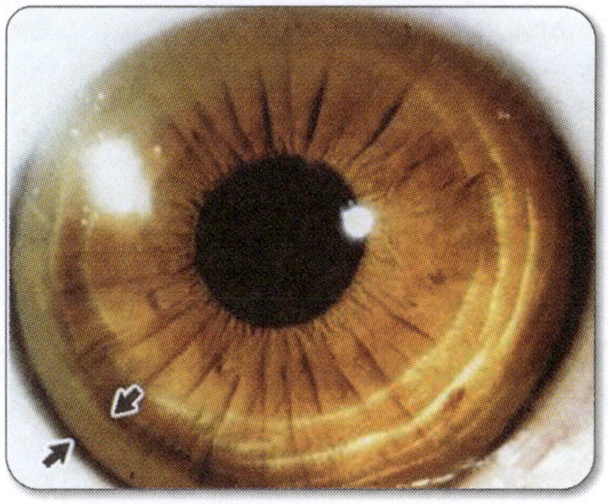

KF ring

- Brown discoloration at the outer margin of the cornea because of the deposition of the copper in the **descemet's membrane**.
- Slit lamp examination is required for secure detection.
- KF ring indicates long-standing disease. Common with neurological (96%), hepatic (60%), asymptomatic (10–20%).
- **Diagnosis:**
  - **Gold standard**: Hepatic copper by liver biopsy.
  - Decreased ceruloplasmin levels (<20mg/dL) (n = 20–35 mg/dL)

- 24-hour urinary copper excretion: >100 µg/day—can go up to 1000 mg/day (n ≤40 µg/dL)
- During a 24-hour urine collection—give 2 doses of 500 mg D-penicillamine 12 hours apart; affected patients excrete >1,600 µg/24 hours
- Panda sign

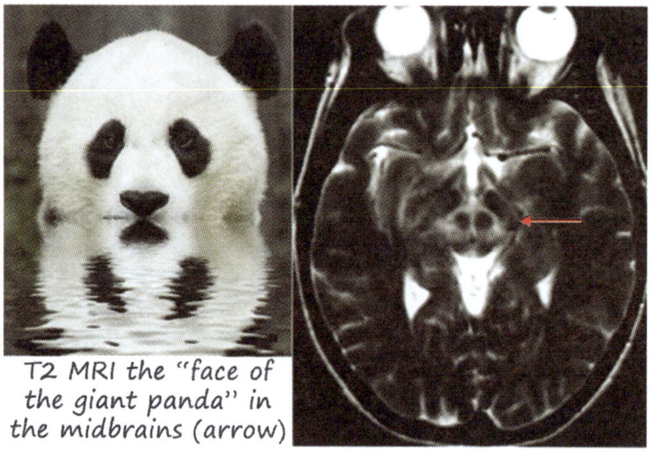

T2 MRI the "face of the giant panda" in the midbrains (arrow)

- **Treatment:**
  - Restrict dietary copper intake to <1 mg/day.
  - Demineralize the water if copper content exceeds 0.1 mg/L.
  - **Cu chelating agents**: Oral D-penicillamine* (b-dimethyl cysteine) 1g/day in 2 doses before meal (adults), 20 mg/kg/day (children).
  - Triethylenetetramine dihydrochloride (trientine) 0.5–2.0 g/day (adults), 20 mg/kg/day (children)

Key Points

- **Best screening test**: Serum ceruloplasmin level which is decreased
- **Most specific screening test:** Urinary 24-hour copper*
- **Gold standard**: Liver biopsy*
- Urinary copper is >100 µg/day (normal is <40 µg/day)

DISORDERS OF AMINO ACID METABOLISM

- Essential amino acid (mnemonic: private tim hall)
- Phenylalanine
- Valine
- Tryptophan
- Threonine
- Isoleucine
- Methionine
- Histidine
- Arginine
- Lysine
- Leucine

Disorder of Phenylalanine Metabolism

- Deficiency of phenylalanine hydroxylase.
- Increased level of phenylalanine.
- Decreased level of tyrosine.
- Metabolism shifted to the alternative pathway.
- Increased concentration of phenylalanine and its metabolites—phenylpyruvate, phenylacetic acid.
- The main organ damaged by PKU is brain.
- Autosomal recessive condition

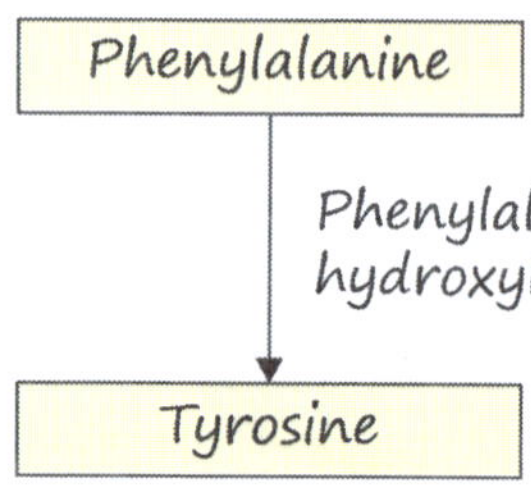

- ***Clinical features***:
  - Microcephaly
  - Normal at birth later intellectual disability
  - Blonde hair: Yellowish discoloration of hair
  - Blue iris
  - Fair skin
  - Musty/mousy body odor (like damp corner without any air for too long)

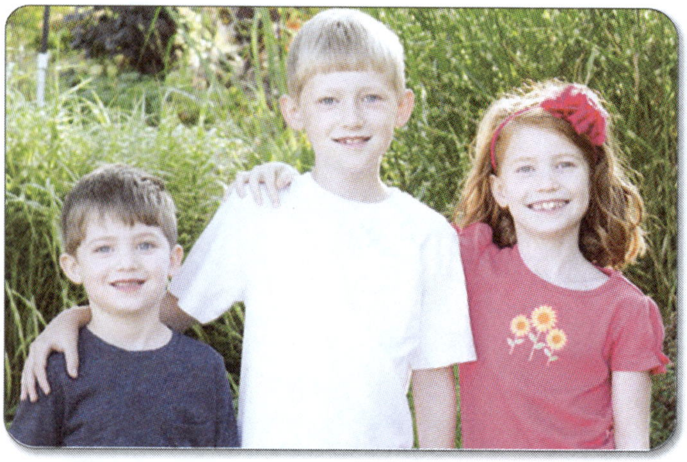

Blonde hair, fair skin

- **Diagnosis:**
    - Ferric chloride test

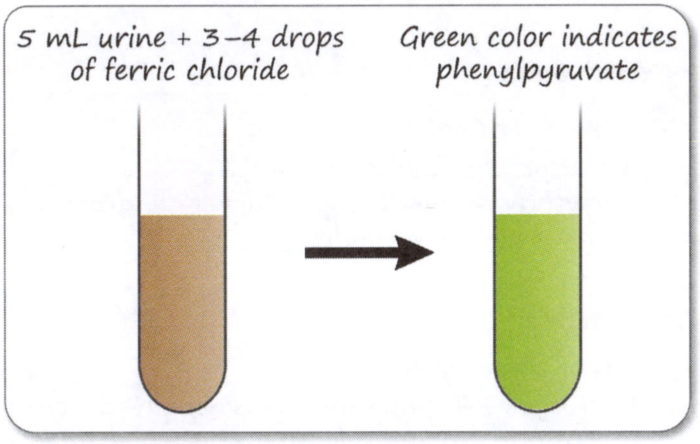

- **Treatment:**
    - Low phenylalanine diet
    - Adequate intake of tyrosine
    - Sapropterin hydrochloride

Maple Syrup Urine Disease

- Autosomal recessive inheritance.
- It is a disorder of amino acid metabolism.
- Deficiency in ability to metabolize branch chain amino acids.
- Branch chain amino acids:
    - Leucine
    - Isoleucine
    - Valine
- **Clinical features:**
    - Normal at birth
    - Hypoglycemia because these branched-chain amino acids later will give glucose to my body.
    - Therefore they end up with hypoglycemia leading to convulsions.
    - Hypertonia
- **Diagnosis:**
    - Antenatal diagnosis of the enzyme activity in the chorionic villi sampling.
    - DMPH – Dinitrophenylhydrazine Test.
    - Take a test tube and take 2 mL of urine and add DNPH reagent.
    - Mix and wait
    - If the test is +ve then you will have yellow precipitate.
    - It will tell us the presence of ketoacetate.

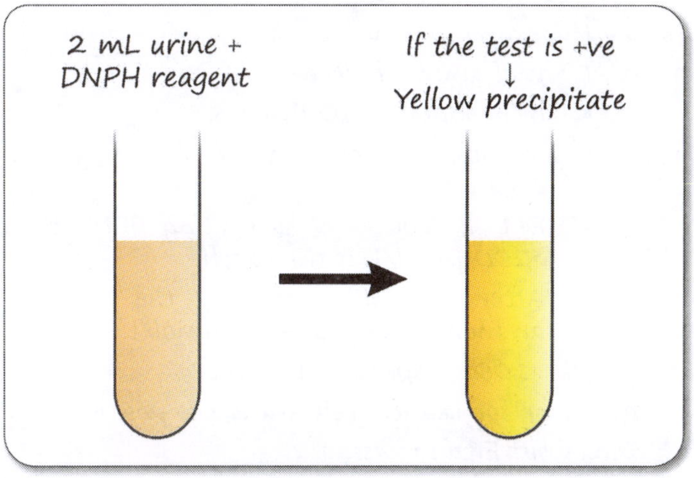

- Levels of leucine (highest amount), isoleucine, valine will be very high in the urine because they are not able to metabolize by the body.
- GCMS – Gas Chromatography Mass Spectrometry.
- **Treatment**:
    - IV glucose
    - Restriction of protein intake
    - Diet devoid of branch chain amino acid
    - Thiamine trial therapy @ 10 mg/kg/day
    - Hemodialysis to reduce branch chain amino acid level in the body.

Extra Points

- Swimming pool odor urine: Hawkinsinuria
- Cat urine odor: 3 hydroxy 3 methyl glutaric aciduria
- Sweat feet odor urine: Isovaleric acidemia
- Boiled cabbage odor urine: Tyrosinemia, hypermethioninemia
- Mousy odor urine: Phenylketonuria
- Rotting fish urine odor: Trimethylaminuria
- Tom cat urine odor (sexually active cat): Multiple carboxylase deficiency

Multiple Carboxylase Deficiency

Enzyme "multiple carboxylase" is an amino acid and it converts into proteins and which gives glucose to the body.

- **Clinical features:**
    - Feeding problem
    - Seizures
    - Alopecia*
    - Tom cat urine odor

- **Lab findings:**
  - Metabolic Acidosis
  - Hyperammonemia
  - Normal ammonia levels
    - In neonate: <110 µmol/L
    - In sick newborn the level can go till 180 µmol/L.
    - But if you are suspecting IEM then >200 µmol/L is the cutoff.
    - After neonatal period the normal ammonia levels: 50–80 µmol/L.
    - >100: Suspect IEM
  - Urine for reducing substances is positive
- **Diagnosis:** Enzyme assay
- **Treatment:** Biotine 10 mg/day because biotin is good for skin.

Alkaptonuria

- Autosomal recessive
- Deficiency of enzyme homogentisic acid oxidase
- Leading to increase levels of homogentisic acid

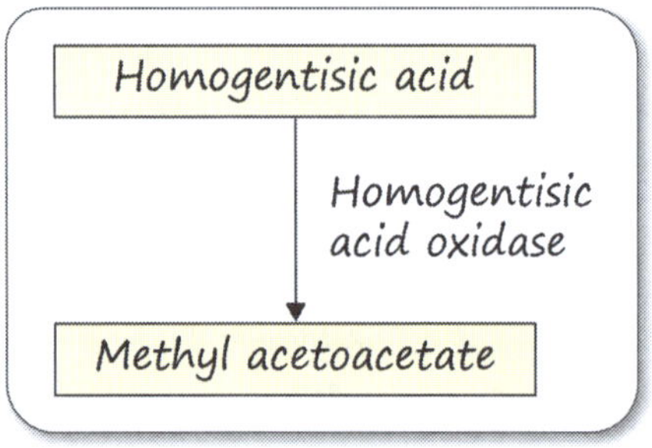

- **Triad:**
  1. Ochronotic arthritis
  2. Ochronotic pigmentation
  3. Darkening of urine on standing

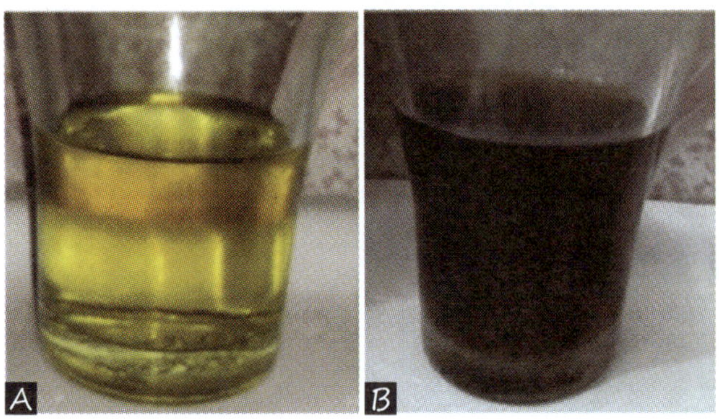

Darkening of urine on standing—Alkaptonuria

- **Treatment:**
  - Nitisinone
  - Vitamin C

> **Extra Points**
>
> **Treatment of Choice**
> - Ivacaftor: Cystic fibrosis
> - Growth hormone therapy: Turner syndrome
> - Losartan: Marfan syndrome

Tyrosinemia

- It is of three types:
  1. In type 1/hepatorenal tyrosinemia—deficient enzyme is fumarylacetoacetate hydroxylase (FAH) which converts fumarylacetoacetic acid to fumarate + acetoacetate.
  2. In type 2/Richner-Hanhart syndrome—deficient enzyme is aminotransferase (pointer A in the image) which helps in converting tyrosine into phenyl hydroxy pyruvic acid.
  3. In type 3—deficient enzyme is phenyl hydroxy pyruvate dioxygenase (pointer B in the image) PHPA helps in conversion of phenylhydroxy pyruvic acid to homogentisic acid.

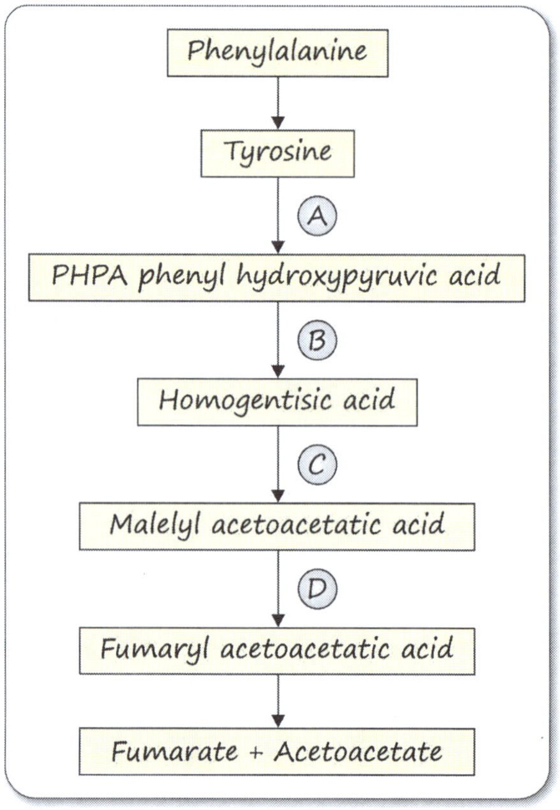

- **Clinical features**:
  - Oculocutaneous problem
    - Ocular: Corneal ulcer
    - Cutaneous: Palmar plantar hyperkeratosis
  - It affects the liver, kidneys and peripheral nerves
  - Cabbage urine odor is seen
  - Developmental delay, seizure
  - Self-destructive behavior*
- **Treatment**: Nitisinone

Hartnup Disorder

- SLC6A19 gene mutation.
- Defect in the transport of the neutral amino acid.
- Pellagra like rash.

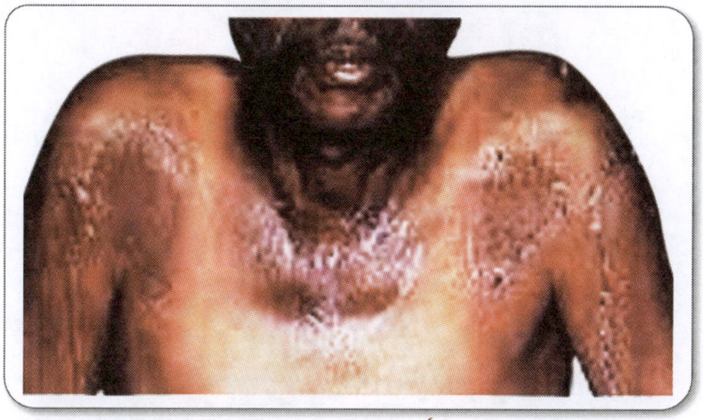

Pellagra like rash

- **Treatment**: Nicotinic acid

Homocystinuria

- Deficiency of enzyme cystathionine beta-synthase.
- Leading to deficiency of cystathionine and accumulation of homocysteine.
- The features are similar to Marfan syndrome. The only difference is in homocystinuria we see inferomedial subluxation of lense (mnemonic – him)
- In Marfan syndrome we see superotemporal subluxation of lense.
- **Treatment:**
  - Vitamin B_6 is a coenzyme of cystathionine beta-synthase
  - Restriction of methionine intake.

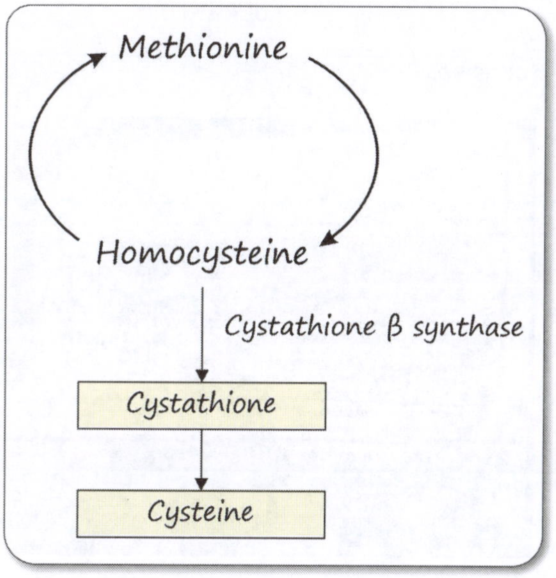

"Life teaches you a new lesson every day, only if you are attentive enough in the class."

100 IMAGES

"Work for it more than you hope for it!!"

1. Vernix Caseosa

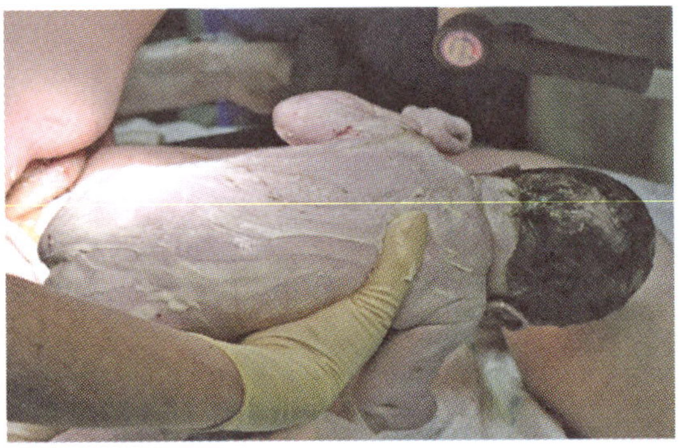

To prevent hypothermia

2. Deferasirox

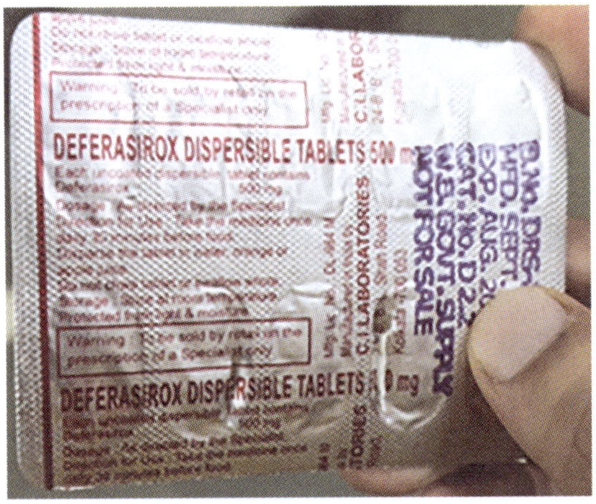

Iron chelator in thalassemia

3. Ascaris lumbricoides

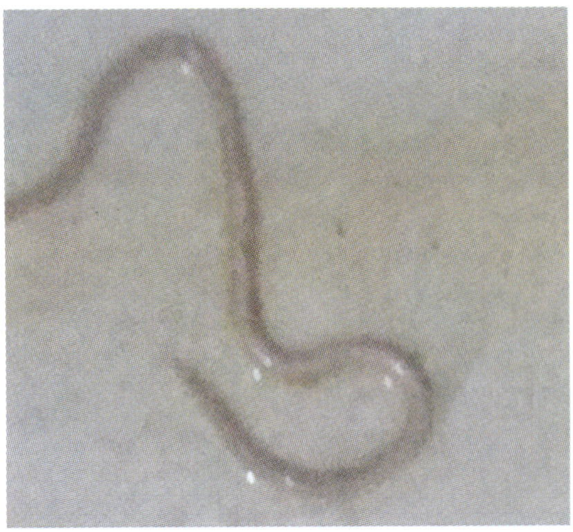

- For deworming
  - <2 years—200 mg
  - >2 years—400 mg

4. Tinea Corporis

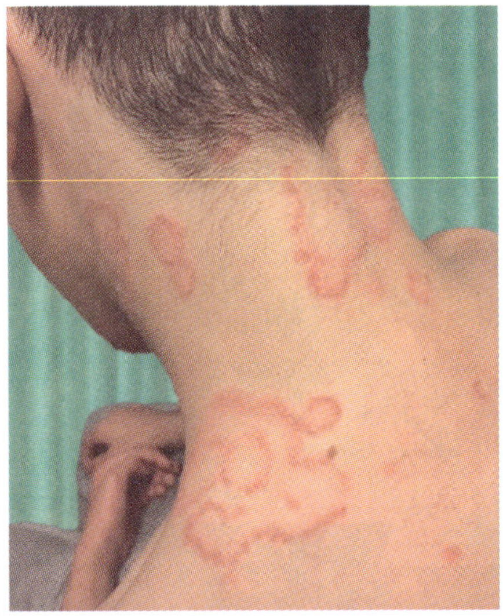

- Ring-like/raised/erythematous border with central clearing

5. Ichthyosis

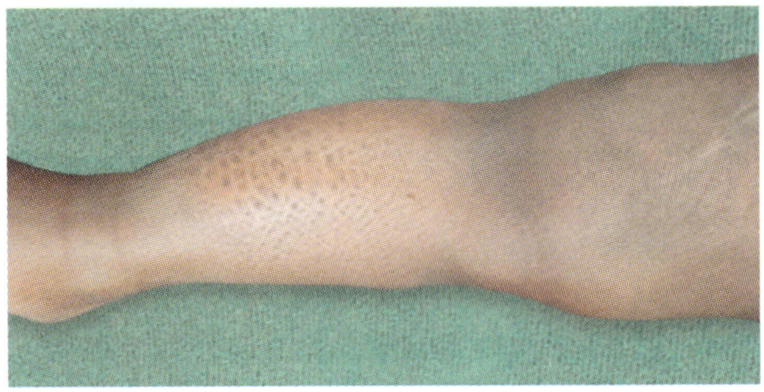

- Fish-like scales
- R_x: Coconut oil

6. Phrynoderma

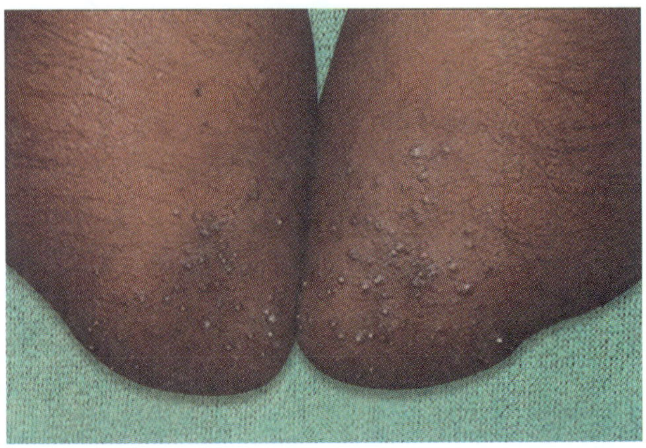

Toad-like skin

7. Pfeiffer syndrome

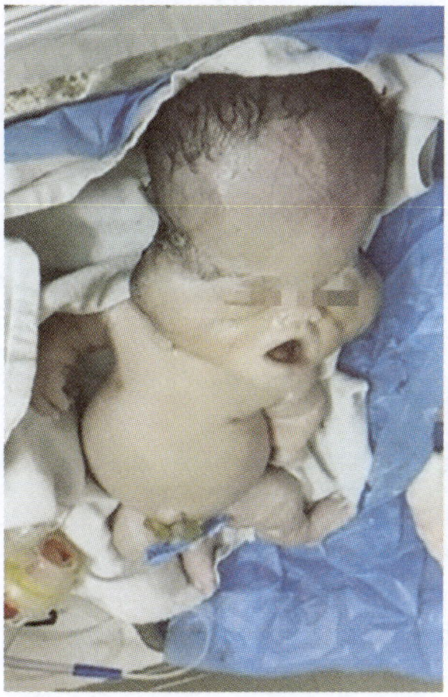

- Cloverleaf shape skull
- FGFR1 Gene mutation

8. Encephalocele with anencephaly

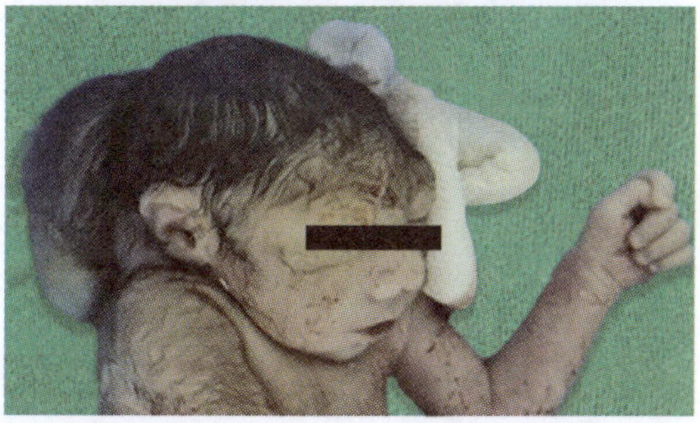

9. Holoprosencephaly

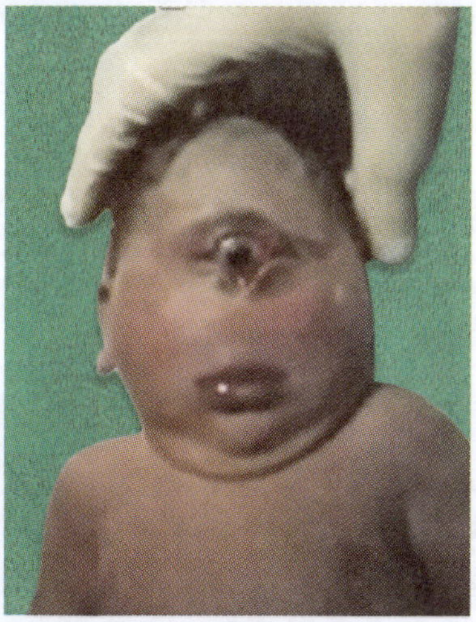

It is not a neural tube defect, it is a forebrain anomaly

10. Meningomyelocele

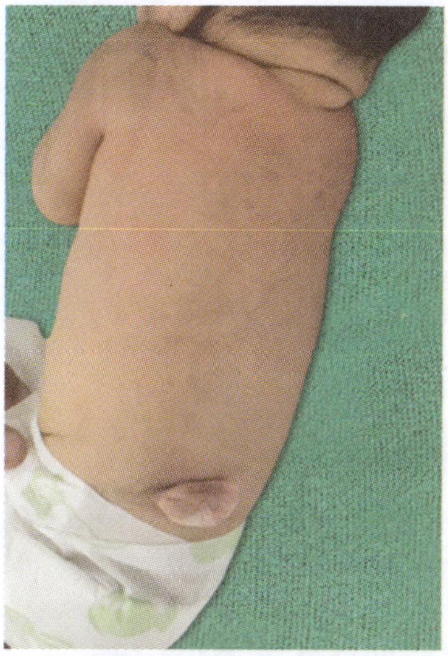

11. Craniorachischisis (NTD with worst prognosis)

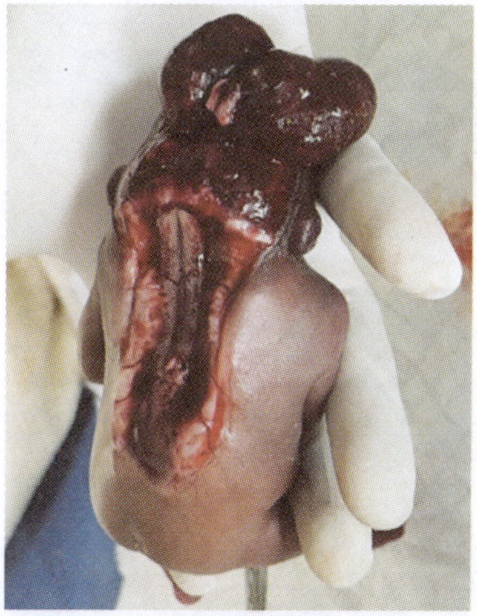

Worst prognosis

12. Dandy-Walker Malformation

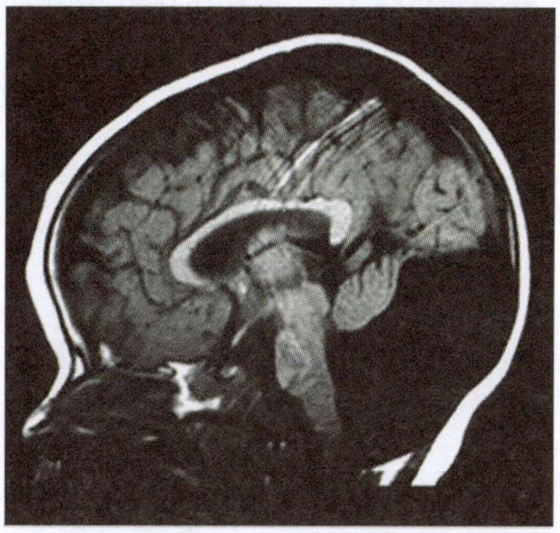

Dandy walker malformation: cerebellar hypoplasia with hydrocephalus

13. Vein of Galen malformation

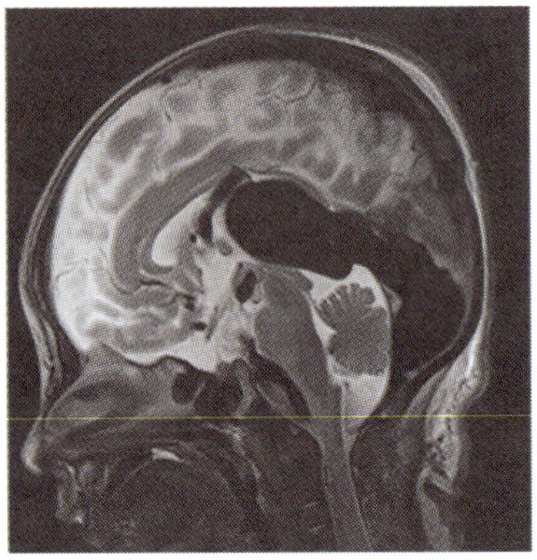

Open anterior fontanelle, mid line lesion on ultrasound with Macrocephaly

14. Arnold-Chiari malformation

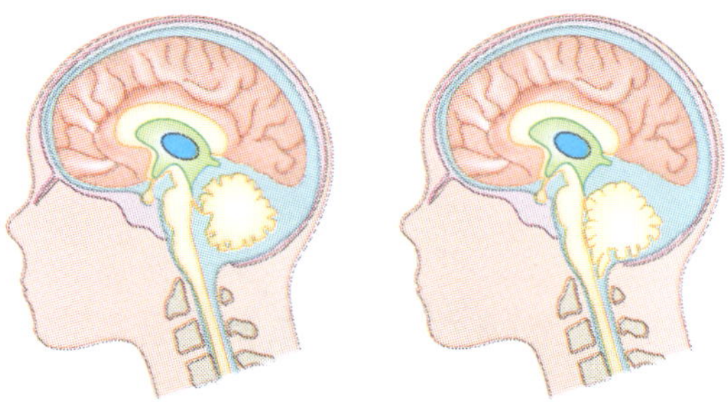

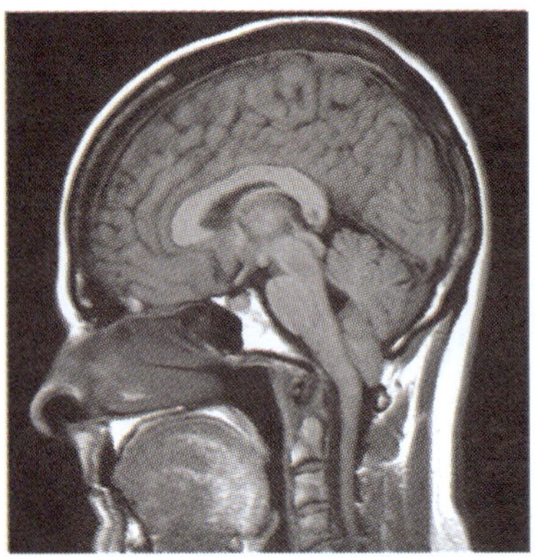

Classical arnold chiari malformation—herniation of cerebellum and brainstem

15. Hydrocephalus

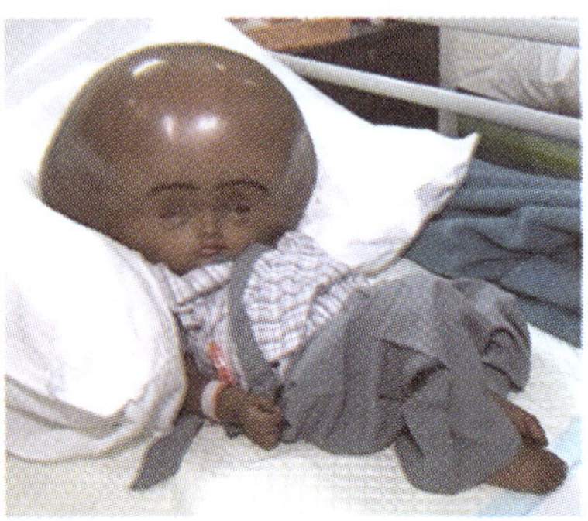

Treatment: VP shunt (ventriculoperitoneal shunt)

16. Poland syndrome

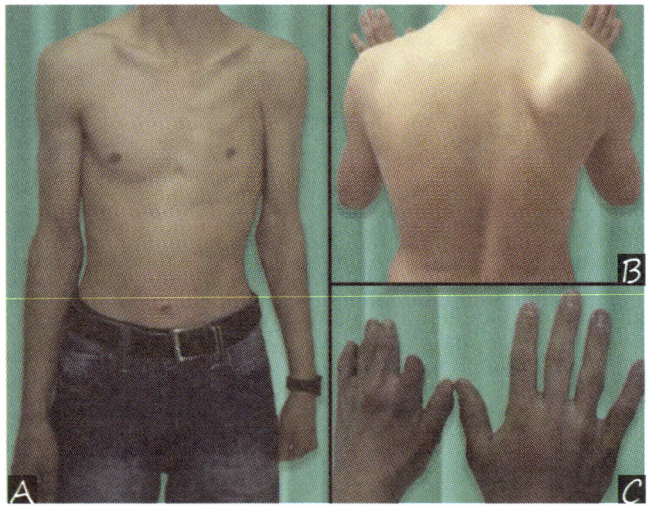

- Aplasia of the pectoralis muscles
- Rib deformities, webbed fingers
- Radial nerve aplasia

17. Cornelia de Lange syndrome

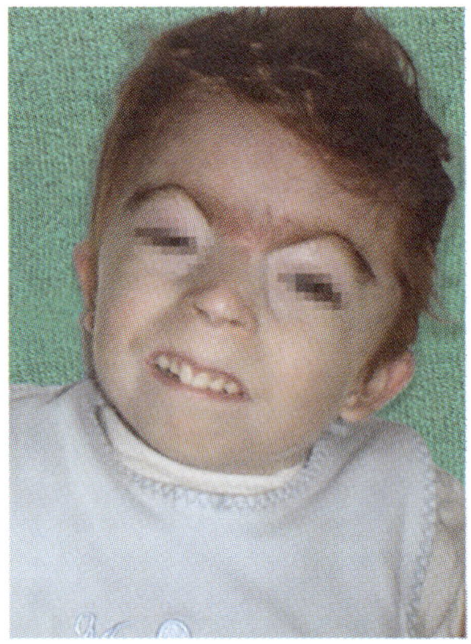

- Thin eyebrows with high arches
- Hirsutism

18. Knuckle Knuckle Dimple Knuckle sign

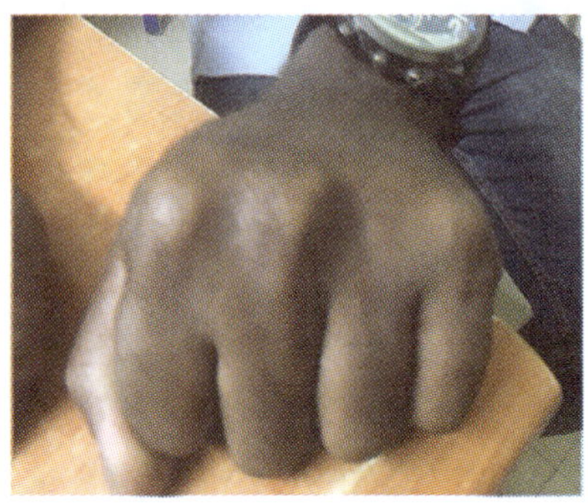

Seen in turner syndrome (short 4th metacarpal)

19. Dose of zinc in diarrhea

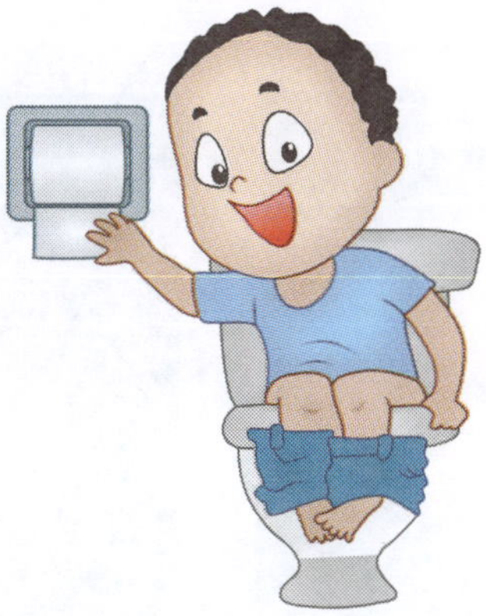

- <6 months = 10 mg
- >6 months = 20 mg
- Given for 14 days

20. Thumb sign: Acute epiglottis

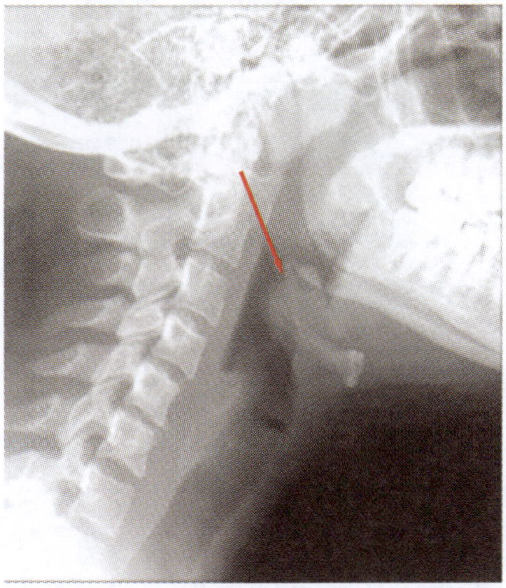

21. Steeple sign: Croup

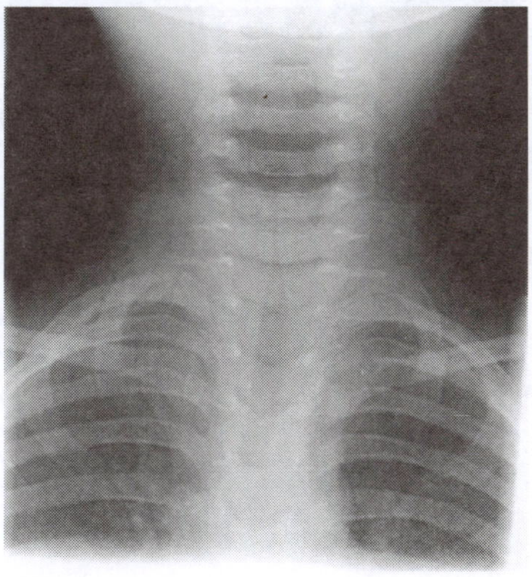

22. Dose of vitamin k in newborn is 1 mg
<1 kg – 0.5 mg

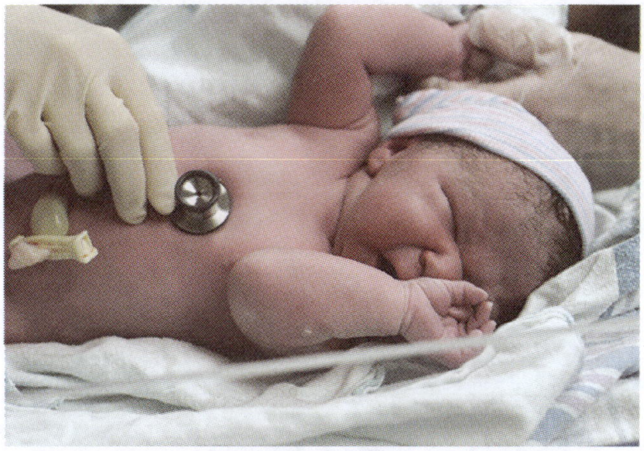

23. Neonatal jaundice

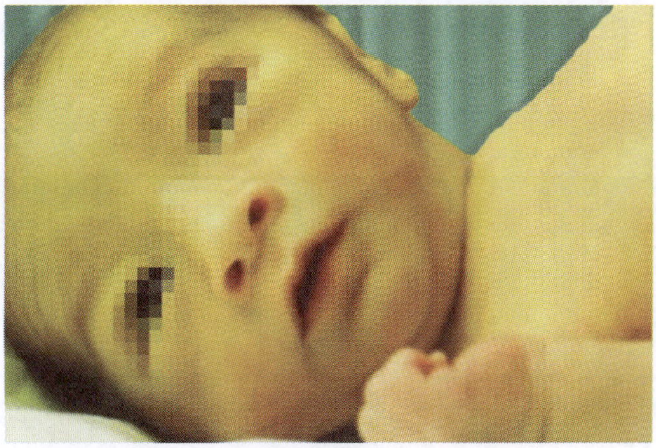

- **Treatment:** Phototherapy (460–490 nm wavelength)

24. Drug of choice in neonatal seizure: Phenobarbitone. Repeated eye blinking in newborns is known as subtle seizure.

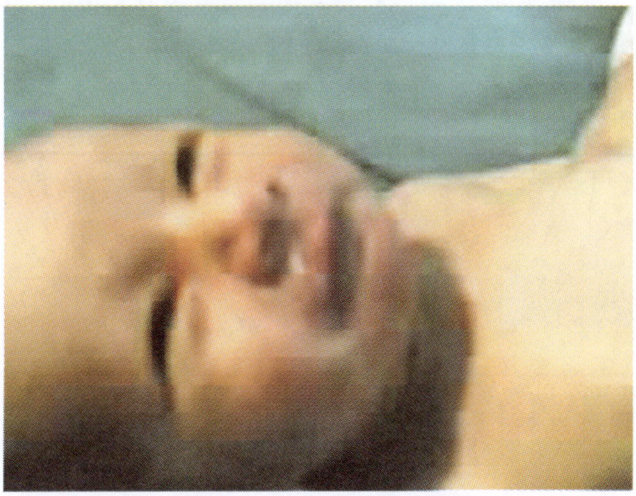

25. Anasarca—Nephrotic syndrome

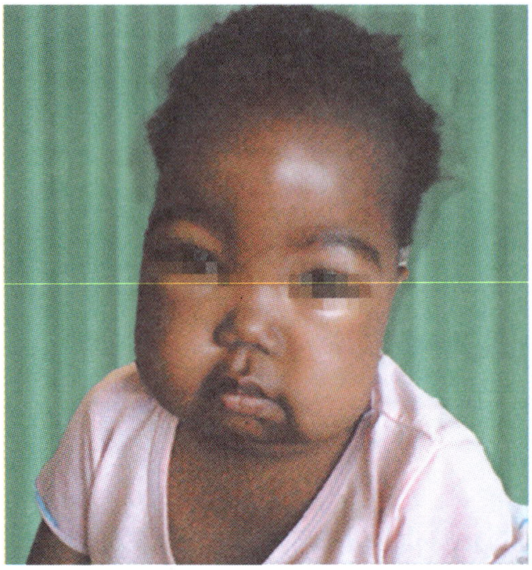

- DOC: Prednisolone

26. Syndactyly (Fusion of Fingers)

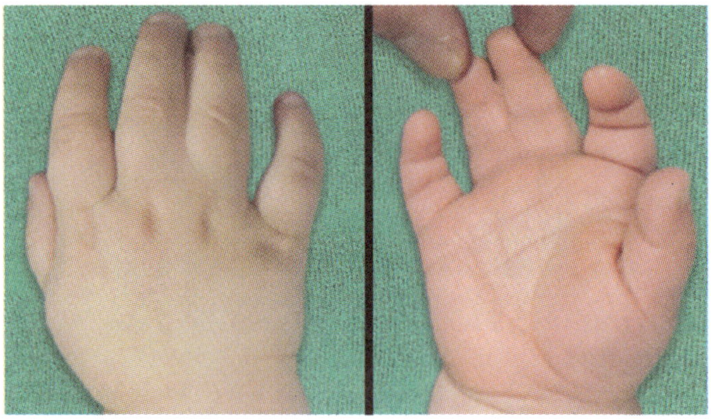

27. Polydactyly (>5 Fingers)

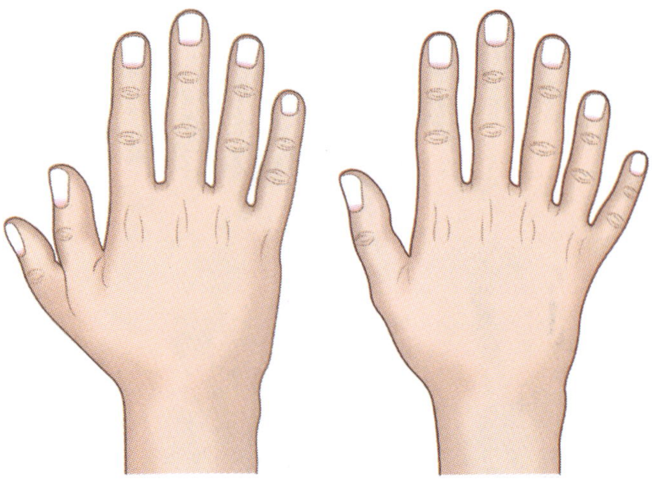

28. Brachydactyly (Small Fingers)

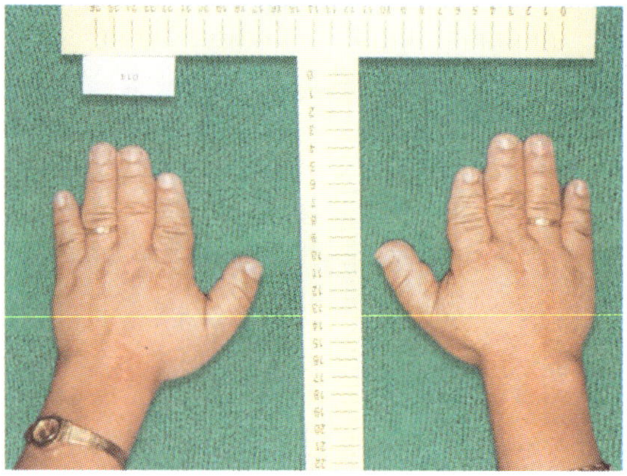

29. Rickets (Bowing of Legs)

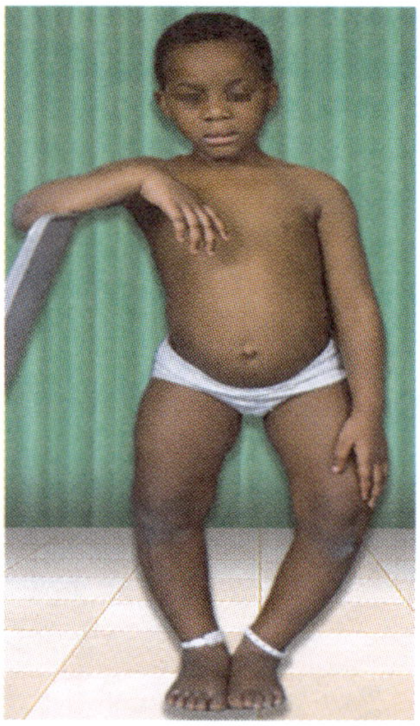

30. White out lung hyaline membrane disease/ Respiratory distress syndrome

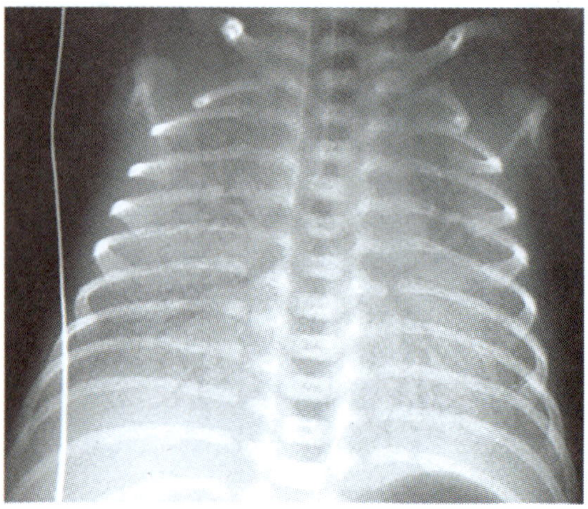

Treatment: Intratracheal surfactant

31. Nasogastric tube (black arrow)

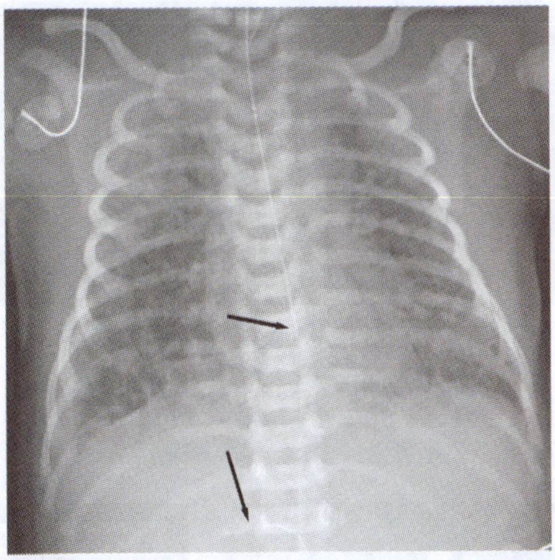

32. Chest X-ray showing patchy infiltrates: Meconium aspiration syndrome

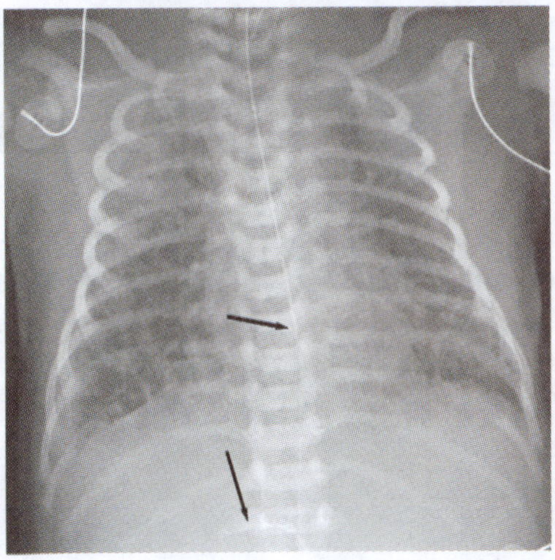

33. Wilson disease (KF ring in the descemet membrane of cornea)

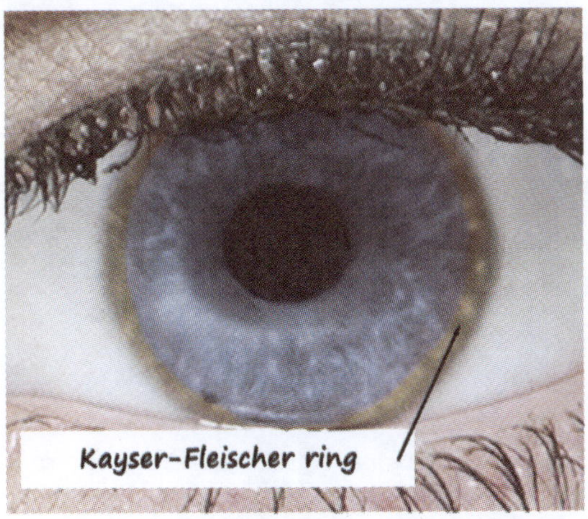

Treatment: Zinc trientine D-penicillamine

34. Boot shape heart—Tetralogy of Fallot

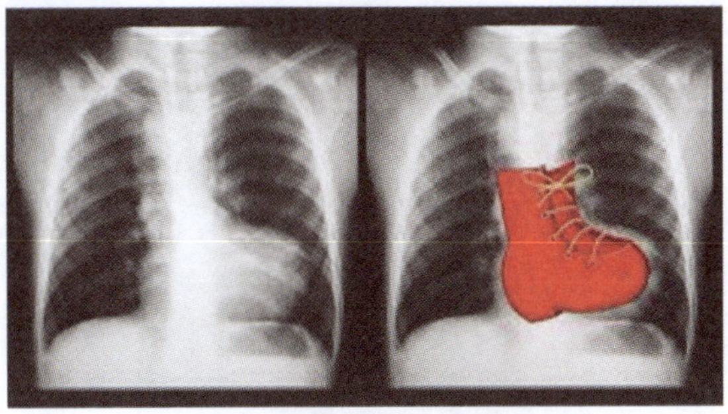

35. Waardenburg syndrome

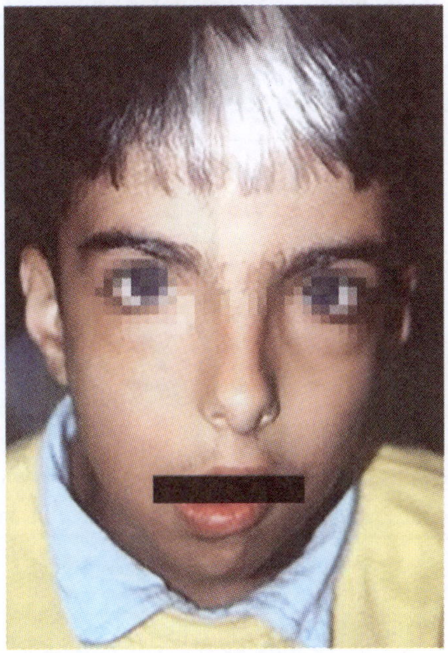

- White bunch of hair
- Hearing loss
- Intellectual disability

36. Turner syndrome (Female with webbed neck)

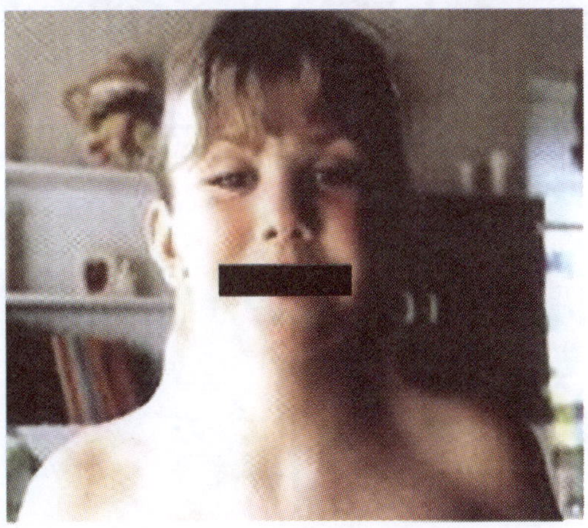

Short stature, normal IQ

37. Edward syndrome (Rocker bottom feet)

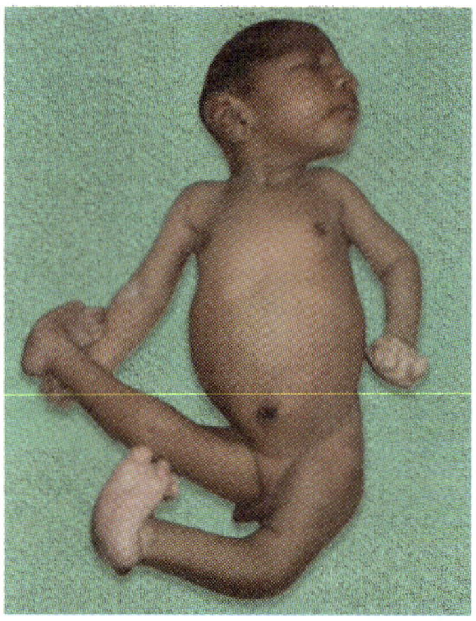

38. Coarctation of the aorta (Figure of 3 appearance)

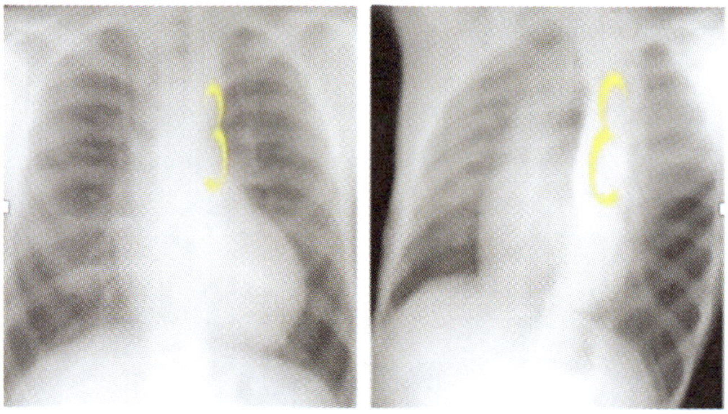

39. Endocardial cushion defect (Gooseneck sign)

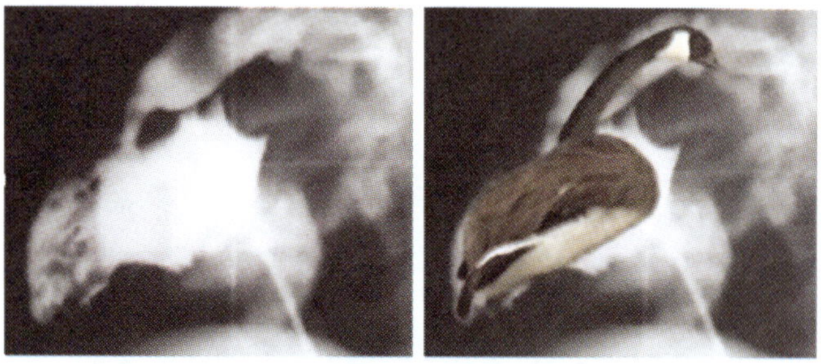

40. Scimitar sign ("Scimitar" means "sword")

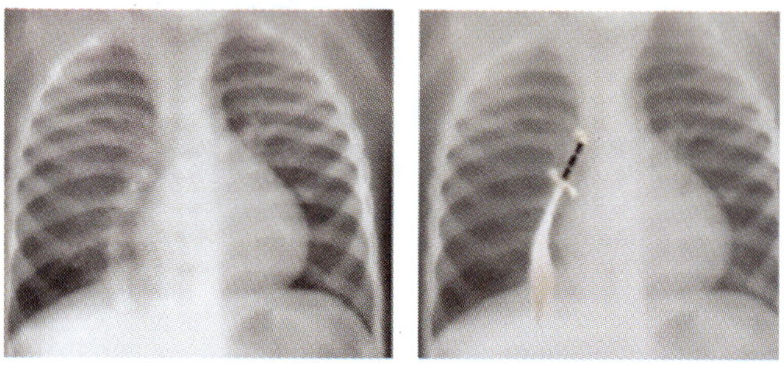

Partial anomalous pulmonary venous connection (PAPVC)

41. Egg on string appearance

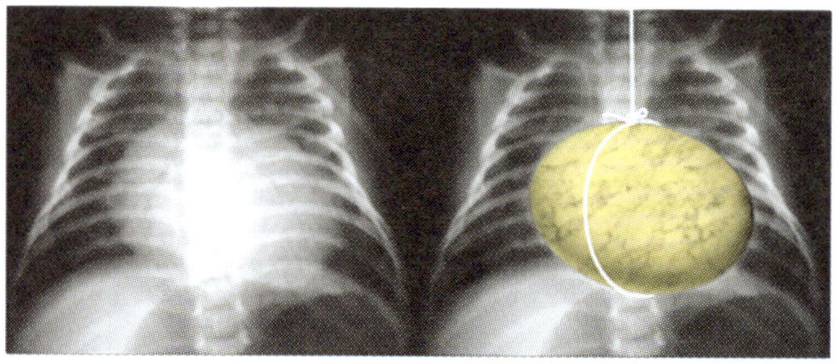

Transposition of great arteries (TGA)

42. Signet ring sign: Bronchiectasis

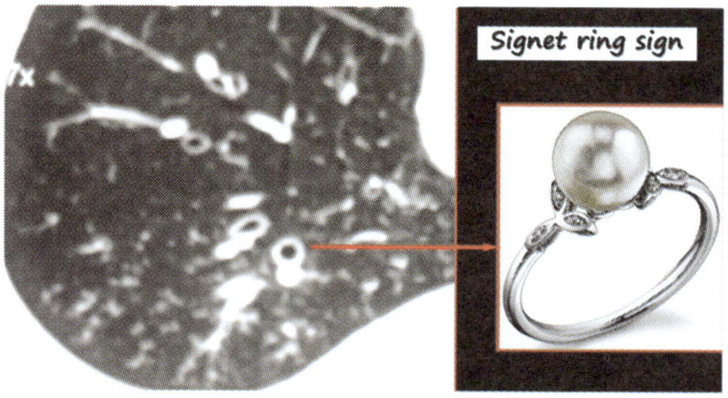

43. Figure of 8 appearance/Snowman sign Supracardiac TAPVC (Total Anomalous Pulmonary Venous Connection)

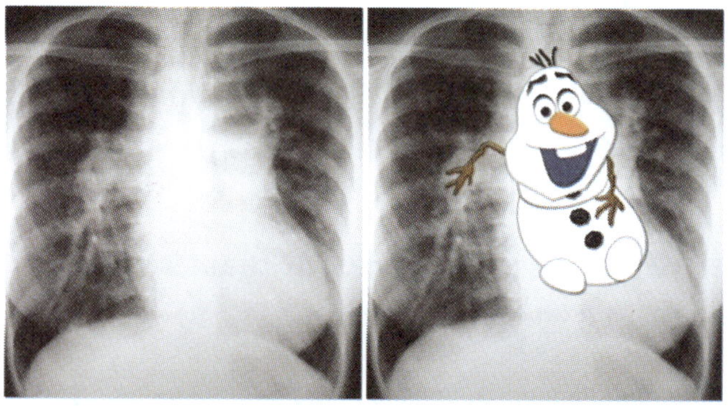

44. Box shape heart—Ebstein anomaly

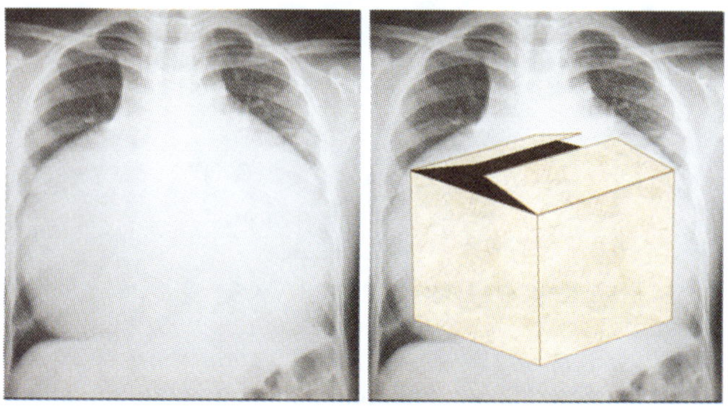

45. Shmoo sign—Left ventricular enlargement

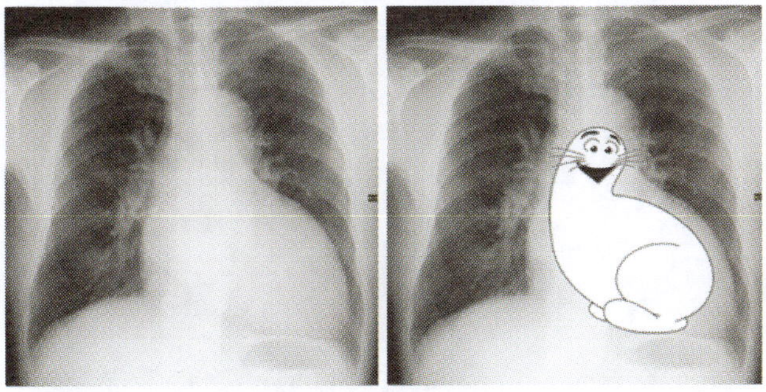

46. Panda sign: Wilson disease

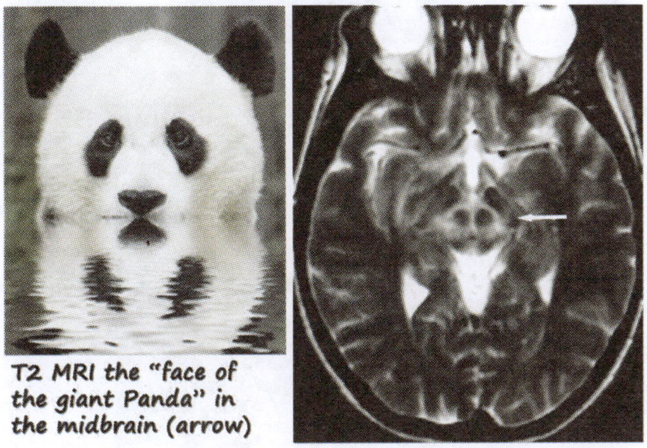

T2 MRI the "face of the giant Panda" in the midbrain (arrow)

47. Water bottle shape heart: Pericardial effusion

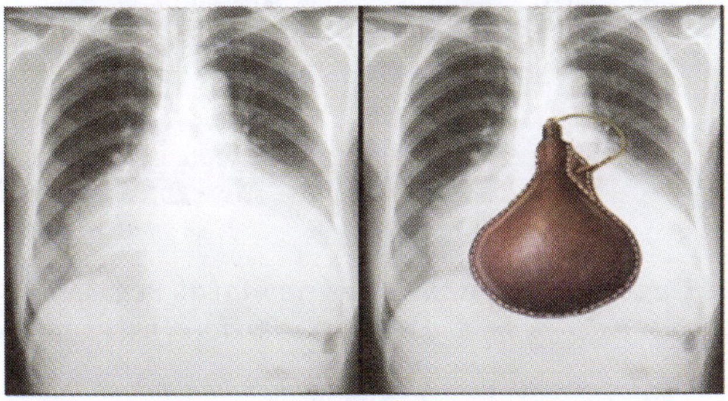

48. Champagne glass pelvis: Achondroplasia

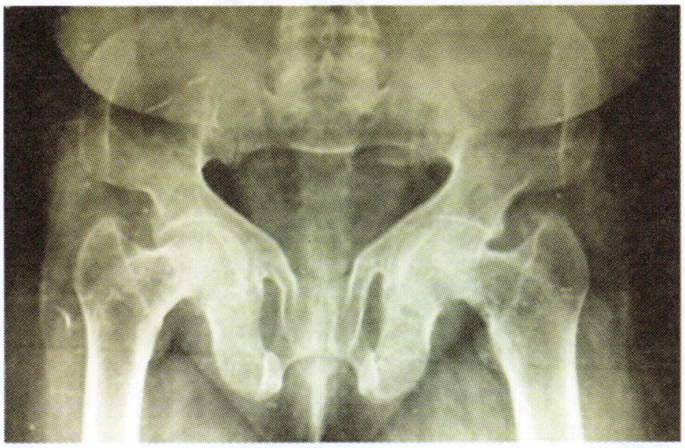

49. Claw sign or coiled spring sign: Intussusception

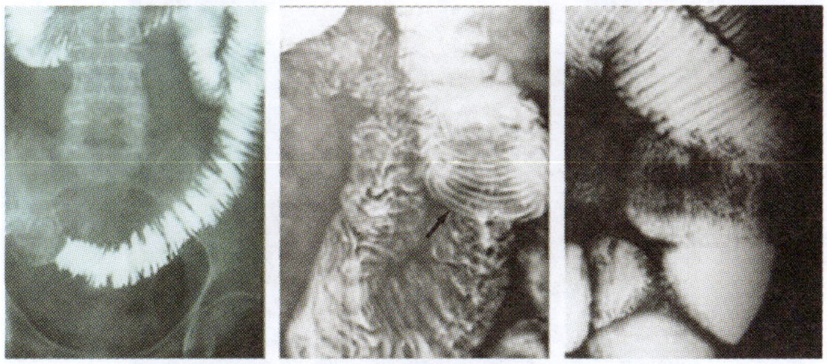

50. Cupping, Fraying, Splaying (Rickets)

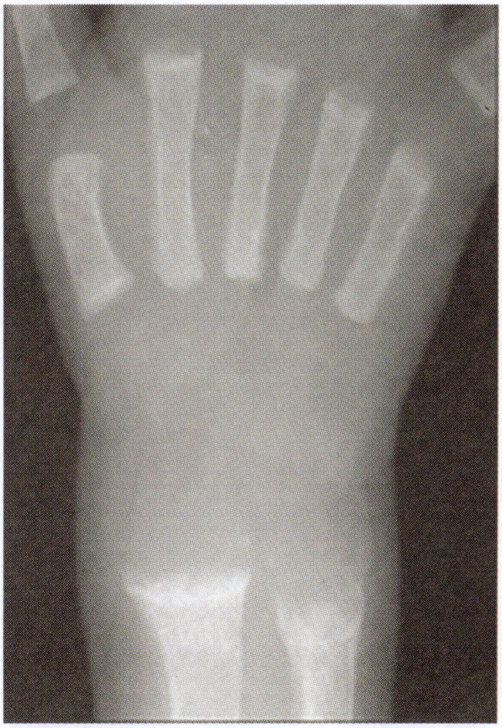

51. Football sign: Pneumoperitoneum stage 3 NEC

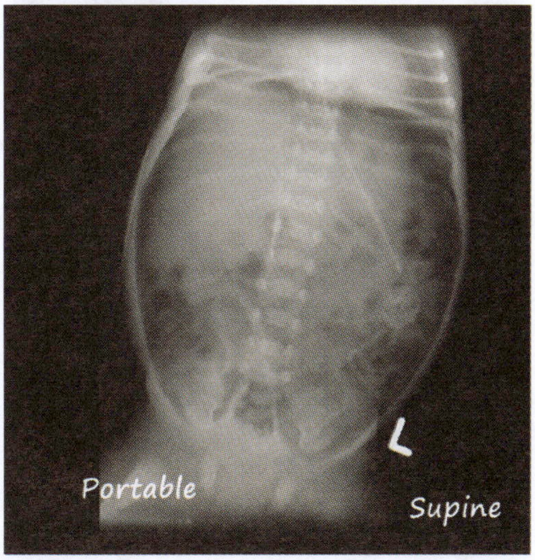

52. Hair on end appearance: Thalassemia

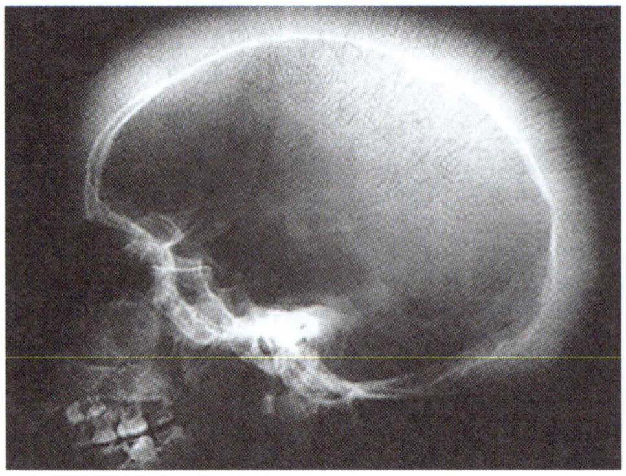

53. Puff of smoke appearance: Moyamoya disease

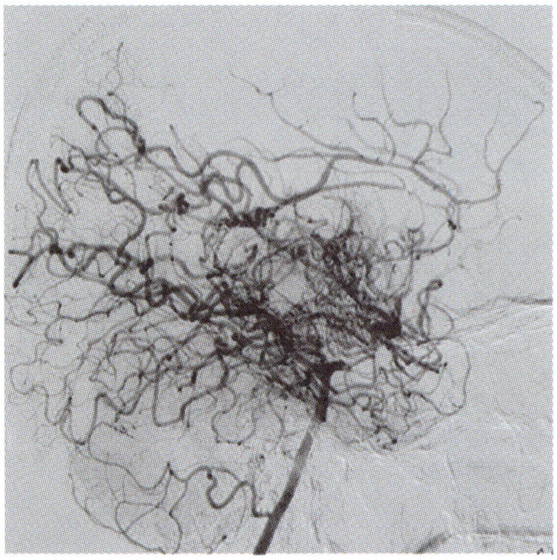

54. Bitot spots (XIB classification of vit. A def.)

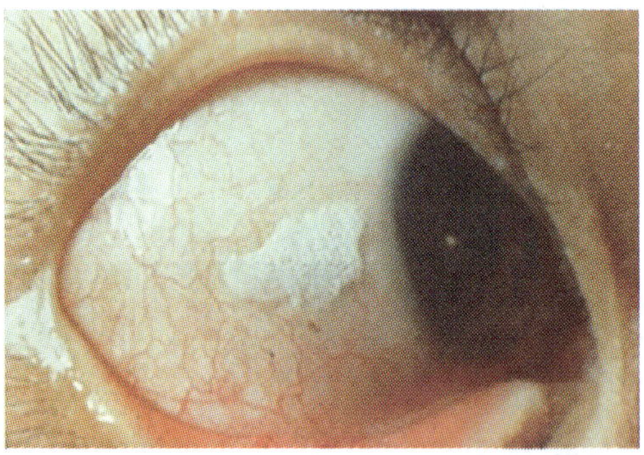

55. Blue sclera + recurrent fracture + deafness = Osteogenesis Imperfecta

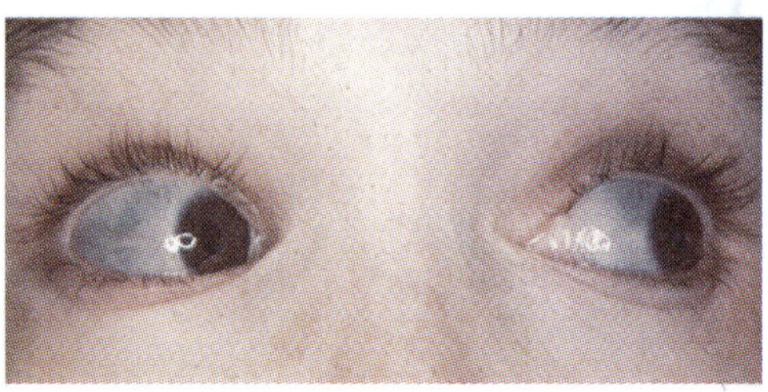

56. Beaded appearance at the costochondral junction known as rachitic rosary seen in Rickets

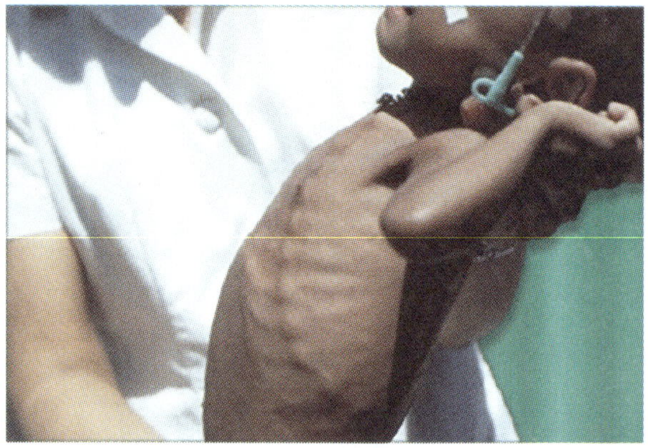

57. Casal's necklace seen due to vitamin B3 Niacin deficiency (Pellagra)

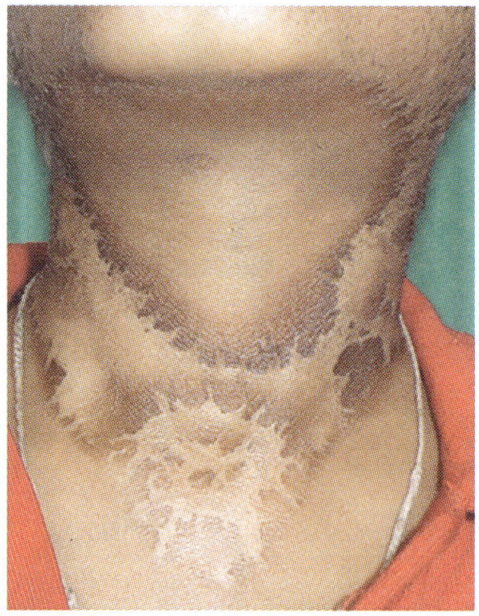

58. Dose of Adrenaline in neonatal resuscitation 0.2 mL/kg In 1:10,000 dilution (Intravenous)

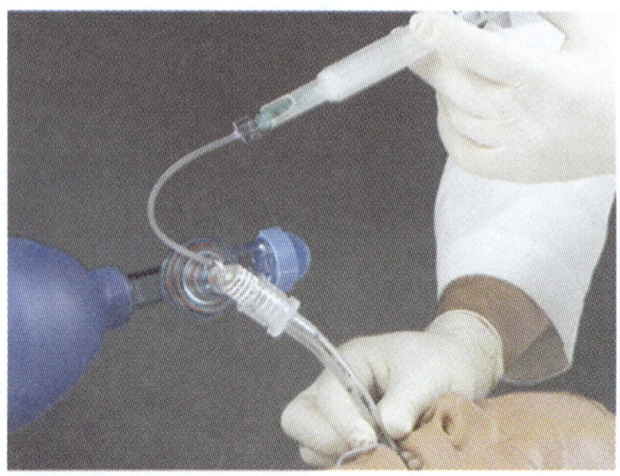

- 0.2 mL/kg means 0.02 mg/kg
- Intratracheal dose: 0.1 mg/kg undiluted (1:1000 dilution)

59. Sitting with support comes in 6 months

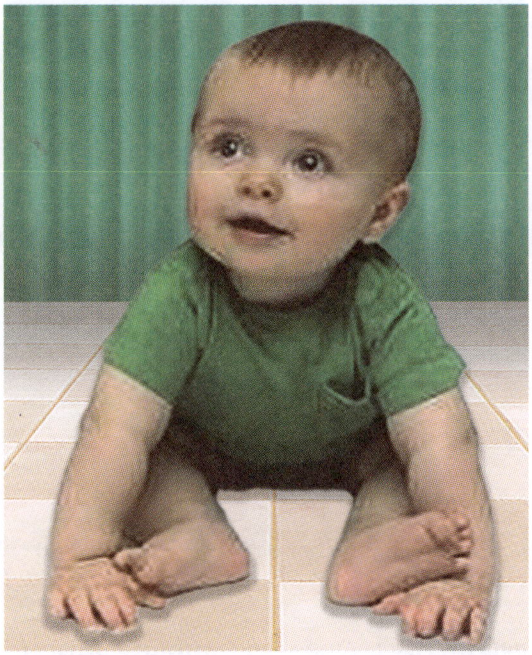

60. Sotos syndrome: Macrocephaly + flushed cheeks + pointed chin

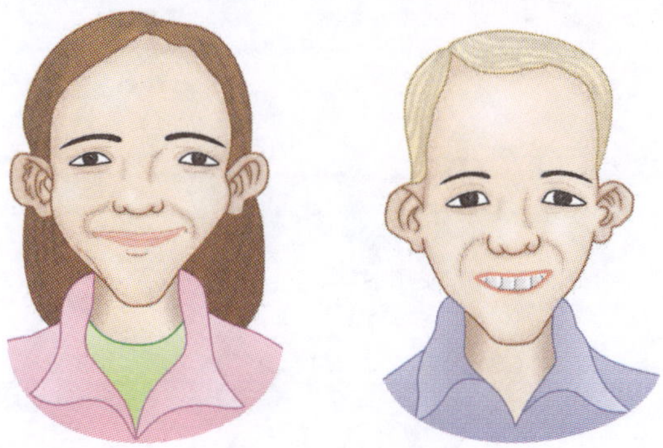

61. Telephone receiver femur: Thanatophoric Dysplasia Type 1

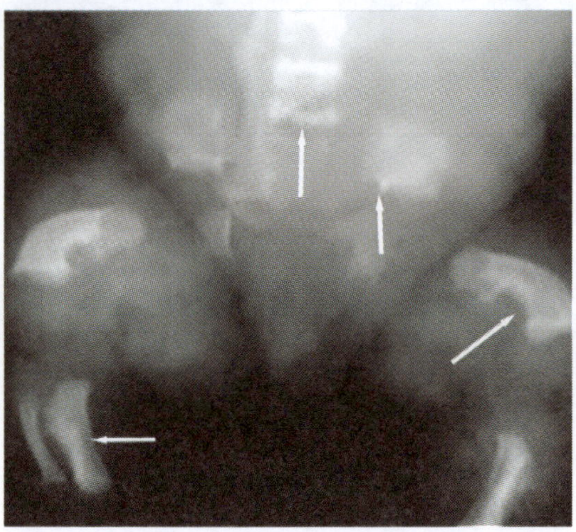

62. Molar tooth sign = Joubert syndrome

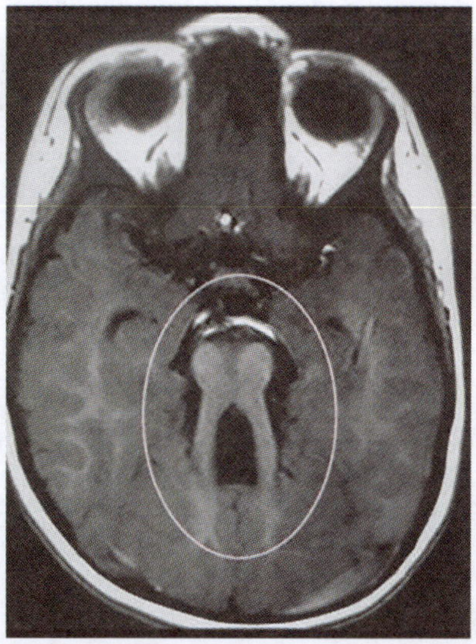

63. Eye of Tiger sign: Pantothenate Kinase-Associated neurodegeneration

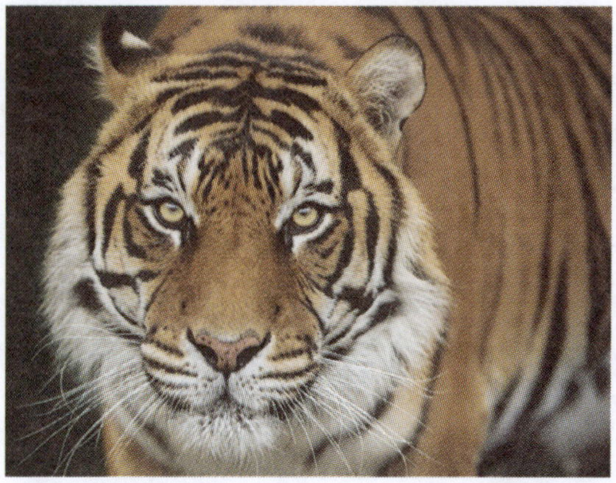

64. Tram Track appearance = Sturge-Weber syndrome

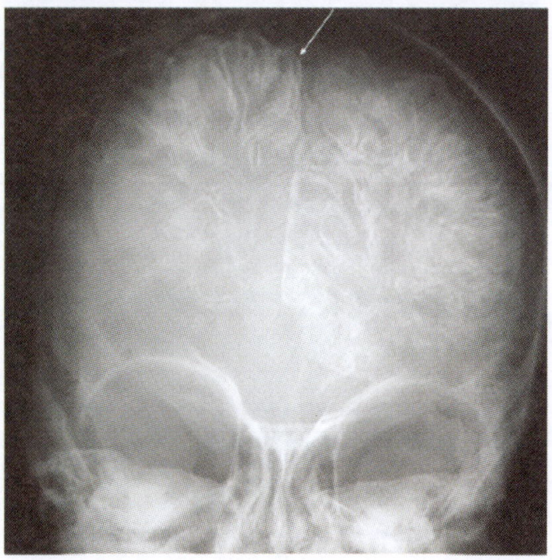

65. Bowel in the chest: Congenital diaphragmatic hernia

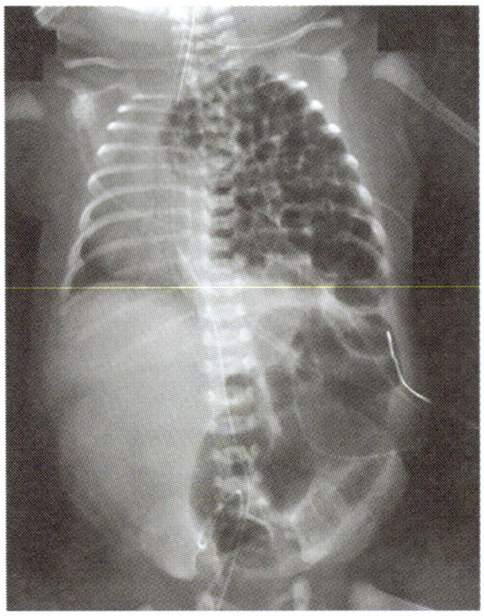

66. Mongolian Spot

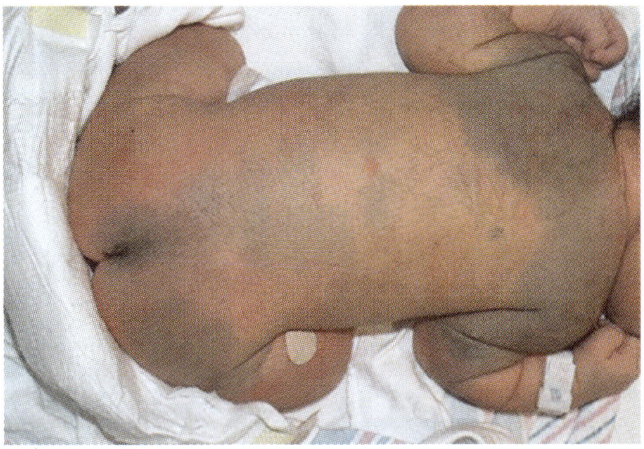

67. Pectus carinatum (pigeon shape chest) and Pectus excavatum (funnel shape chest)

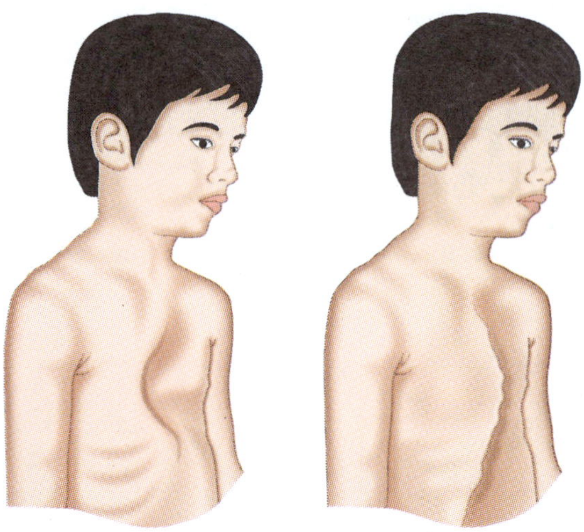

68. Phocomelia due to maternal intake of thalidomide

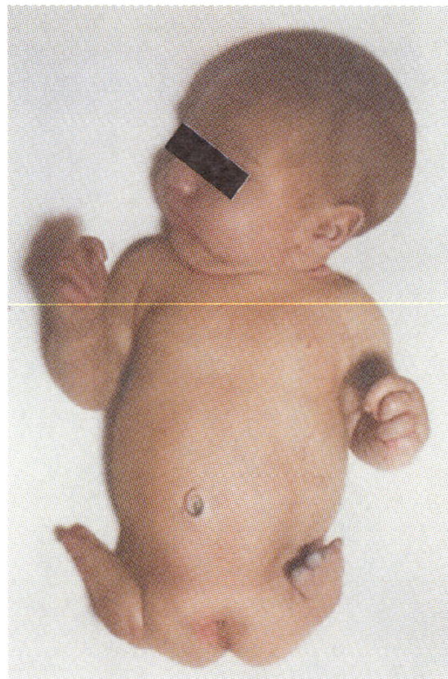

69. Gastroschisis: Open abdominal contents

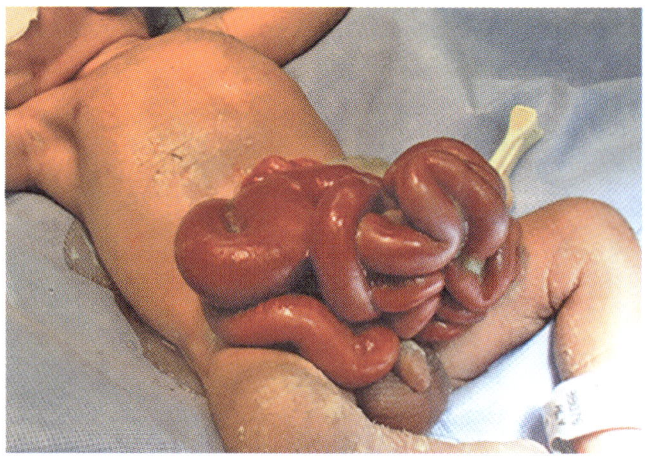

70. Blue color cannula is 22 number

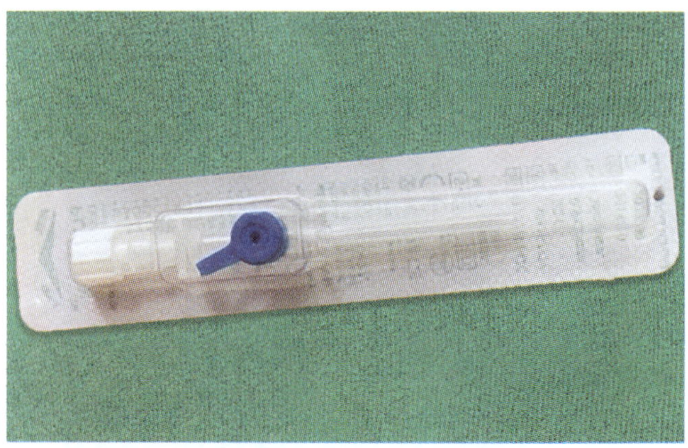

[Yellow = 24, Purple = 26, Orange = 14, Grey = 16, Green = 18, Pink = 20, White = 17]

71. Important strawberry conditions

Strawberry

- Strawberry scrotum = Multiple sebaceous cysts
- Strawberry gallbladder = Cholesterolosis
- Strawberry skull = Antenatal USG in edwards
- Strawberry tongue = Kawasaki
- Strawberry vagina = Trichomoniasis
- Strawberry gingiva = Wegener's granulomatosis

72. Trousseau sign: Seen in latent tetany

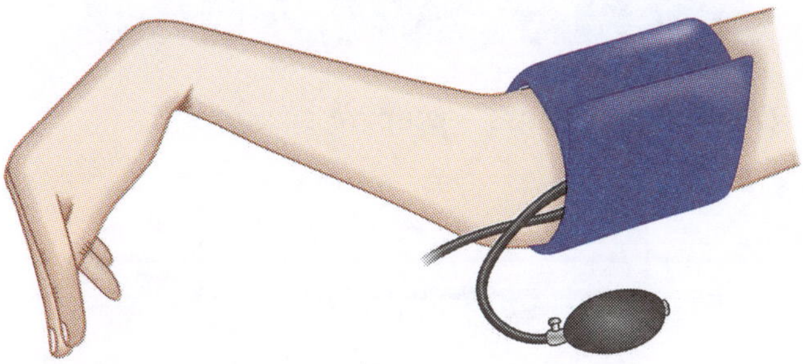

73. Arachnodactyly: Long fingers

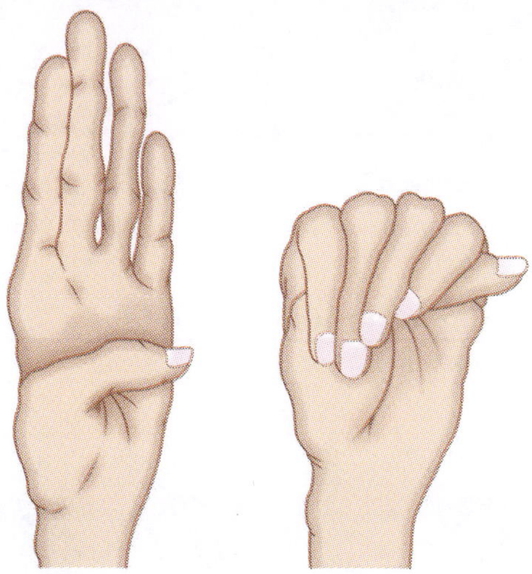

Seen in marf an syndrome

74. Wrist and Thumb signs seen in Marfan syndrome

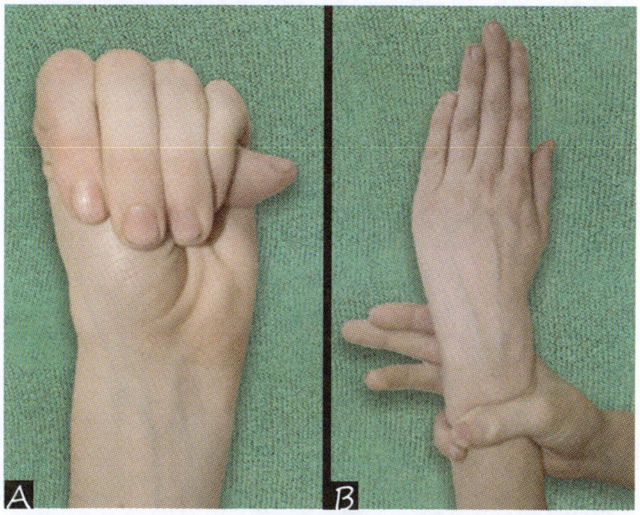

75. Craniopagus—joined at the head

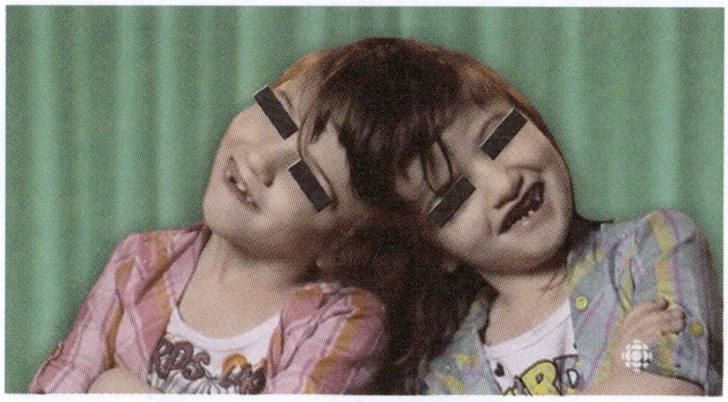

76. SNHL + Anterior lenticonus + Hematuria = Alport Syndrome

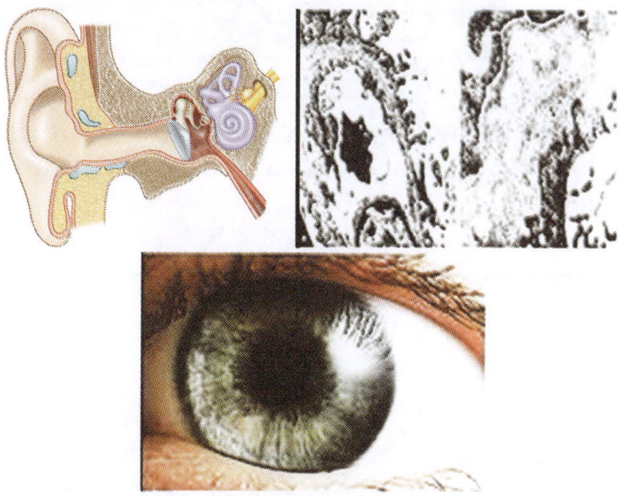

77. Loose abdominal muscles = Prune belly syndrome

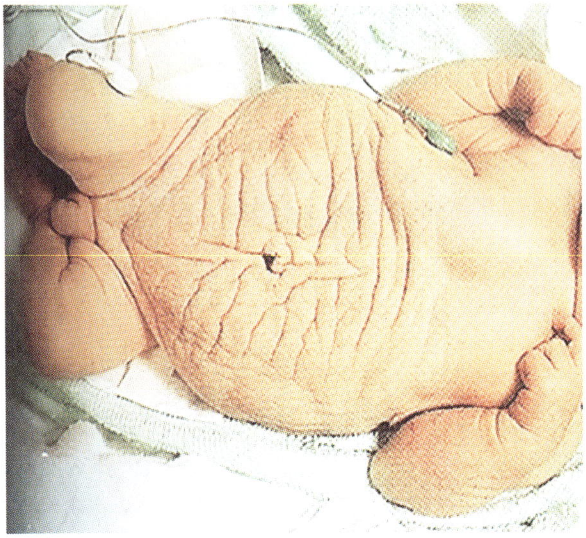

78. Coffee bean sign = Sigmoid volvulus

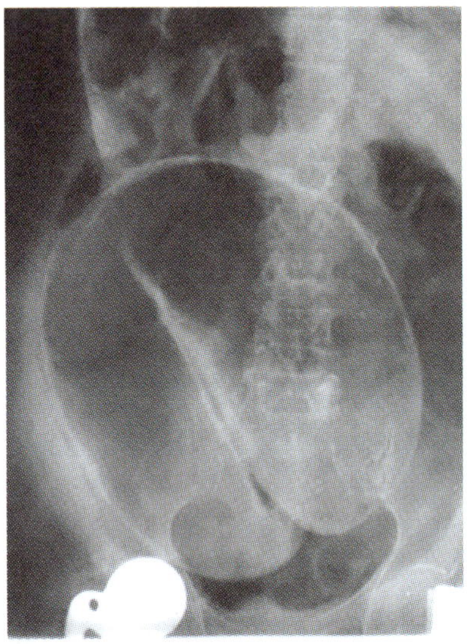

79. Cephalohematoma is confined to the suture line. Caput Succedaneum crosses the suture line

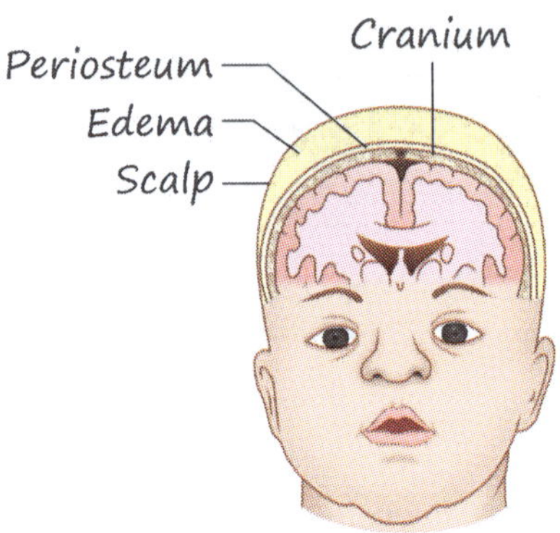

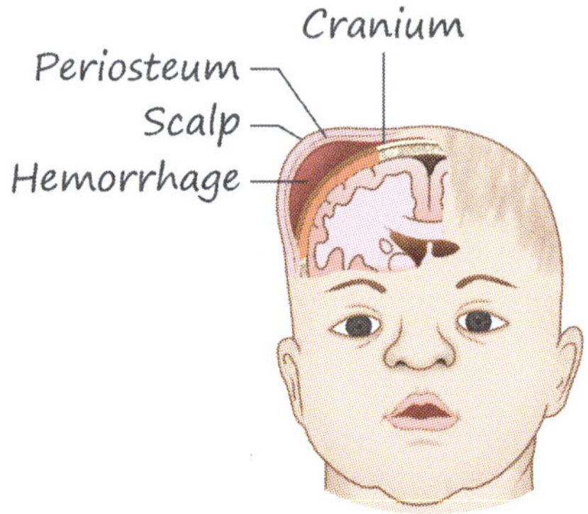

80. Caudal regression syndrome/sacral agenesis

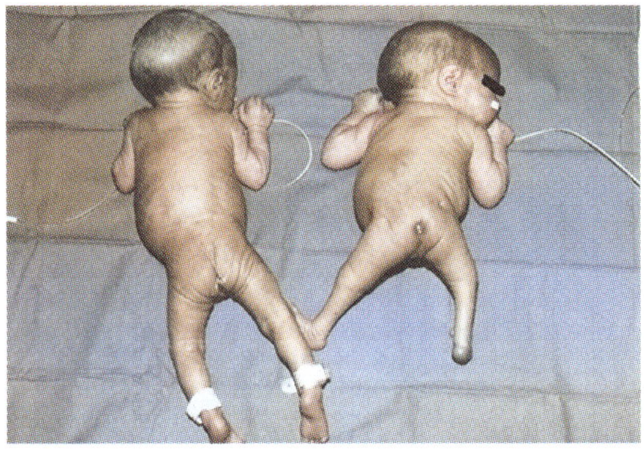

81. Olive shape mass—pyloric stenosis

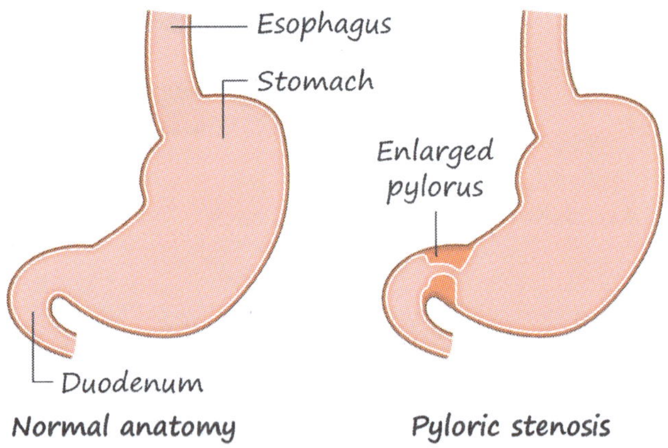

Treatment surgery: Ramstedt's pyloromyotomy

82. Darkening of urine on standing = Alkaptonuria

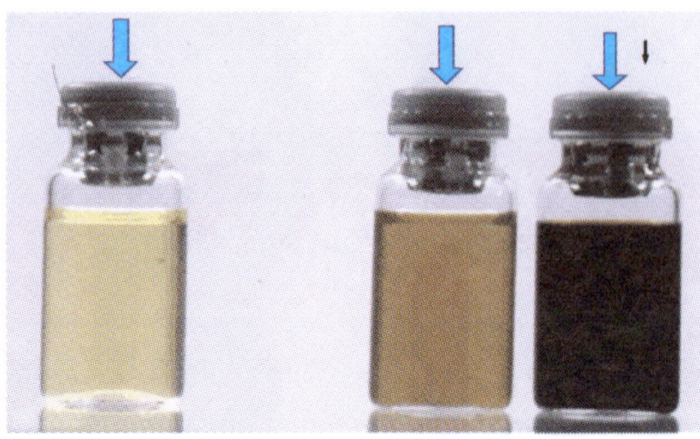

83. Most common type of tracheoesophageal fistula is type C

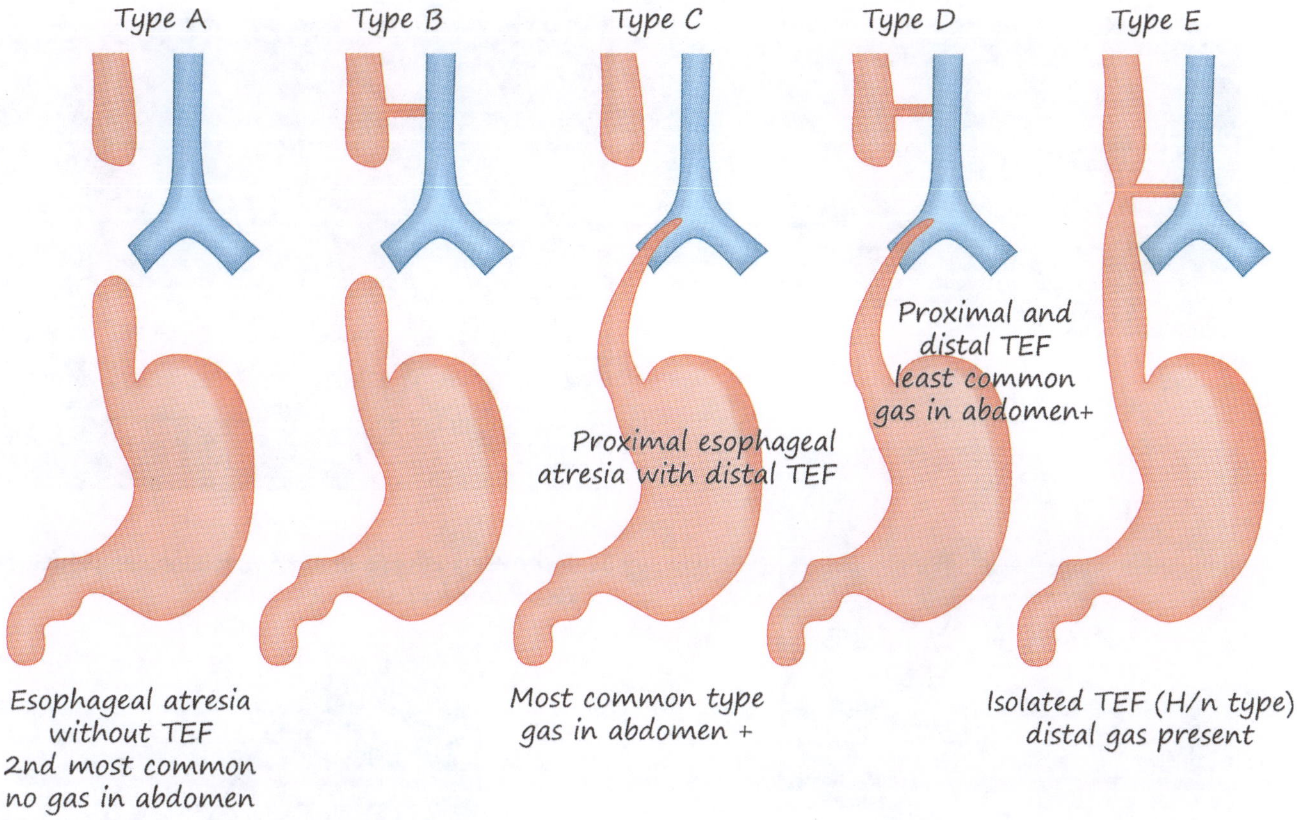

84. Most common congenital anomaly of GI tract is: Meckel's diverticulum

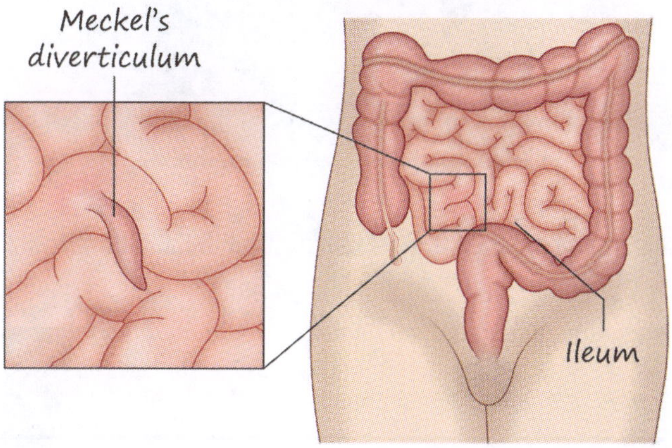

85. Black legged tick/deer tick

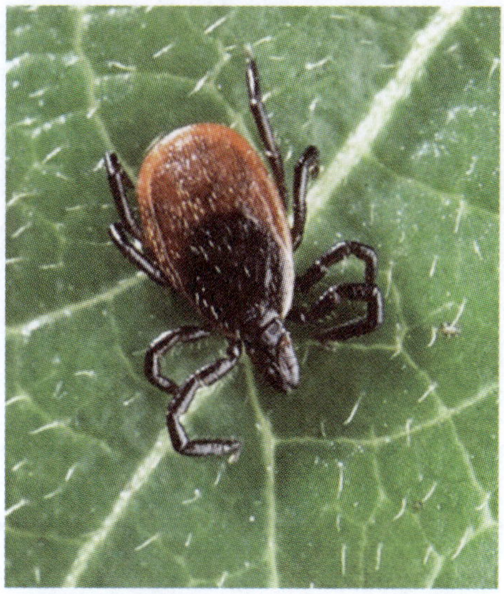

Causes Lyme disease

86. Anemia is a sign not a symptom

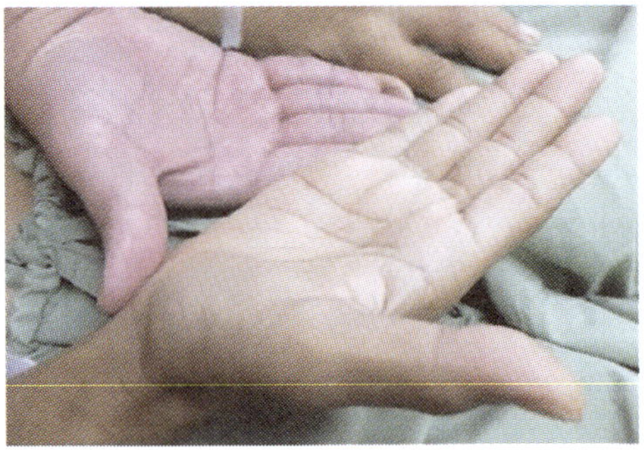

87. Koplik's Spots seen in measles

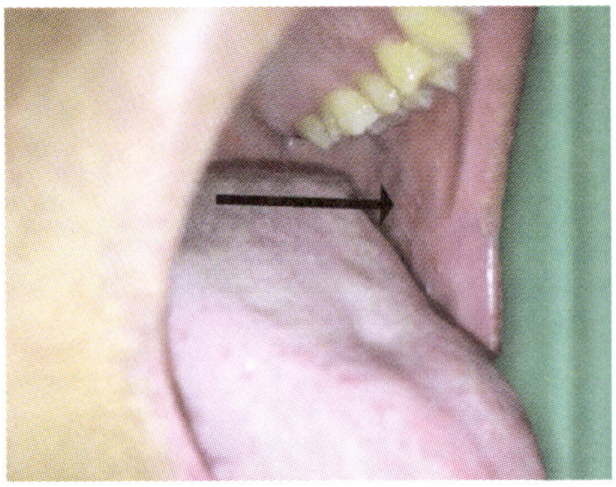

88. Strawberry tongue: Kawasaki and scarlet fever

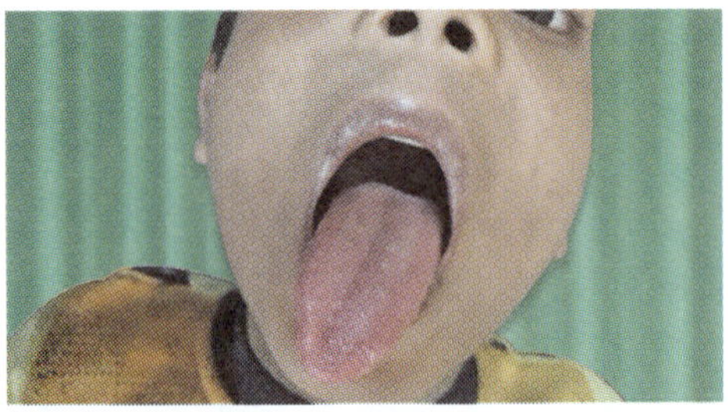

89. Slapped cheek appearance: Erythema infectiosum

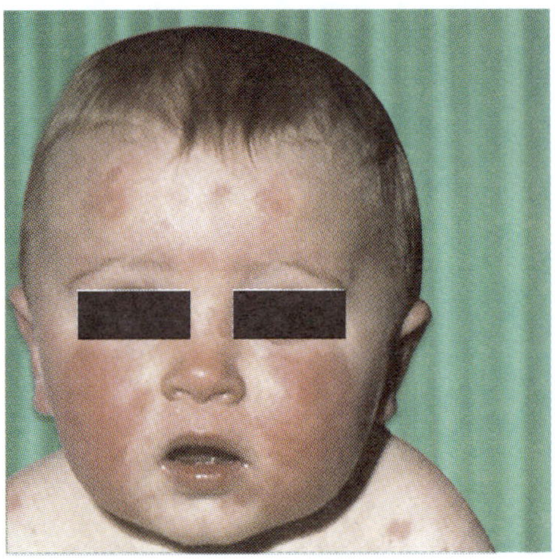

90. Nagayama spot seen in roseola infantum

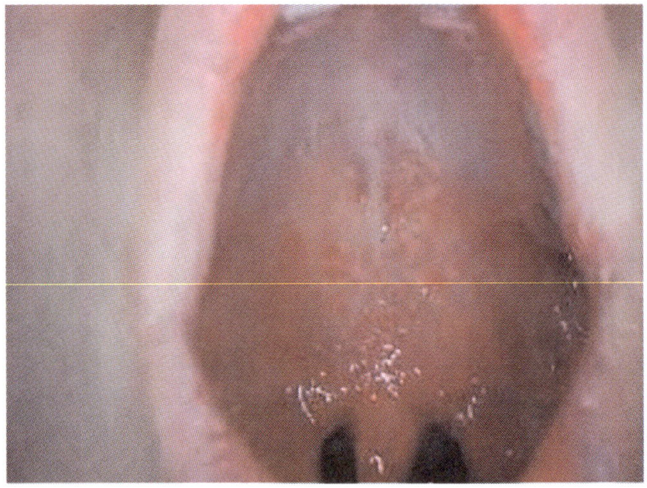

91. Recovery phase of dengue: Isles of white in the sea of red

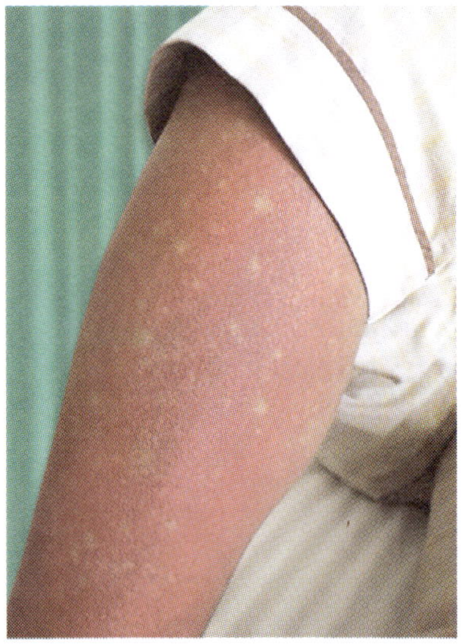

92. It takes 6-12 weeks for the BCG scar to appear

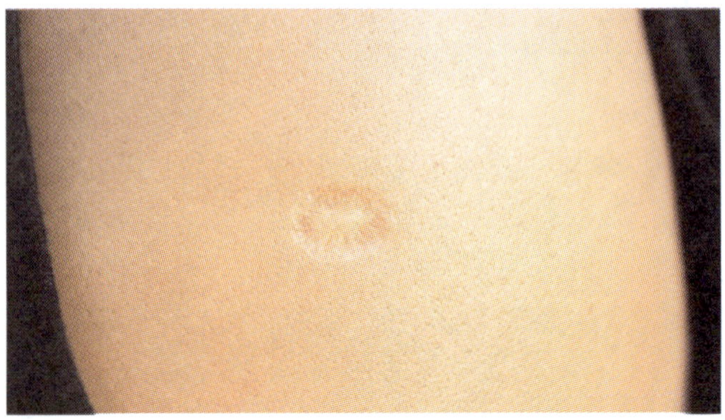

93. Great toe deviated and broad thumbs = Rubinstein-Taybi syndrome – CBP* mutation

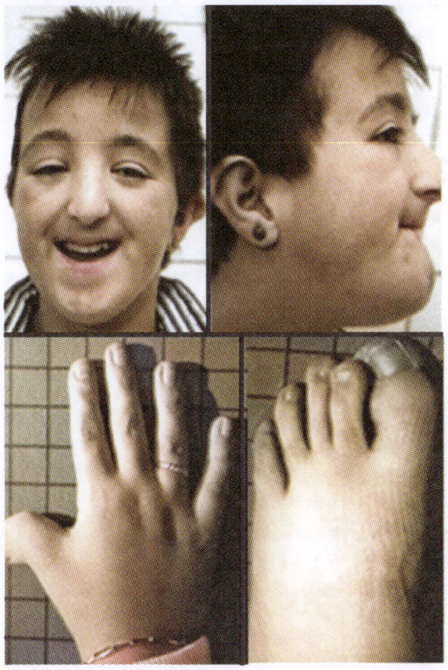

94. Sandal gap: Down syndrome

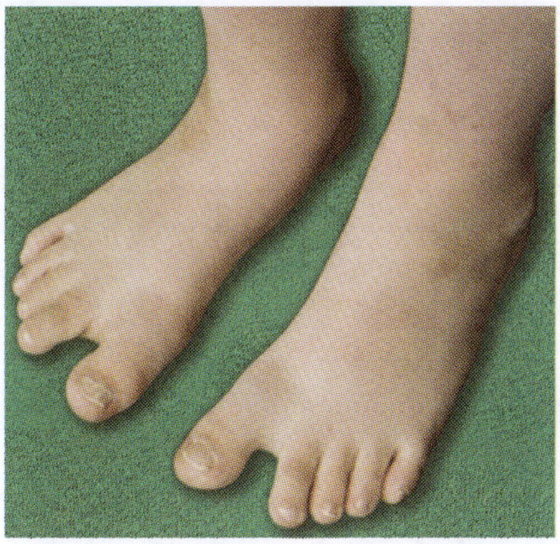

95. Single palmar crease: Down syndrome

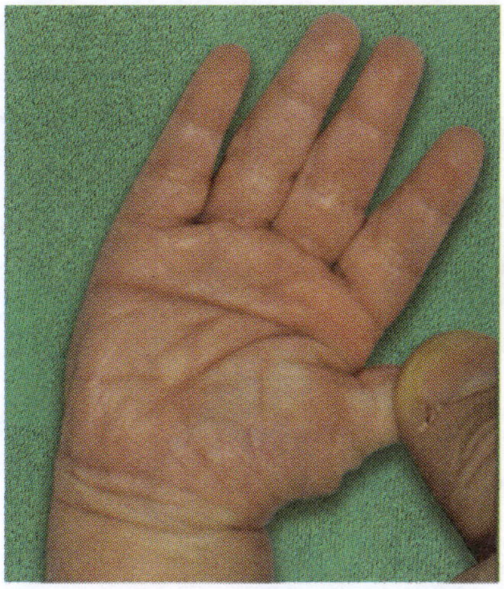

96. Single bubble sign: Congenital hypertrophic pyloric stenosis

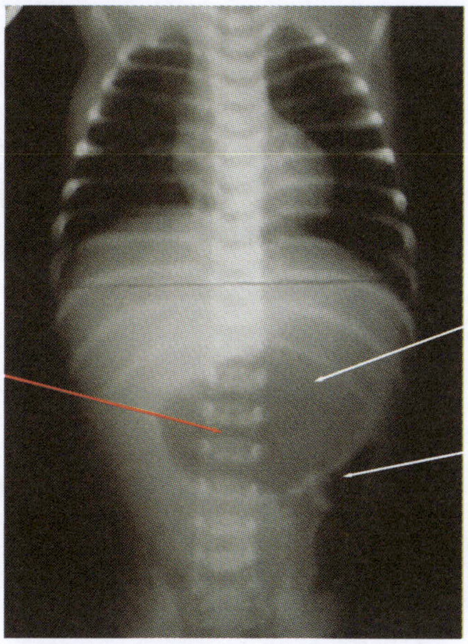

97. Double bubble sign: Duodenal atresia

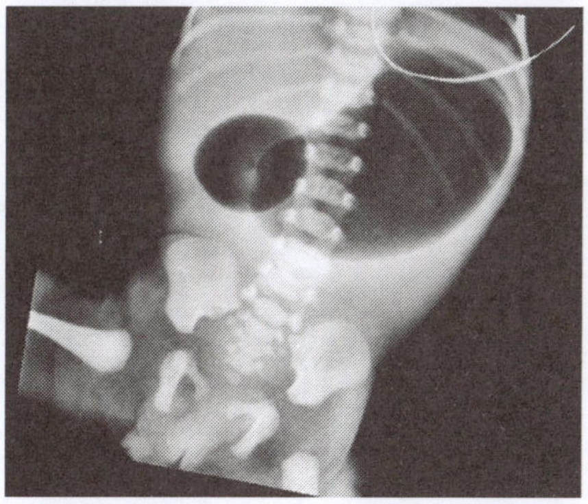

98. Triple bubble sign: Jejunal atresia

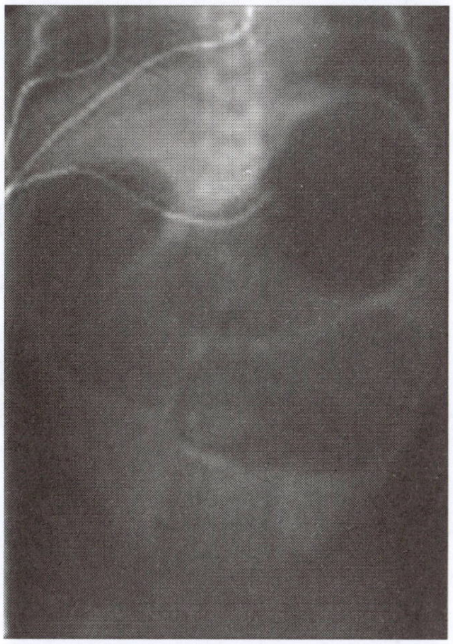

99. Sinus which is absent in a newborn is frontal sinus

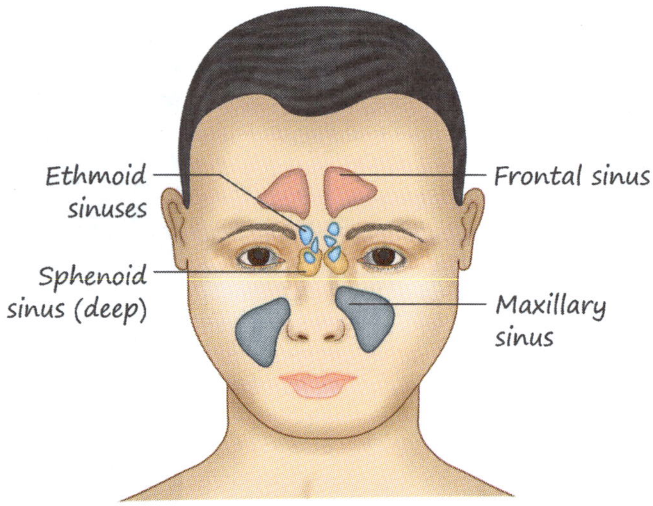

100. Image

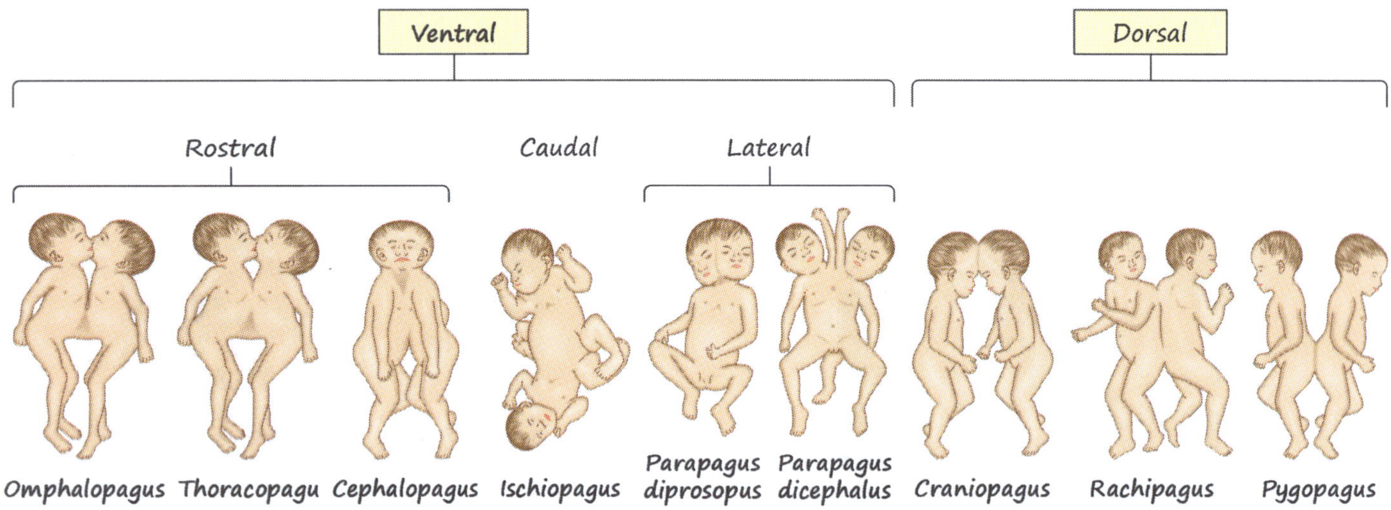

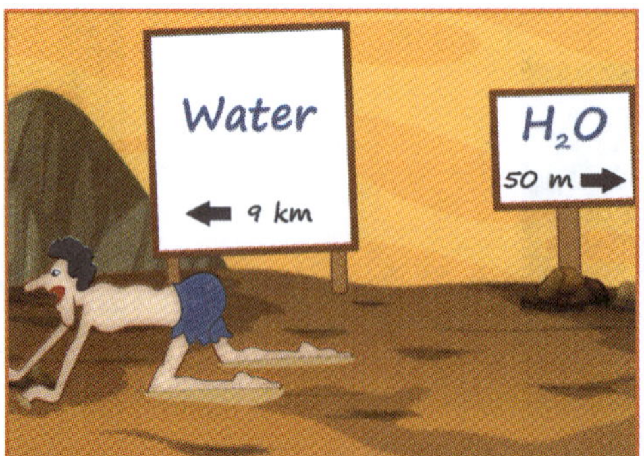

"Knowledge is power"

"The more you learn, the better you will be able to make decision about the direction of your life."

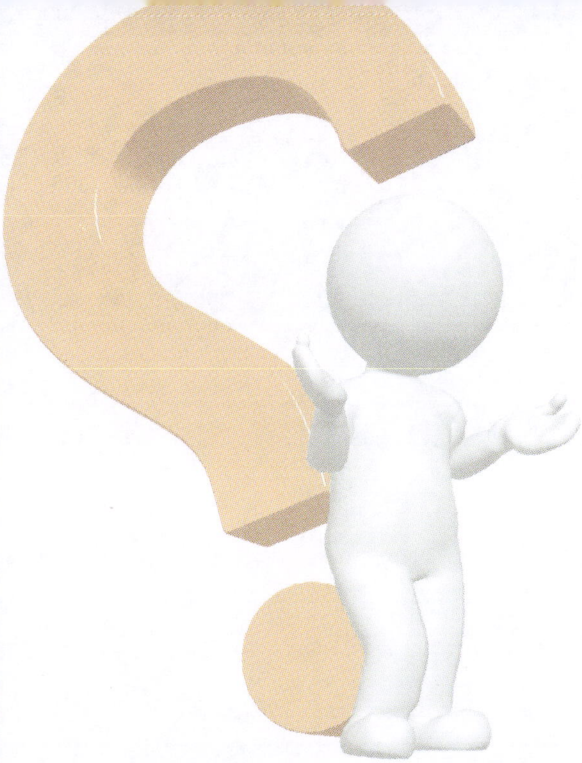

Latest Question Papers

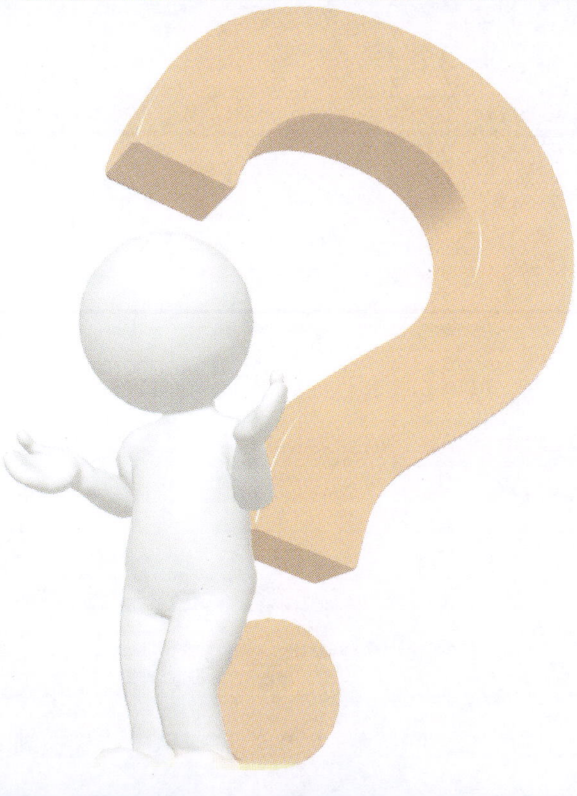

- → NEET 2023-2021
- → INI-CET 2023-2021
- → FMGE 2023 (JULY AND JANUARY)
- → FMGE 2022

NEET 2023-2021

"No one is you and that is your power."

1. **A newborn presented with chest retractions, dyspnea, and lethargy. The pediatrician diagnosed the baby with respiratory distress syndrome. This occurs due to the deficiency of:**
   a. Dipalmitoyl inositol
   b. Lecithin
   c. Sphingomyelin
   d. Dipalmitoylphosphatidylethanolamine

Ans. b. Lecithin

2. **A 10-year-old child weighing 30 kg presents with a history of loose stools for 2 days. On examination, there is severe dehydration. Laboratory investigations are as follows. What is the initial management as per ISPAD guidelines?**

RBS	550 mg/dL
pH	7.01
Na+	158 mEq/L
Urine glucose	3+

   a. Manage ABC, NS 20 mL/kg and start insulin after 1 hour
   b. Manage ABC, NS 20 mL/kg along with insulin 0.1 IU/kg/hr
   c. Manage ABC, NS 10 mL/kg along with insulin 0.1 IU/kg/hr
   d. Manage ABC, NS 10 mL/kg and start insulin after 1 hour

Ans. b. Manage ABC, NS 20 mL/kg along with insulin 0.1 IU/kg/hr

3. **Which of the following is the best sign to indicate adequate growth in an infant with a birth weight of 2.8 kg?**
   a. Increase in length of 25 centimeters in the first year
   b. Weight gain of 300 grams per month till 1 year
   c. Anterior fontanel closure by 6 months of age
   d. Weight under 75th percentile and height under 25th percentile

Ans. a. Increase in length of 25 centimeters in the first year

4. **A child is brought to the hospital with respiratory distress and biphasic stridor. The radiograph is shown below. What is the diagnosis?**

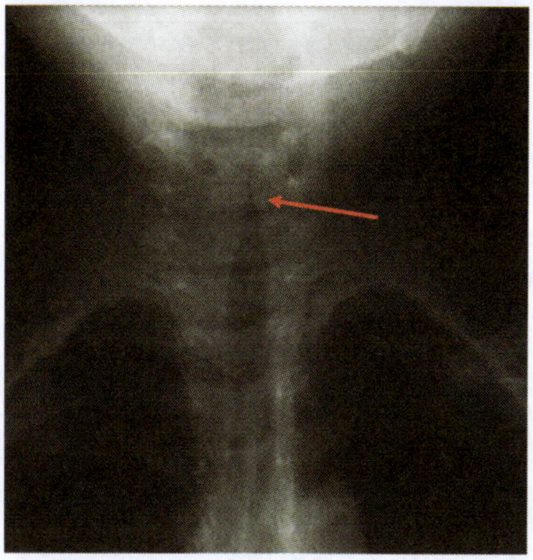

   a. Acute epiglottitis
   b. Acute laryngotracheobronchitis
   c. Foreign body aspiration
   d. Laryngomalacia

Ans. b. Acute laryngotracheobronchitis

5. **A 3-month-old baby comes with complaints of deafness, cataract, and patent ductus arteriosus. Which of the following is the most likely diagnosis?**
   a. Congenital herpes simplex virus infection
   b. Congenital toxoplasmosis
   c. Congenital cytomegalovirus infection
   d. Congenital rubella syndrome

Ans. c. Congenital cytomegalovirus infection

6. **Chloride level in sweat is used in the diagnosis of which disease?**
   a. Phenylketonuria
   b. Cystic fibrosis
   c. Gaucher's disease
   d. Osteogenesis imperfecta

Ans. b. Cystic fibrosis

7. **A 3-month-old baby presents with jaundice and clay-colored stools. Lab investigation reveals that the baby has conjugated hyperbilirubinemia. The liver biopsy shows periductal proliferation. What is the most likely diagnosis?**

a. Crigler-Najjar syndrome
b. Rotor syndrome
c. Dubin-Johnson syndrome
d. Biliary atresia

Ans. c. Dubin-Johnson syndrome

8. A child presents with fever and a rash spreading from the face, behind cheeks, and buccal mucosa to other body parts. On examination, Koplik's spot is present. What is the likely diagnosis?
a. Measles b. Rubella
c. Varicella d. Mumps

Ans. a. Measles

9. An infant presents with hepatosplenomegaly and thrombocytopenia. Neuroimaging with CT shows periventricular calcifications. What is the most likely diagnosis?
a. Congenital rubella syndrome
b. Congenital herpes simplex virus infection
c. Congenital toxoplasmosis
d. Congenital cytomegalovirus infection

Ans. d. Congenital cytomegalovirus infection

10. A 3-week-old infant presents with a cough and sore throat. The mother reports that the infant develops a paroxysm of cough followed by apnea. The total leucocyte count is >50,000 cells/μL. Which of the following drugs will you prescribe for this patient?
a. Azithromycin
b. Amoxicillin
c. Cotrimoxazole
d. Clarithromycin

Ans. a. Azithromycin

11. A 1-day-old neonate has not passed urine since birth. What is the next step in management?
a. Continue breastfeeding and observe
b. Admit to NICU
c. Start artificial feeding
d. Start intravenous fluids

Ans. a. Continue breastfeeding and observe

12. A 7-year-old boy presented with abdominal pain, vomiting, oliguria, and periorbital puffiness following chemotherapy. Investigations reveal hyperuricemia, raised creatinine levels, and hyperkalemia. What is the next best step in the management of this condition?
a. Hydration b. Probenecid
c. Allopurinol d. Rasburicase

Ans. a. Hydration

13. A baby presented with abdominal pain. On examination, a mass is palpated in the right lumbar region. A barium enema is done, and the image is given below. What is the likely diagnosis?

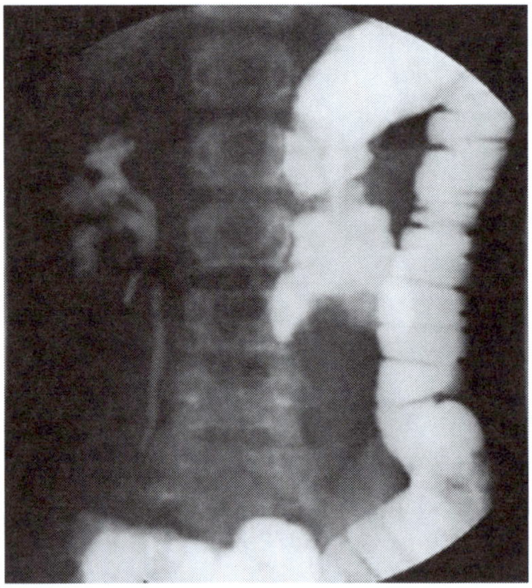

a. Intussusception
b. Volvulus
c. Duodenal atresia
d. None of the above

Ans. a. Intussusception

14. An 8-day-old newborn was found to have thyroid-stimulating hormone level of more than 100 mIU/L. Which of the following will be the next best investigation?
a. Urine iodine excretion
b. Serum thyroid receptor antibody
c. Radiotracer uptake with technetium
d. Perchlorate secretion test

Ans. b. Serum thyroid receptor antibody

15. A 10-month-old infant was brought with complaints of jerking movement of limbs toward the body. On examination, there is a regression of developmental milestones. Electroencephalogram shows hypsarrhythmia. Which of the following is the drug of choice in this condition?

a. Phenytoin
b. Adrenocorticotropic hormone (ACTH)
c. Levetiracetam
d. Phenobarbitone

Ans. b. Adrenocorticotropic hormone (ACTH)

16. A 2-month-old infant born to an HIV-positive mother presents with recurrent diarrhea. What is the next best step?

a. Test stool for giardia and give antibiotics
b. Dried spot sample for HIV DNA PCR
c. Antibody tests for HIV
d. Aerobic culture

Ans. b. Dried spot sample for HIV DNA PCR

17. An 8-year-old child has difficulty walking and getting up from a squatting position. A muscle biopsy was done and is as shown in the image. Which of the following is true about this condition?

a. Death occurs in 3rd decade
b. Previous history of viral prodrome
c. It is a mitochondrial storage disorder
d. Early treatment has excellent prognosis

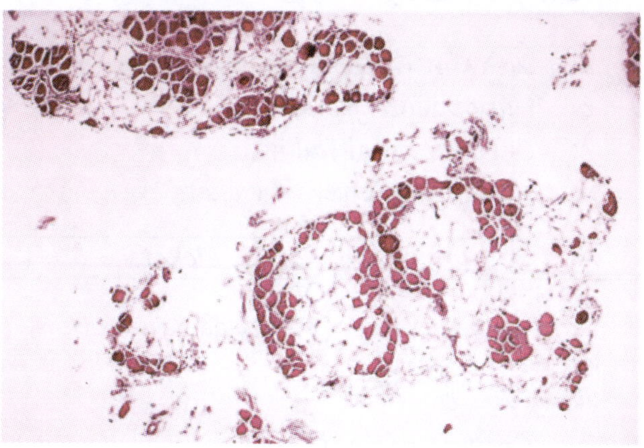

Ans. a. Death occurs in 3rd decade

18. A child presented with a history of loose stools with an increase in frequency for 4 days. On examination, he is drowsy, unable to feed, and skin on pinching goes back very slowly. According to the Integrated Management of Neonatal and Childhood Illness (IMNCI), this child will be classified as having:

a. Mild dehydration
b. Some dehydration
c. Severe dehydration
d. Moderate dehydration

Ans. c. Severe dehydration

19. Which of the following children are considered at-risk babies?

1. Baby with a birth weight of 2.5 kg
2. Baby on artificial feeds
3. Baby of working mother/single parent
4. Baby with weight <85% of expected weight
5. Birth order of 3 or more

a. 2, 3
b. 1, 2, 3, 4
c. 4, 5
d. 1, 4

Ans. a. 2, 3

20. Identify the condition.

a. Bladder exstrophy
b. Omphalocele
c. Persistent vitellointestinal duct
d. Gastroschisis

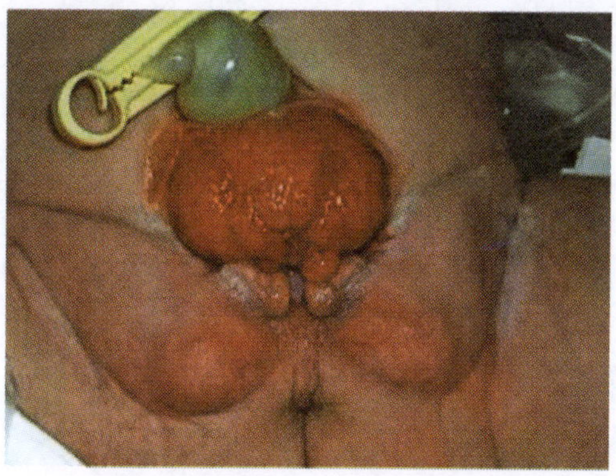

Ans. a. Bladder exstrophy

21. A previously healthy child presented with acute-onset dyspnea. A chest X-ray shows unilateral hyperinflation of the lungs. What is true for this patient?
   a. Focal area of decreased air entry will be suggestive of foreign body
   b. Flexible bronchoscopy used for removal
   c. In complete obstruction, ball and valve mechanism causes hyperinflation
   d. The child has developed acute laryngotracheobronchitis

Ans. a. Focal area of decreased air entry will be suggestive of foreign body

22. A male child presented with arthralgia and abdominal pain. On examination, there was palpable purpura over the lower limbs. There is past history of upper respiratory tract infection prior to the onset of presenting symptoms. Which of the following is the treatment for this condition?
   a. Azathioprine
   b. Methotrexate
   c. Cyclosporine
   d. Glucocorticoids

Ans. d. Glucocorticoids

23. A 10-year-old presents with edema and anasarca. A diagnosis of minimal change disease is made. Which of the following is true about this condition?
   a. Light microscopy shows effacement of podocytes
   b. Good response to steroids
   c. Most common in adults
   d. Non-selective proteinuria

Ans. b. Good response to steroids

24. A 10-year-old child presents with diarrhea and weight loss. On examination, the height and weight are lesser than expected. Laboratory investigations were positive for class II HLA-DQ2. Which of the following will you advise the child?
   a. Fat-free diet
   b. Lactose-free diet
   c. Low carbohydrate diet
   d. Gluten-free diet

Ans. d. Gluten-free diet

25. A child with infantile hypertrophic pyloric stenosis has multiple episodes of nonbilious vomiting. Which of the following metabolic abnormality is likely to be seen in this condition?
   a. Hypochloremic, hypokalemic acidosis
   b. Hypochloremic, hypokalemic alkalosis
   c. Hypokalemic hyperchloremic alkalosis
   d. Hyperchloremic hypokalemic acidosis

Ans. b. Hypochloremic, hypokalemic alkalosis

26. A 6-year-old girl born out of nonconsanguineous marriage presented with rachitic changes in limbs since 1½ years of age for which she has received multiple courses of vitamin D. Investigations showed the following. What is the most likely diagnosis?

Parameter	Lab determined value
Calcium	9.5 mg/dL
Phosphate	1.6 mg/dL
Alkaline phosphatase (ALP)	814 IU
Serum Parathyroid hormone (PTH)	Normal Levels
Serum electrolytes	Within Normal Limits (WNL)
Serum creatinine	Within Normal Limits (WNL)
Arterial Blood Gas analysis (ABG)	Within Normal Limits (WNL)

   a. Vitamin D dependent rickets
   b. Hypoparathyroidism
   c. Chronic renal failure
   d. Hypophosphatemic rickets

Ans. d. Hypophosphatemic rickets

27. During the anthropometric evaluation, the height for age of a child is <- 2SD. This is most likely due to:
   a. Chronic malnutrition
   b. Acute malnutrition
   c. Recent infection
   d. No malnutrition

Ans. a. Chronic malnutrition

28. A child presents with generalized edema and was found to have hypercholesterolemia. Urine analysis shows protein 3+ and fat bodies. What is the likely diagnosis?

a. Nephrotic syndrome
b. Nephritic syndrome
c. Goodpasture syndrome
d. IgA nephropathy

Ans. a. Nephrotic syndrome

29. A young child with congenital hydrocephalus was treated with a successful ventriculoperitoneal (VP) shunt. Four months' postsurgical repair, the child presented with fever, nuchal rigidity and irritability. You suspect meningitis. What is the next best step?

a. Wait and watch
b. Check shunt patency by nuclear study
c. Blood culture and take CSF sample from shunt tap
d. Blood culture and take CSF sample by lumbar puncture

Ans. c. Blood culture and take CSF sample from shunt tap

30. In fetal circulation, which vessel carries deoxygenated blood back to the placenta?

a. Umbilical Vein
b. Umbilical artery
c. Descending aorta
d. Pulmonary Artery

Ans. b. Umbilical artery

31. A 10-year-old boy presented with seizures. His past history is significant for an episode of fever with rash at 1 year of age which resolved spontaneously. What is the most helpful investigation to diagnose his condition?

a. IgG measles in CSF
b. MRI mesial temporal lobe sclerosis
c. IgM measles in CSF
d. C1Q4 antibodies in the CSF

Ans. a. IgG measles in CSF

32. A 16-month-old boy is found to weigh 8 kg. A WHO growth chart (weight-for-age) is provided as follows. What is the most appropriate advice based on the plotted graph?

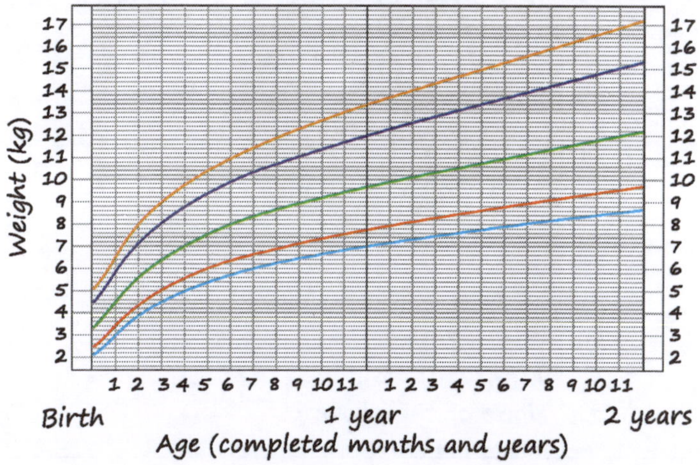

a. No malnutrition—assure the mother
b. Mild malnutrition—home treatment
c. Severe malnutrition—refer to nutrition rehabilitation center
d. Moderate malnutrition—teach the mother on how to feed

Ans. c. Severe malnutrition—refer to nutrition rehabilitation center

33. A day-old newborn with hepatosplenomegaly with periventricular calcifications and hearing loss. What is the best possible diagnosis?

a. Toxoplasmosis
b. CMV
c. Syphilis
d. Rubella

Ans. b. CMV

34. A 10-year-old came for routine vaccination, which vaccine should be given to the child?

a. Pentavalent
b. DPT
c. MMR
d. TT/TD

Ans. d. TT/TD

35. Water lily sign is seen in:

a. Amoebic liver abscess
b. Biliary atresia
c. Hydatid liver cyst
d. None of the above

Ans. c. Hydatid liver cyst

36. Identify the image and choose the best answer.

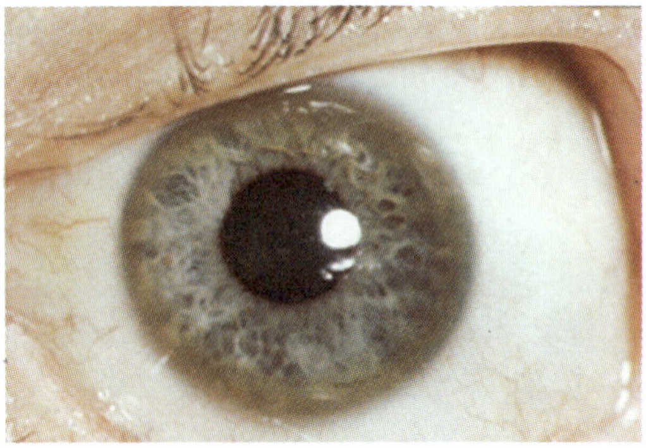

a. KF ring is seen in Wilson disease
b. Bitot spots
c. Trantas spots
d. None of the above

Ans. a. KF ring is seen in Wilson disease

37. A 4-year-old child came with complaints of bowing of legs and widening of wrist. On further examination, the child appears to have low serum calcium with the image shown as follows. Choose the best answer.

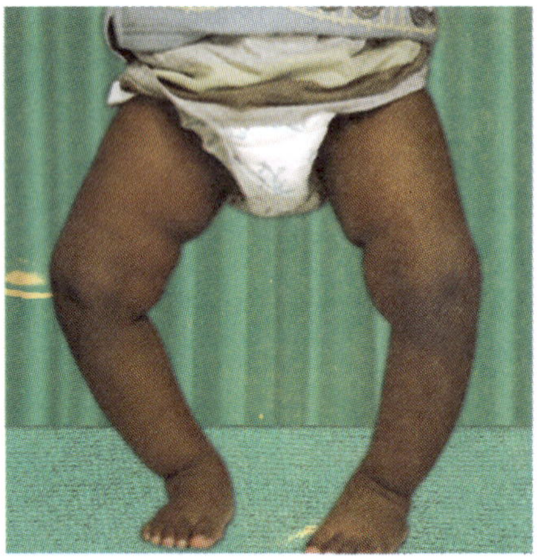

a. Osteogenesis imperfecta
b. Rickets
c. Scurvy
d. Pellagra

Ans. b. Rickets

38. A 10-day-old baby came with blue cornea. On further ophthalmologic evaluation, baby found to have blue cornea with photophobia and lacrimation. What is the diagnosis?

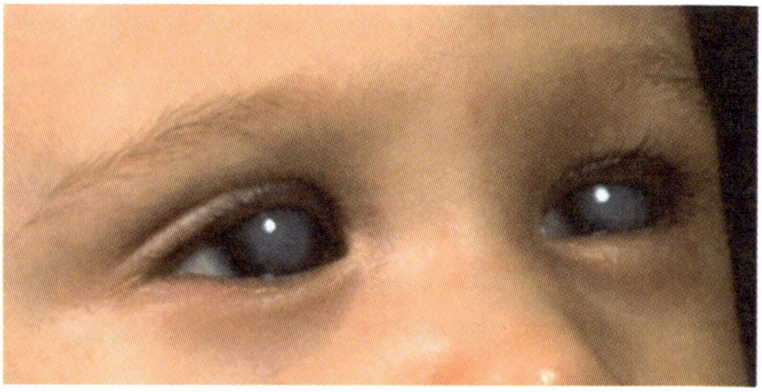

a. Congenital glaucoma
b. Galactosemia
c. Wilson disease
d. Alkaptonuria

Ans. a. Congenital glaucoma

39. A 3-year-old female baby came with cough and fast breathing for 5 days. Chest X-ray was done which showed a finding in the image. What is the diagnosis?

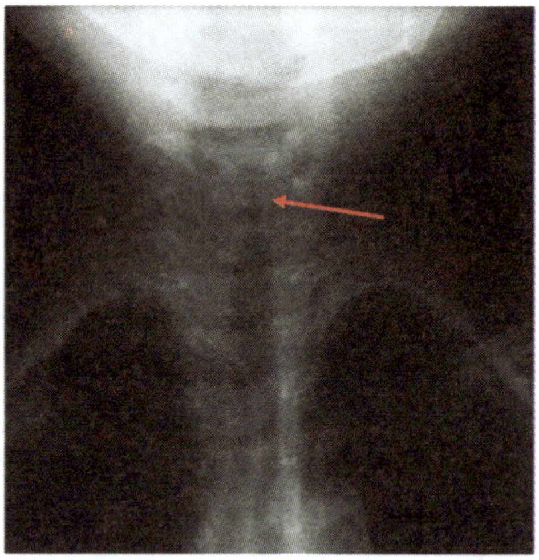

a. Laryngomalacia
b. Pneumonia
c. Croup
d. Subglottic stenosis

Ans. c. Croup

40. What are the vitamin K dependent clotting factors?

a. II, VII, IX, X
b. II, VII, IX, XI
c. II, VII, IX, XII
d. II, VII, IX, XIII

Ans. a. II, VII, IX, X

41. A child has been diagnosed with scurvy. The reason for bleeding manifestations/ecchymosis in vitamin C deficiency is due to:
   a. Defective mineralization of bone
   b. Due to lack of sunlight exposure
   c. Due to raised alkaline phosphatase
   d. Defective collagen formation

Ans. d. Defective collagen formation

42. Elevated sweat chloride test is done in which disease?
   a. Gaucher disease
   b. Cystic fibrosis
   c. Niemann-Pick disease
   d. Tyrosinemia

Ans. b. Cystic fibrosis

43. A 5-year-old baby came with suspected case of IEM. During the urine workup, the junior resident on duty found that there was darkening of urine on standing. What is the best possible diagnosis?

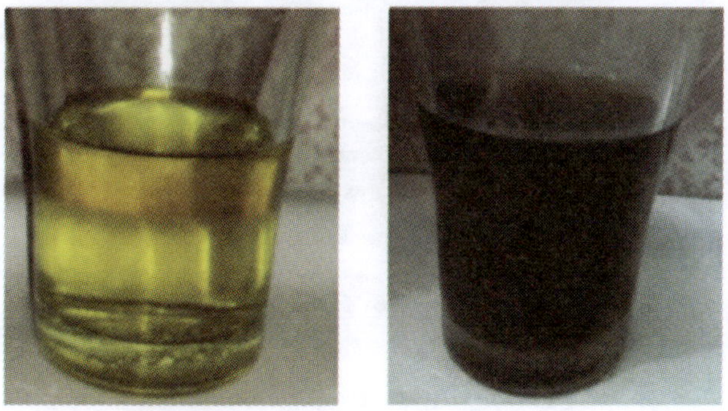

   a. Alkaptonuria
   b. Tyrosinemia
   c. Hartnup disease
   d. None of the above

Ans. a. Alkaptonuria

44. A 10-month-old baby presented with perioral rash/perivaginal rash with history of delayed wound healing. Which is the most common nutrient deficiency in this case?
   a. Selenium
   b. Zinc
   c. Copper
   d. Lead

Ans. b. Zinc

45. A 7-year-old child came dehydrated with blood sugar 550 mg/dL with fruity odor breath. Urine for ketones was advised which came out to be 3+. Which is the best possible diagnosis?
   a. Moderate dehydration
   b. Urinary tract infection
   c. Diabetic ketoacidosis
   d. Severe acute malnutrition

Ans. c. Diabetic ketoacidosis

46. Which of the following is the correct option?
   a. Height increases by 25 cm by 1st year
   b. Height remains at 25th percentile
   c. Weight remains at 75th percentile
   d. Baby's weight increases by 300 grams per month

Ans. a. Height increases by 25 cm by 1st year

INI-CET 2023-2021

47. Which of the following is the most effective indicator of successful ventilatory effort in neonatal resuscitation?
   a. Color change
   b. Rise in heart rate
   c. Air entry
   d. Chest rise

Ans. b. Rise in heart rate

48. Which can be used as an alternative to mother's milk in a low birth weight (LBW) baby?
   a. Cow's milk
   b. Preterm formula
   c. Term formula
   d. Human donor milk

Ans. d. Human donor milk

49. A 4-year-old male child with a body weight of 15 kg and height of 100 cm is admitted with renal failure. His blood urea was 100 mg/dL and serum creatinine was 1 mg/dL. What is the closest calculated eGFR in the patient?
   a. 33 mL/min/1.73 m^2 BSA
   b. 40 mL/min/17.3 m^2 BSA
   c. 55 mL/min/1.73 m^2 BSA
   d. 80 mL/min/1.73 m^2 BSA

Ans. b. 40 mL/min/17.3 m^2 BSA

50. **Adrenocorticotropic hormone is the drug of choice in which of the following conditions?**
   a. Juvenile myoclonic epilepsy
   b. Rolandic epilepsy
   c. West syndrome
   d. Lennox-Gastaut syndrome

Ans. c. West syndrome

51. **Regarding urinary tract infection (UTI) in children, which of the following is true?**
   1. Most common cause of UTI is streptococcus pneumoniae.
   2. Bowel, bladder dysfunction increases the risk of recurrence
   3. Cotrimoxazole is not given
   4. Micturating cysto-urethrogram (MCU) is done in children with recurrence of UTI

   a. 1, 3, 4 b. 2, 4
   c. 2, 3, 4 d. 1, 4

Ans. b. 2, 4

52. **Handedness is seen at the age of______________.**
   a. 1 year b. 2 years
   c. 3 years d. 4 years

Ans. c. 3 years

53. **Which of the following cyanotic heart disease causes increased pulmonary blood flow?**
   1. Ebstein anomaly
   2. Tetralogy of Fallot
   3. Transposition of the great arteries (TGA)
   4. Total anomalous pulmonary venous communication (TAPVC)

   a. 1, 4 b. 1, 2
   c. 3, 4 d. 2, 4

Ans. c. 3, 4

54. **An 11-year-old boy was brought to the outpatient clinic with intentional tremors, and poor scholastic performance. His sister has similar complaints. On examination, hepatomegaly is seen. The eye findings are shown in the following image. What is the probable diagnosis?**
   a. Wilson's disease
   b. Huntington's chorea
   c. Glutaric aciduria
   d. Hepatitis A

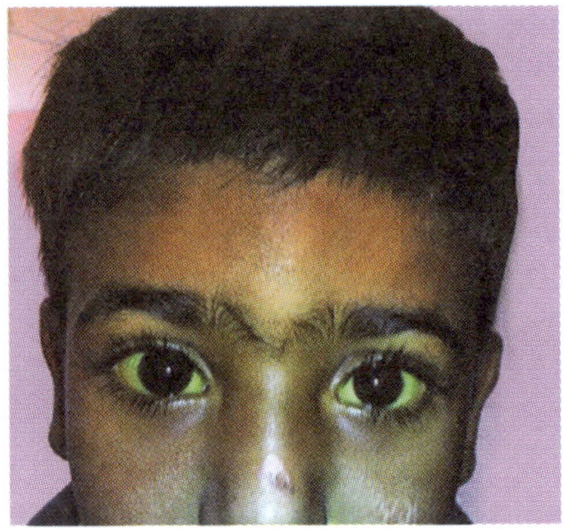

Ans. a. Wilson's disease

55. **Which alternative method can be used for the procedure shown in the following image?**

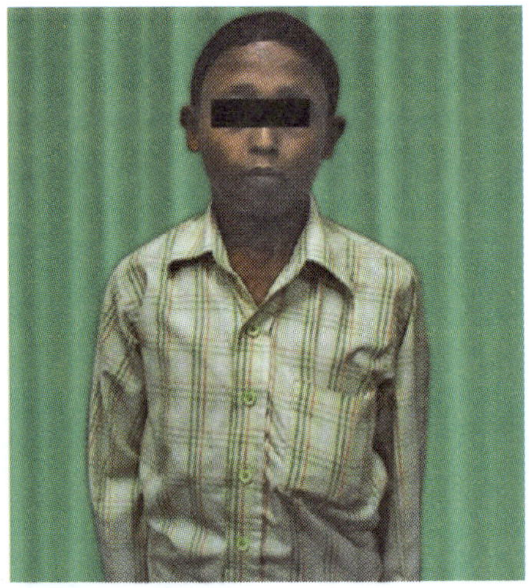

   a. Head circumference
   b. Arm span
   c. Crown-rump length
   d. Knee height

Ans. b. Arm span

56. **A child presents with acute exacerbation of asthma. Which of the following would you do?**
   1. Chest X-ray
   2. Oxygen administration
   3. Salbutamol nebulization three times in 60 minutes
   4. Administration of oral corticosteroids

   a. 3, 4
   b. 1, 4
   c. 1, 3, 4
   d. 2, 3, 4

Ans. d. 2, 3, 4

57. A young man is brought to the hospital with high-grade fever and altered consciousness. On examination, the patient had neck rigidity and pain when bending the neck. A lumbar puncture was performed and it showed a WBC count of 1500 cells/μ, majority being neutrophils, elevated pressure with protein of 120 mg/dL, and a glucose level of 70 mg/dL (blood glucose level – 300 mg/dL). How will you manage the index case?

a. Piperacillin + tazobactum
b. Amphotericin + flucytosine
c. Vancomycin + ceftriaxone
d. Antitubercular therapy

Ans. c. Vancomycin + ceftriaxone

58. Which of the following increases the risk of recurrence of febrile seizures?

1. Age < 1 year
2. Temperature of 38°-39°C
3. Duration of fever <24 hours
4. Duration of fever >48 hours

a. 1, 2, 4 b. 1, 4
c. 1, 2, 3 d. 1, 3, 4

Ans. c. 1, 2, 3

59. Choose the most appropriate answer.

Assertion: In phenylketonuria, the urine has a mousy odor.

Reason: The serum levels of tyrosine, dopamine, and norepinephrine are decreased in phenylketonuria.

a. Both assertion and reason are independently false statements.
b. The assertion is independently a true statement, but the reason is independently a false statement.
c. Both assertion and reason are independently true statements, but the reason is not the correct explanation for the assertion.
d. Both assertion and reason are independently true statements, and the reason is the correct explanation for the assertion.

Ans. c. Both assertion and reason are independently true statements, but the reason is not the correct explanation for the assertion.

60. A child is brought to the casualty with a history of choking. On examination, there is decreased air entry in the left lung. What would be the correct management?

1. Bronchoscopy
2. Computed tomography scan
3. ICD insertion
4. Chest X-ray

a. 1, 2, and 4 b. 1 and 2
c. 3 and 4 d. 1 and 4

Ans. d. 1 and 4

61. A 9-month-old boy presents with progressive pallor and abdominal distension. The peripheral smear done is as shown in the following image, and the Mentzer index was found to be less than 13. What are the investigations to be done in this patient?

1. High-performance liquid chromatography (HPLC)
2. PT and APTT
3. Bone marrow
4. Peripheral blood smear

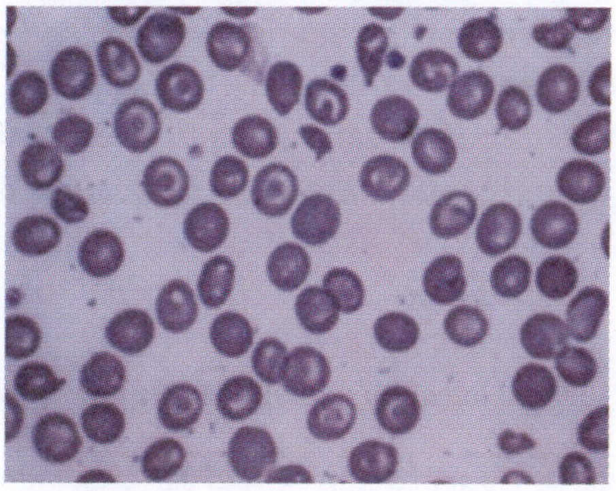

a. 1, and 2
b. 1, 3, and 4
c. 1 and 4
d. 1, 2, 3, and 4

Ans. c. 1 and 4

62. A child presents with complaints of fever, rash, body ache, and throat ache. He has a history of thorn prick injury a week back. What antibiotics would you give empirically to this child?

a. Ceftriaxone
b. Amoxicillin + clavulanate
c. Vancomycin
d. Meropenem

Ans. b. Amoxicillin + clavulanate

63. A child with thalassemia is undergoing multiple blood transfusions. What is the best method to detect iron overload?
   a. Liver iron concentration
   b. MRI T2 myocardium
   c. Serum ferritin
   d. NTBI

Ans. a. Liver iron concentration

64. How would you manage a child with status epilepticus?
   1. Airway and breathing
   2. IV Lorazepam
   3. Midazolam, Propofol, Thiopentone
   4. IV Fosphenytoine
   a. 1, 2, 3, 4
   b. 2, 1, 4, 3
   c. 1, 3, 4, 2
   d. 1, 2, 4, 3

Ans. d. 1, 2, 4, 3

65. A child presents with cold feet and a history of wearing socks even in the summers. On examination, lower limb pulses are diminished as compared to the radial pulse. Prominent radio femoral delay is present. What is the underlying condition?
   a. There is hypertrophy of ductus arteriosus.
   b. Coarctation distal to the origin of the left subclavian artery
   c. Supply is from posterior to anterior thoracic artery.
   d. Collaterals develop to supply upper limb.

Ans. b. Coarctation distal to the origin of the left subclavian artery

66. An unconscious child is brought to the casualty. What is the correct sequence of management?
   1. Assess breathing
   2. Assess pulse
   3. Assess response
   4. Start compressions
   5. Bag and mask ventilation
   a. 3-1-2-5-4
   b. 1-2-3-4-5
   c. 3-1-2-4-5
   d. 1-2-4-3-5

Ans. c. 3-1-2-4-5

67. Which of the following statements are true regarding cytomegalovirus (CMV) infection?
   1. Neonates who are asymptomatic at birth have a lesser risk of later sequelae.
   2. 20-40% are symptomatic at birth.
   3. In developing countries, the rate of transmission of CMV infection to the infant is more common from primary maternal infection than reactivation.
   4. Diagnosis by urine specimen at 4 weeks of age
   a. 3, 4
   b. 1, 2
   c. 2, 4
   d. 1, 3

Ans. d. 1, 3

68. The hormone that does not play a role in the growth of the fetus is:
   a. Insulin
   b. Growth hormone
   c. Thyroxine
   d. Glucocorticoids

Ans. b. Growth hormone

69. Which of the following statements is true regarding the tape shown in the image?
   1. It is called Shelter's tape.
   2. It is used to assess severe acute malnutrition.
   3. Reading of 13.5 to 14.5 cm is considered undernourished.
   4. It is mainly useful for frontline field workers.

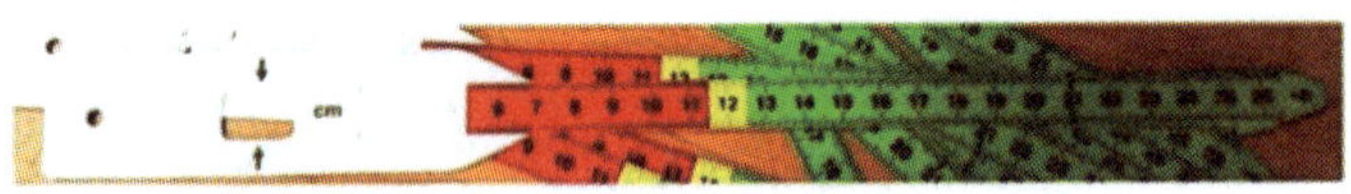

   a. 1,3
   b. 2, 4
   c. 2, 3
   d. 1, 4

Ans. b. 2, 4

70. Which of the following is a true statement about congenital CMV infection?
   a. About 20-30% of the infections are symptomatic
   b. Triad of SNHL, periventricular calcification and enamel hypoplasia

c. Most children asymptomatic at birth can develop conductive hearing loss later in life
d. If mother is IgG positive for CMV, the child is unlikely to develop infection

Ans. d. If mother is IgG positive for CMV, the child is unlikely to develop infection

71. Which of the following are components of kangaroo mother care?

a. Early discharge, skin to skin contact, prevent infection
b. Early discharge, skin to skin contact, exclusive breastfeeding
c. Skin to skin contact, exclusive breastfeeding, prevent infection
d. Early discharge, exclusive breastfeeding and prevent infection

Ans. b. Early discharge, skin to skin contact, exclusive breastfeeding

72. Which of the following is given as a part of the therapy for a child with severe COVID?

a. Corticosteroids
b. Ivermectin
c. Remdesivir
d. All of the above

Ans. a. Corticosteroids

73. Which of the following is seen in physiological jaundice?

a. Increased indirect bilirubin, increased urobilinogen, absent bilirubin in urine
b. Increased indirect bilirubin, absent urobilinogen, absent bilirubin in urine
c. Increased direct bilirubin, increased urobilinogen, absent bilirubin in urine
d. Increased direct bilirubin, absent urobilinogen, absent bilirubin in urine

Ans. a. Increased indirect bilirubin, increased urobilinogen, absent bilirubin in urine

74. A child presents with fever and vesicular lesions on the upper limb and the lower limb. Neck stiffness was present. Similar lesions were present on the palms, soles, and oral cavity. CSF analysis revealed normal glucose levels and elevated lymphocytes and protein. What is the most likely diagnosis?

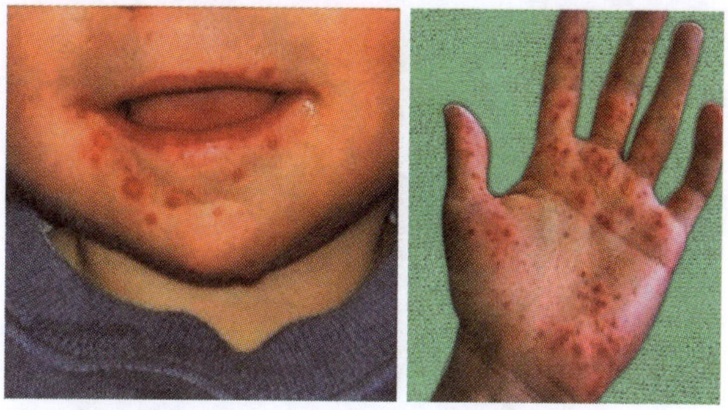

a. Bacterial meningitis with sepsis
b. Coxsackie viral meningitis and Hand Foot Mouth disease
c. Herpes simplex gingivostomatitis and meningoencephalitis
d. Tuberculous meningitis

Ans. b. Coxsackie viral meningitis and Hand Foot Mouth disease

75. Match the following developmental milestones:

1. Transfers objects	A. 1-2 months
2. Social smile	B. 6-7 months
3. Pincer grasp	C. 12-15 months
4. Walks 1-2 steps	D. 9-12 months

a. 1-A, 2-B, 3-C, 4-D
b. 1-B, 2-A, 3-D, 4-C
c. 1-C, 2-B, 3-A, 4-D
d. 1-D, 2-C, 3-B, 4-A

Ans. b. 1-B, 2-A, 3-D, 4-C

76. Which of the following congenital heart disease has equal saturation in all the chambers of the heart?

a. Tetralogy of Fallot
b. Total anomalous pulmonary venous circulation
c. Tricuspid atresia
d. Transposition of great arteries

Ans. b. Total anomalous pulmonary venous circulation

77. Which of the following marked structure is damaged in respiratory distress syndrome?

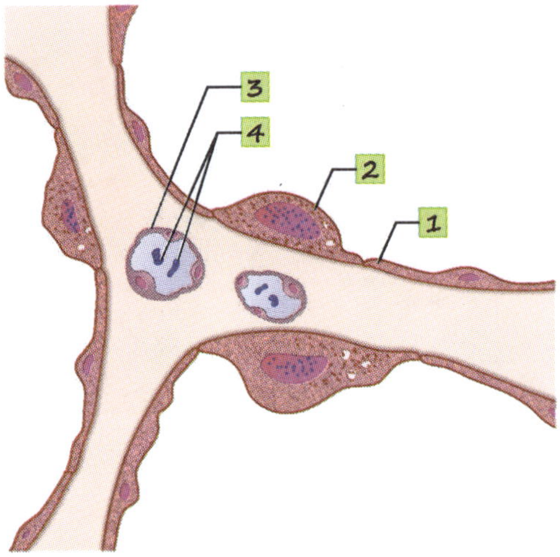

a. 1 b. 2
c. 3 d. 4

Ans. b. 2

78. Which of the following are causes of neonatal seizures?

1. Hyponatremia 2. Hypomagnesemia
3. Hypocalcemia 4. Hypernatremia

a. 1, 2, 3 only
b. 1, 2, 3, and 4
c. 1, 3, 4 only
d. 2, 4 only

Ans. b. 1, 2, 3, and 4

79. A neonate is found to have increased irritability, poor feeding, and two episodes of seizures. Lumbar puncture was done and the findings were suggestive of meningitis. What is the most likely causative organism?

a. Streptococcus agalactiae
b. Escherichia coli
c. Neisseria meningitidis
d. Listeria monocytogenes

Ans. a. Streptococcus agalactiae

80. At what age does a child attain half-height of the adult height?

a. 12-18 months
b. 20-24 months
c. 32-36 months
d. 40-48 months

Ans. b. 20-24 months

81. Nada's Minor Criteria include:

1. Systolic murmur Grade 3 - Major
2. Diastolic murmur - Major
3. Abnormal second heart sound - Minor
4. Abnormal BP - Minor

a. 1, 2 and 3
b. 1, 2, 3 and 4
c. 3 and 4
d. 2, 3, and 4

Ans. c. 3 and 4

82. An 18-month old child with 3 days' history of watery diarrhea and vomiting presented with altered sensorium. Which of the following are differential diagnoses?

1. Severe dehydration
2. HUS X 5-10 days: dysentery
3. Cerebral Venous Thrombosis dehydration
4. Hyponatremia

a. 1, 2, 3, 4 b. 1, 2, 3
c. 1, 3, 4 d. 2, 3, 4

Ans. c. 1, 3, 4

83. The causative agent of the condition shown in the following image is associated with which of the following disorders?

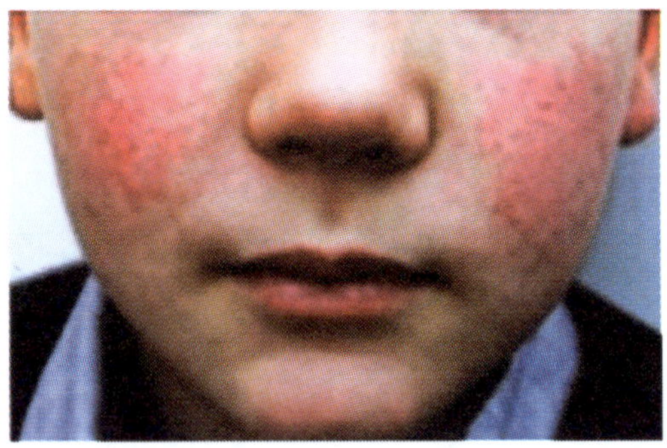

a. Gingivostomatitis
b. Pure red cell aplasia
c. Molluscum contagiosum
d. Kaposi sarcoma

Ans. b. Pure red cell aplasia

84. Which of the following has the least risk of perinatal transmission?

a. HSV b. CMV
c. Hepatitis B d. Rubella

Ans. d. Rubella

85. A 6-year-old boy was brought with history of chronic cough, and foul smelling stools. His sibling who had similar complaints died a few years back. Sweat chloride test and CFTR gene studies were done. CFTR gene encodes proteins that are involved in transport of which ions?

a. Cl^- b. Na^+

c. HCO_3^- d. K^+

Ans. a. Cl^-

86. A 4-year-old boy presented with history of fever, conjunctival congestion and erythematous desquamation of skin. 2D echo shows coronary aneurysm. First line treatment is:

a. Aspirin b. Clopidogrel

c. IVIG d. LMWH

Ans. c. IVIG

87. A 4-year-old boy presented with history of fever, conjunctival congestion and erythematous desquamation of skin. 2D echo shows Kawasaki disease. First line treatment is:

a. Aspirin
b. Clopidogrel
c. IVIG 2 g/2 kg
d. LMWH

Ans. c. IVIG 2 g/2 kg

88. Regarding a baby born with Meconium-stained liquor (MSL), which of the following are recommended as per neonatal resuscitation guidelines?

1. Intrapartum suction of nose and mouth before delivery of shoulder
2. Intratracheal suction in case of nonvigorous baby
3. Gentle suction of nose and mouth in case of vigorous baby
4. PPV in case of nonvigorous baby after early steps

a. 1, 2, 3, 4
b. 1, 3, 4
c. 2, 4
d. 3, 4

Ans. d. 3, 4

89. The perinatal transmission of an infection shows the spectrum of anemia, possibly myocarditis, high output cardiac failure, and ascites. Identify the causative agent.

a. Parvovirus B19
b. CMV - microcephaly, periventricular $C4^{2+}$
c. Treponema pallidum
d. Toxoplasma gondii

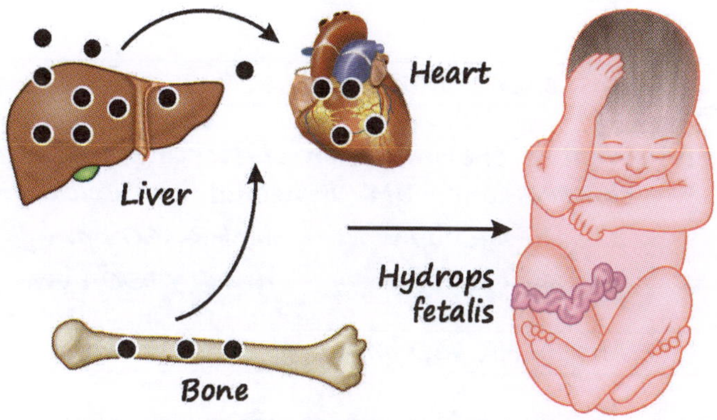

(Microcephaly Diffuse calcification)

Ans. a. Parvovirus B19

90. Match the following:

1. Trisomy 18	A. Sickle cell anemia
2. Trisomy 13	B. Edwards syndrome
3. Trinucleotide repeats	C. Patau syndrome
4. 6th position of HB chain (Glu → Val)	D. Huntington's disease (CAG)

a. 1-A, 2-B, 3-C, 4-D
b. 1-B, 2-A, 3-C, 4-D
c. 1-B, 2-C, 3-D, 4-A
d. 1-C, 2-A, 3-B, 4-D

Ans. c. 1-B, 2-C, 3-D, 4-A

91. Pompe disease is due to the deficiency of?

a. Alpha glucosidase
b. Phosphofructokinase
c. Myophosphorylase
d. Glucose-6-phosphatase

Ans. a. Alpha glucosidase

FMGE 2023 (JULY AND JANUARY)

92. A newborn baby born through cesarean section did not cry immediately after birth. On further evaluation, baby had HR <60 bpm. What will be the next best step?

a. Chest compressions
b. Bag and mask ventilation
c. CC + BMV
d. Adrenaline

Ans. c. CC + BMV

93. What is the indication of starting the chest compressions + BMV in neonatal resuscitation?

a. HR <40 bpm b. HR <60 bpm
c. HR <80 bpm d. HR <100 bpm

Ans. b. HR <60 bpm

94. How much percentage of oxygen should be given to a newborn baby INITIALLY in neonatal resuscitation if the baby is having apnea or HR <100 bpm?

a. 20% b. 21%
c. 15% d. 17%

Ans. b. 21%

95. A 2-day-old neonate came with complaints of distress, frothing of secretions, dribbling of saliva and mother having history of polyhydramnios. According to the following X-ray, what is the best possible diagnosis?

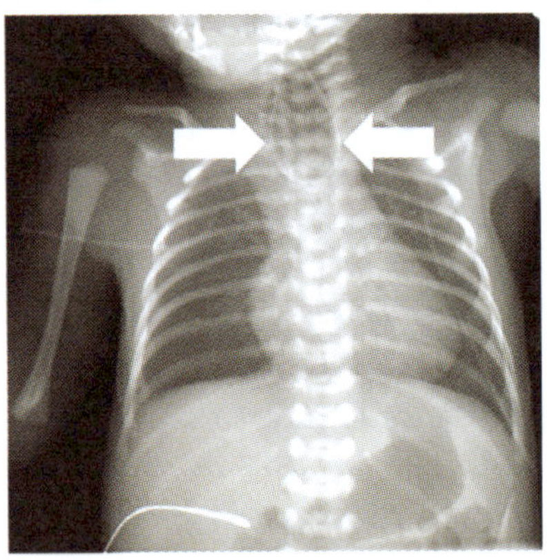

a. Hyaline membrane disease
b. Respiratory distress syndrome
c. Transient tachypnea of newborn
d. Tracheoesophageal fistula

Ans. d. Tracheoesophageal fistula

96. A 4-year-old boy with periorbital swelling, facial puffiness and pedal edema was on steroid therapy. On further evaluation in the electron microscopy: effacement of the foot processes of the podocytes was seen. Patient proteinuria was > 40 mg/m²/h. What is the possible diagnosis?

a. FSGN
b. Nephritic syndrome
c. Nephrotic syndrome
d. Hemolytic uremic syndrome

Ans. c. Nephrotic syndrome

97. A 7-year-old female child comes with cough, coryza, conjunctivitis with centripetal rash. The diagnosis is:

a. Measles
b. Mumps
c. Erythema infectiosum
d. Chicken pox
e. Roseola infantum

Ans. a. Measles

98. What is D in pediatric emergency care?

a. Disability b. Defibrillation
c. Deafness d. Deworming

Ans. a. Disability

99. What is the dose of vitamin A required for a 11-month-old female child?

a. 50,000 IU b. 1 lakh IU
c. 2 lakh IU d. 3 lakh IU

Ans. b. 1 lakh IU

100. A one-month-old doll-like facies baby with hepatomegaly is diagnosed with von Gierke's disease. Which is the most common enzyme deficient in children?

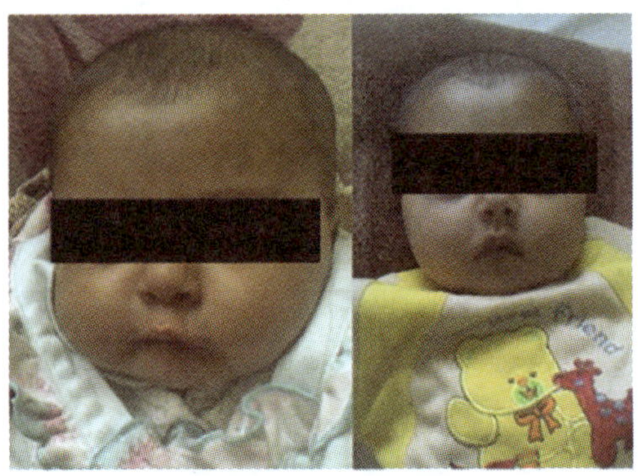

a. Fructose-6-phosphate
b. Glucokinase
c. Glucose-6-phosphate
d. Glucose-6-phosphatase
e. Debranching enzyme

Ans. d. Glucose-6-phosphatase

101. A 5-year-old boy has consumed multiple iron tablets and parents are worried for the treatment of the baby. What is the next best approach?

a. Deferasirox/desferrioxamine
b. D penicillamine
c. Zinc
d. N acetyle cysteine

Ans. a. Deferasirox/desferrioxamine

102. A post-term neonate is defined as born >:

a. 40 weeks b. 41 weeks
c. 42 weeks d. 43 weeks

Ans. c. 42 weeks

103. Which vitamin is responsible for the collagen formation/collagen defect?

a. Vitamin A b. Vitamin B
c. Vitamin C d. Vitamin D
e. Vitamin E

Ans. c. Vitamin C

104. A 10-year-old male child came with fever, irritability and meningeal signs. His CSF picture showed low sugar high protein lymphocytic predominance. What is the best diagnosis?

a. Viral meningitis
b. Tubercular meningitis
c. Bacterial meningitis
d. Encephalitis
e. Cerebral malaria

Ans. b. Tubercular meningitis

105. Identify the following image:

a. Mongolian spot
b. Milia
c. Harlequin color change
d. Hemangioma
e. Cavernous hemangioma

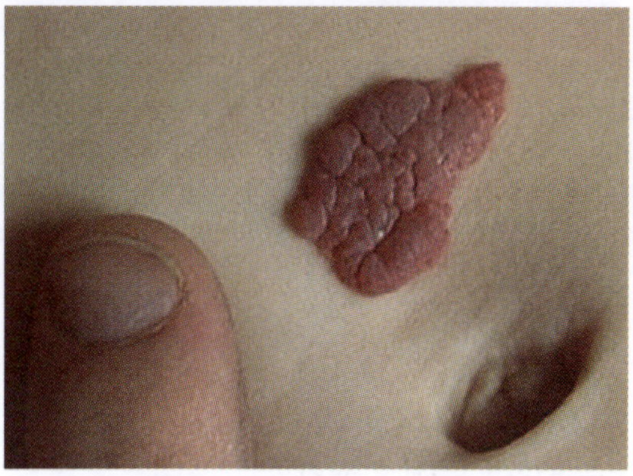

Ans. d. Hemangioma

106. Breastfeeding should be started in how many hours of life?

a. 1 hour b. 2 hours
c. 3 hours d. 4 hours

Ans. a. 1 hour

107. A 4-year-old patient came with decreased weight for height < -3 SD with MUAC <11.5 cm with anasarca and abdominal distension. What is the best interpretation?

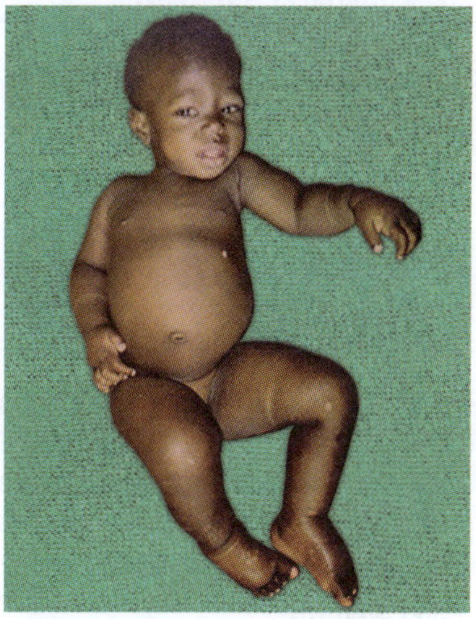

a. Marasmus is due to deficiency of calories + hypoalbuminemia + proteins
b. Kwashiorkor is due to deficiency of proteins
c. Marasmus is due to deficiency of calories + proteins
d. Marasmus is due to deficiency of calories only

Ans. b. Kwashiorkor is due to deficiency of proteins

108. The mother of a 5-year-old boy complains that he is not growing as compared to other siblings. On further evaluation, the boy's height was <3rd percentile and bone age was < chronological age. The parent's height was NORMAL. What is your best interpretation?
   a. Familial short stature
   b. Constitutional delay in growth and puberty
   c. Hypothyroidism
   d. None of the above

Ans. b. Constitutional delay in growth and puberty

109. A 28-year-old couple is trying to conceive a child. They present to OPD for routine examination. During the checkup, husband had small testis and gynecomastia. The most likely diagnosis is:
   a. Noonan syndrome
   b. Down syndrome
   c. Turner syndrome
   d. Klinefelter syndrome

Ans. d. Klinefelter syndrome

110. When does the handedness come?
   a. 18 months
   b. 24 months
   c. 36 months–38 months
   d. 48 months

Ans. c. 36 months–38 months

111. A 2-year-old child on regular OPD visit seems to have growth chart showing BMI between 90th–95th percentile. What is the best possible option for this child in terms of obesity?
   a. BMI needed for the interpretation
   b. Overweight
   c. Obesity
   d. SAM
   e. Short stature

Ans. b. Overweight

112. A term baby has 2.5 kg weight at the time of delivery. On examination, the baby was limp/gasping. What is your next best step?
   a. Antenatal counseling, team briefing, equipment check
   b. Check whether the baby is term, tone and crying
   c. Routine care
   d. Warmth, Position, suction, stimulation, reposition
   e. Bag and mask ventilation

Ans. d. Warmth, Position, suction, stimulation, reposition

113. Which of the following vaccines are given at birth?
   a. BCG OPV Hep B
   b. DPT OPV Hep B
   c. Rotavirus BCG OPV
   d. BCG OPV Hep C

Ans. a. BCG OPV Hep B

114. First dose of hepatitis B is given at:
   a. 6 weeks
   b. 10 weeks
   c. 14 weeks
   d. Birth

Ans. d. Birth

115. A 4-year-old with severe acute malnutrition has decreased height for age. Which parameter will be affected?
   a. Wasting
   b. Stunting
   c. Normal
   d. None of these

Ans. b. Stunting

116. A 2-month-old patient came with complaints of darkening of urine on standing/color of the diaper became black. Which enzyme is responsible for the aforementioned condition?
   a. Transaminase
   b. Ketoacid decarboxylase
   c. Phenylalanine hydroxylase
   d. Homogentisic acid oxidase

Ans. d. Homogentisic acid oxidase

117. A 6-year-old child came with abdominal pain with rashes over the lower limbs. On further examination, patient had hematuria and proteinuria. What is your best possible diagnosis?
   a. HUS
   b. Henoch-Schonlein purpura (HSP)
   c. Nephrotic syndrome
   d. SLE

Ans. b. Henoch-Schonlein purpura (HSP)

118. A 2.5-year-old male patient came with cough and fever for the last 4 days. He also had chest indrawing with RR of 38/min. What is the next best step?
   a. Ampicillin and gentamicin and refere immediately
   b. Oral antibiotics and refer immediately
   c. No antibiotics needed
   d. Home treatment

Ans. b. Oral Antibiotics and refer immediately

119. A 4-year-old baby came with complaints of chest pain. On detailed evaluation, baby had irregularly irregular radial pulse with absent P wave. What is the best diagnosis?
   a. Atrial fibrillation
   b. Supraventricular tachycardia
   c. Ventricular fibrillation
   d. None of the above

Ans. a. Atrial fibrillation

120. In which of the following conditions you will see macrocytic anemia?
   a. Sideroblastic anemia
   b. Iron deficiency anemia
   c. Thalassemia
   d. Anemia of chronic disease
   e. Lead poisoning
   f. Liver disease

Ans. f. Liver disease

FMGE 2022

121. Which disease shows multifactorial inheritance?
   a. Neural tube defect
   b. Cleft clip and palate
   c. Hirschsprung disease
   d. CHPS
   e. All of the above

Ans. a. Neural tube defect

122. Which vitamin is rich in breast milk?
   a. Vitamin A
   b. Vitamin D
   c. Vitamin B_{12}
   d. Vitamin K

Ans. a. Vitamin A

123. Which vitamin is DEFICIENT in breast milk?
   a. Vitamin D: present in very less amount
   b. Vitamin K
   c. Vitamin A
   d. Vitamin C

Ans. b. Vitamin K

124. Newborn who are exclusively breastfed can lead to which of the following condition?
   a. Hemolytic disease of newborn
   b. Hemorrhagic disease of newborn
   c. Icterus
   d. None of the above

Ans. b. Hemorrhagic disease of newborn

125. A 9-month-old baby came for its routine measles vaccination, mother wants to enquire about the next dose of measles vaccination. What should the nurse tell the mother?
   a. 15 months
   b. 20 months
   c. 24 months
   d. 30 months

Ans. a. 15 months

126. During an epidemic, an 8-month-old baby came for its routine measles vaccination, mother wants to enquire about the next dose of measles vaccination. What should the nurse tell the mother?
   a. 12 months
   b. 15 months
   c. 20 months
   d. 24 months
   e. 30 months

Ans. a. 12 months

127. Unused measles vaccines should be discarded within how many hours?
   a. 2-4 hours
   b. 4-6 hours
   c. 6-8 hours
   d. 8-10 hours

Ans. b. 4-6 hours

128. Identify the image:

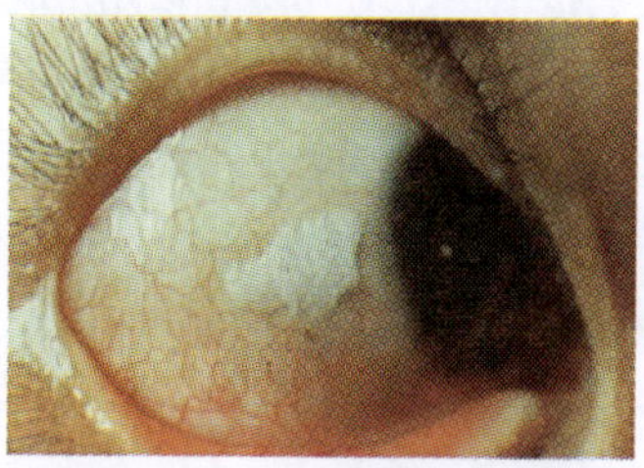

a. Brushfield spots
b. Bitot spots
c. Retinal hemorrhagic spot
d. None of the above

Ans. b. Bitot spots

129. A 5-year-old child shows growth retardation + mental changes + apathy + edema + not growing well. The child has:
a. Kwashiorkor
b. Marasmus
c. SAM
d. All of these

Ans. a. Kwashiorkor

130. A 7-year-old boy came to the clinic with episodes of daydreaming in the class. He also had staring episodes. What is the best management?
a. Sodium valproate
b. Lamotrigine
c. Phenobarbitone
d. Eptoin

Ans. a. Sodium valproate

131. Which is the absolute contraindication of breastfeeding?
a. Hepatitis A
b. Breast abscess
c. Galactosemia
d. Herpes Simplex

Ans. c. Galactosemia

132. Which of the following is not true about colostrum?
a. Rich in IgA
b. Rich in proteins and amino acid
c. Rich in fat and sugar
d. Lemon yellow in color

Ans. c. Rich in fat and sugar

133. An 8-year-old child presented with hematuria with history of sore throat for the last 2 weeks. On further evaluation, there is cola color urine. What is the most probable diagnosis?
a. PSGN
b. Membranous nephropathy
c. IgA Nephropathy
d. Minimal Change Disease

Ans. a. PSGN

134. At what level spinal cord ends in newborn and infants?
a. L1
b. L2
c. L3
d. L4

Ans. c. L3

135. A 5-year-old child presented with fever. After the subsiding of fever, rash appeared as seen in the following image. Which is the most probable diagnosis?

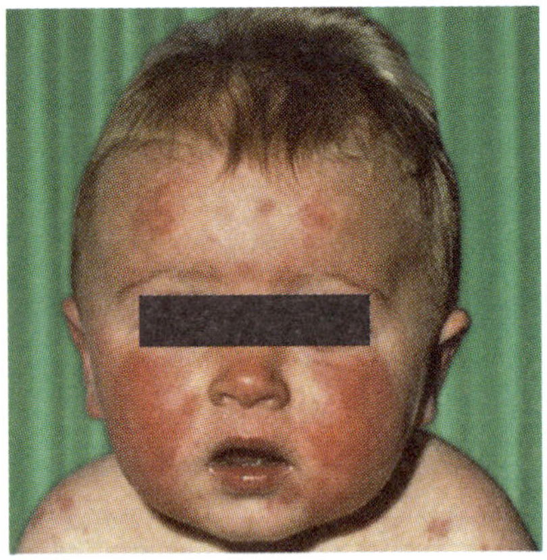

a. 5th disease
b. 6th disease
c. Measles
d. Varicella

Ans. a. 5th disease

136. A 4-year-old baby had fever for the last 5 days. On further evaluation, he had chest indrawing and refusal to feed. His RR was 46/min. What is the best possible diagnosis?
a. No pneumonia
b. Severe pneumonia
c. Very severe pneumonia
d. Pneumonia

Ans. b. Severe pneumonia

137. A 3-year-old boy with syndromic facies is having hypocalcemia with microdeletion in chromosome number 22q11.2. What is the best possible diagnosis?
a. Turner syndrome
b. Patau syndrome
c. DiGeorge syndrome
d. Down syndrome

Ans. c. DiGeorge syndrome

138. Which of the following embryological development is affected in the given image?

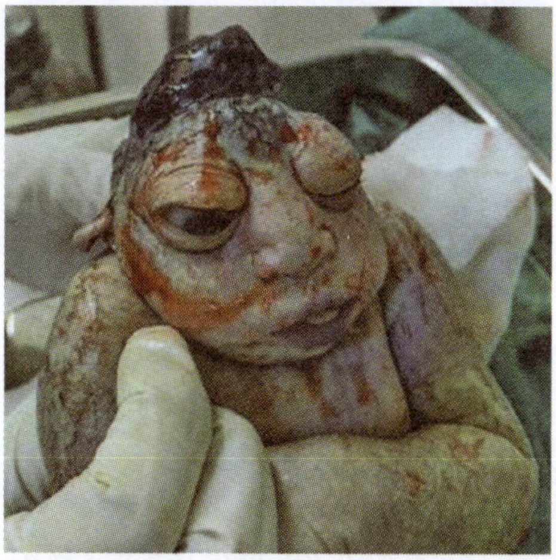

a. Anterior neuropore closure failure—leads to cranial defect
b. Posterior neuropore closure failure–leads to caudal defect
c. Whole neural tube is exposed
d. It is a forebrain anomaly

Ans. a. Anterior neuropore closure failure—leads to cranial defect

139. 4 year baby came with history of cow's milk diluted with water. On further examination, child had anasarca and mid upper arm circumference was <11.5 cm. What is the best possible diagnosis?

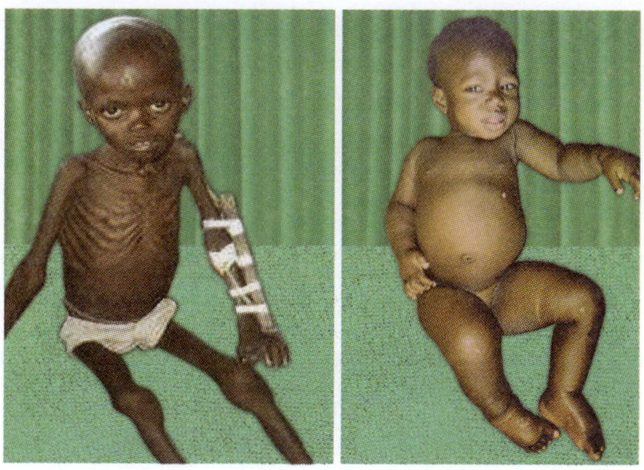

a. Marasmus
b. Kwashiorkor
c. Failure to thrive
d. Rickets

Ans. b. Kwashiorkor

140. A 5-day-old baby passes stool from the umbilicus, what is the nearest possible explanation?

a. Omphalocele
b. Gastroschisis
c. Patent urachus
d. Patent vitellointestinal duct/omphalomesenteric duct
e. Ureterocele

Ans. d. Patent vitellointestinal duct/omphalomesenteric duct

141. Young child with the following red cell indices with history of recurrent blood transfusions. What is your diagnosis?

Hb: 4 g/dL
MCV: 24 fl
MCH: 60 pg
MCHC: 30%

a. Iron deficiency anemia
b. Thalassemia
c. Sickle cell anemia
d. Megaloblastic anemia

Ans. b. Thalassemia

142. A 4-day-old baby has distress which improves on crying. What is the best possible diagnosis?

a. Choanal atresia
b. TEF
c. HMD
d. Cleft lip and palate

Ans. a. Choanal atresia

143. A 10-year-old child came with jaundice which was seen after having stress/strenuous exercise. His liver enzymes were normal and he was having unconjugated hyperbilirubinemia. What is the best possible diagnosis?

a. Dubin-Johnson syndrome
b. Rotor syndrome
c. Gilbert syndrome
d. Viral hepatitis

Ans. c. Gilbert syndrome

144. Gum bleeding is seen in which of the following?

a. Rickets
b. Scurvy
c. Megaloblastic anemia
d. Thalassemia

Ans. b. Scurvy

145. A 25-day-old baby with chronic constipation came with complaint of abdominal distension. On further evaluation, he had history of not passing stool in first 3 days of life. What is the best management?

a. Barium meal
b. Barium swallow
c. Rectal biopsy – MC area is rectum
d. Challenge test

Ans. c. Rectal biopsy – MC area is rectum

146. A 7-year-old baby came with rash in the lower limbs. He also complained of joint pain and hematuria. However, his platelets count was normal. What is the best possible diagnosis?

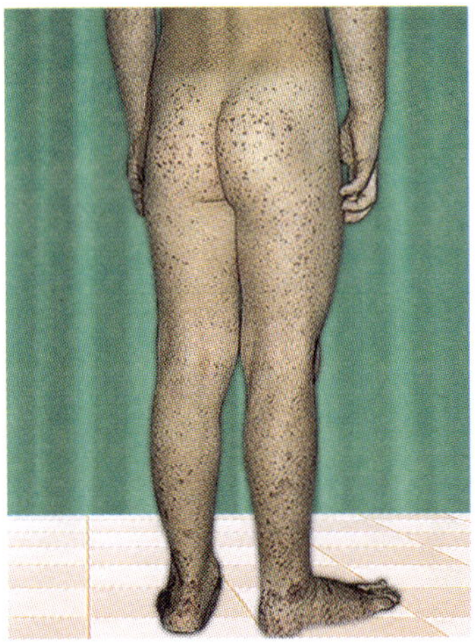

a. ITP
b. HSP
c. Kawasaki
d. Wegener's granulomatosis

Ans. b. HSP

147. A 6-year-old child complains of abdominal pain and red, elevated skin rashes, mainly involving the lower limbs. What is the probable diagnosis?

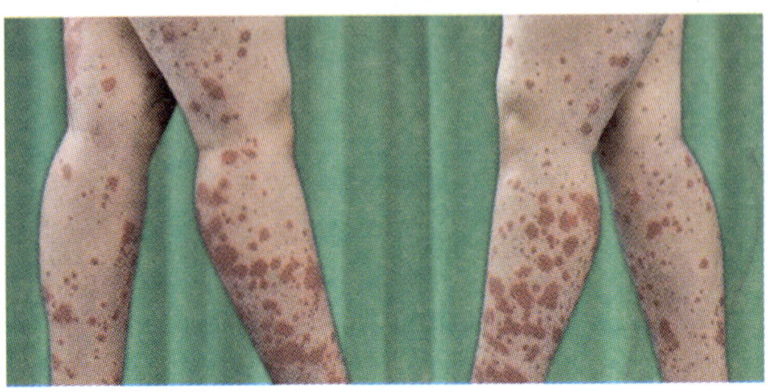

a. Kawasaki
b. HSP
c. Varicella infection
d. Meningococcemia

Ans. b. HSP

148. What is the first line of drug for febrile seizures?

a. Diazepam
b. Midazolam
c. Phenytoin – 2nd line
d. Phenobarbitone

Ans. b. Midazolam

149. Which is the best possible finding seen in infant of diabetic mother?

a. Hyperglycemia
b. Hypoglycemia
c. Hyperthermia
d. IUGR

Ans. b. Hypoglycemia

150. What will be the dose of folic acid for a mother who had a previous baby with neural tube defect?

a. 400 mcg b. 4000 mcg
c. 1 mg d. 0.1 mg

Ans. b. 4000 mcg

151. You are the doctor in the internal ward of Rajagiri Hospital and you meet Mr. Bharath. He responses to strong pain and withdraws his hand, and utters incomprehensible word. GCS is:

a. 6 b. 7
c. 8 d. 9

Ans. c. 8

152. Conjugated hyperbilirubinemia is seen in:

a. Dubin-Johnson syndrome
b. Gilbert's syndrome
c. Breast milk jaundice
d. Crigler-Najjar syndrome
e. None of the above

Ans. a. Dubin-Johnson syndrome

153. 1 gram of Hb liberates how many mg of bilirubin?

a. 40 b. 34
c. 15 d. 55

Ans. b. 34

154. A 4-day-old breastfed, otherwise well, term neonate presents with jaundice. On testing, the bilirubin level was found to be 18 mg/dL. Which of the following is the best step of management?

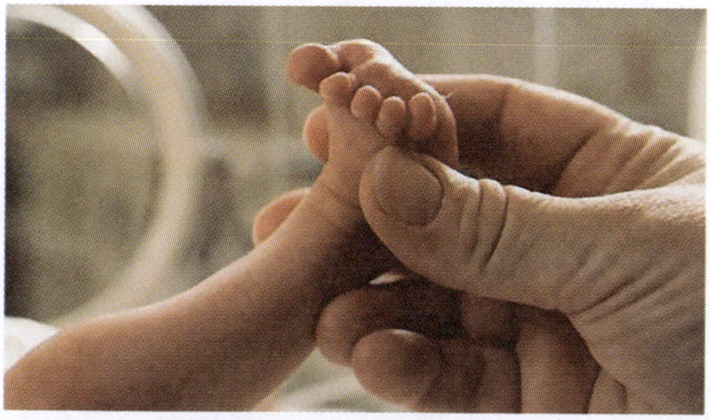

a. Start phototherapy and continue breastfeeding
b. Start IV fluids and give phototherapy
c. Initiate exchange transfusion
d. Stop breastfeeding and do phototherapy

Ans. a. Start phototherapy and continue breastfeeding

155. All of the following are true about breast milk jaundice; except:

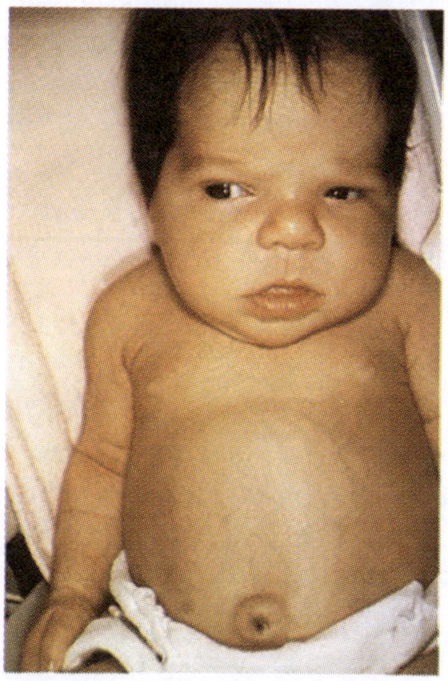

a. Bilirubin is 10-15 mg/dL
b. Occurs between day 5-10 of life
c. Staining of diaper by urine is present
d. Breastfeeding should be stopped to treat it

Ans. d. Breastfeeding should be stopped to treat it

156. A term neonate has jaundice till palm and soles on day 4 of life. What is the expected bilirubin of the baby?

a. 8-10 mg/dL b. 10-12 mg/dL
c. 12-15 mg/dL d. >15 mg/dL

Ans. d. >15 mg/dL

157. A 3-day-old neonate is brought by the mother to the pediatrician and is found to have bilirubin of 17 g/dL. What is the next step?

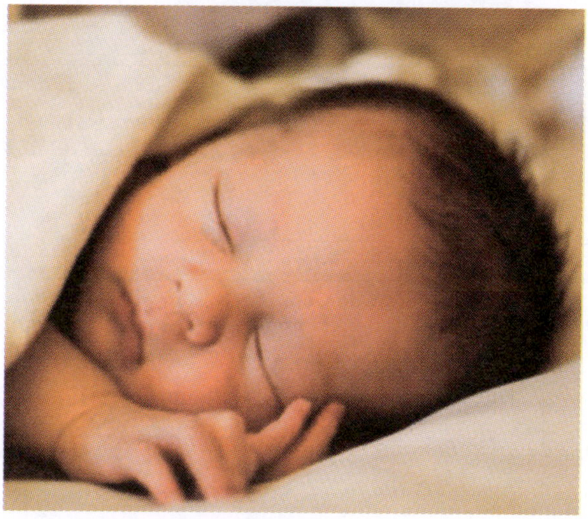

a. Stop breastfeeding
b. Start phototherapy and continue breastfeeding
c. Start phototherapy and stop breastfeeding
d. Exchange transfusion

Ans. b. Start phototherapy and continue breastfeeding

158. Menkes Disease is associated with the metabolism of which of the following minerals?

a. Copper
b. Molybdenum
c. Zinc
d. Calcium

Ans. a. Copper

159. All are seen in HSP (Henoch-Schonlein purpura); except:
   a. Thrombocytopenia
   b. Glomerulonephritis
   c. Arthralgia
   d. Abdominal pain

Ans. a. Thrombocytopenia

160. A 4-year-old baby has blonde hair, blue iris, and developmental delay. On further examination, the child has autosomal recessive condition. All of the following are true statements for this given condition; except:
   a. It is a case of tyrosinemia
   b. Ferric chloride test can be done in this case
   c. Urine odor will be mousy
   d. Enzyme deficiency is phenylalanine hydroxylase

Ans. c. Urine odor will be mousy

161. The main organ damaged by PKU is:
   a. Kidney
   b. Brain
   c. Liver
   d. GIT

Ans. b. Brain

162. Which is the most common organ involved in congenital tuberculosis?
   a. Kidney
   b. Brain
   c. Liver
   d. GIT
   e. Adrenals

Ans. c. Liver

163. All of the following statements are true about human and cow milk; except:
   a. $Ca:PO_4$ ratio is more in human milk
   b. Breast milk is rich in vitamin A
   c. Lactose content is higher in human milk
   d. Casein protein is present in higher quantities in cow milk

Ans. a. $Ca:PO_4$ ratio is more in human milk

164. A long-term and rare complication of Measles is:
   a. Orchitis
   b. Otitis Media
   c. SSPE
   d. Koplik spots

Ans. c. SSPE

165. A 3-year-old child has been suffering from diarrhea for many hours along with two episodes of vomiting, the child is restless and thirsty and is drinking water eagerly. On examination, the skin pinch goes back slowly and oral mucosa is dry. The patient is to be treated with:
   a. 5-10 mL/kg ORS per loose stool
   b. 75 mL/kg ORS over 4 hours
   c. 100 mL/kg IV fluids over 3 hours
   d. 75 mL/kg IV fluids over 4 hours

Ans. b. 75 mL/kg ORS over 4 hours

166. APGAR score includes all of the following parameters; except:
   a. Activity
   b. Pulse rate
   c. Respiratory rate
   d. Grimace

Ans. c. Respiratory rate

167. A 4-year-old patient came with generalised body swelling and decreased urine output. On further examination the patient had massive proteinurea. The urinary protein: urinary creatinine ratio is more than 2. The best treatment option for this child is:
   a. Cyclophosphamide
   b. Cyclosporine
   c. Prednisolone
   d. Levamisole

Ans. c. Prednisolone

168. A patient with 6 days of fever presents with erythematous rashes over trunk and extremities; also complains of watering from eyes. On examination, there are mucosal hyperemia and palpable nodes. The most probable diagnosis is:
   a. Scarlet Fever
   b. Henoch-Schonlein Purpura
   c. Polyarteritis Nodosa
   d. Kawasaki disease

Ans. d. Kawasaki disease

169. A child was suffering from sore throat for which he was given medications but within a few days, the child now presents with hematuria, and proteins on dipstick come positive. What is the diagnosis?
   a. Post streptococcal glomerulonephritis
   b. Berger's disease

c. Rapidly progressive glomerulonephritis
d. Minimal change disease

Ans. c. Rapidly progressive glomerulonephritis

170. Embrace equivalent is exaggerated in case of:

a. HIE Stage 3 b. Erb's Palsy
c. HIE Stage 1 d. None of these

Ans. c. HIE Stage 1

171. A 15-month-old child cannot do the following:

a. Verbalizes word "salad"
b. Feeds self with a cup
c. Makes a tower of two cubes
d. Draws a horizontal line

Ans. d. Draws a horizontal line

172. A child presents with short stature and hyperpigmented café au lait macules on body. The child has microcephaly, small eyes, epicanthic folds, small ears, absent radius and hypoplastic thumb. The most probable diagnosis is:

a. Idiopathic Thrombocytopenic purpura
b. Fanconi anemia
c. Langerhans cell histiocytosis
d. Hodgkin's disease

Ans. b. Fanconi anemia

173. Differential cyanosis is a characteristic feature in cases of:

a. COA b. VSD
c. PDA d. TAPVC

Ans. c. PDA

174. NADAS criteria are used to assess the presence of:

a. Congenital heart diseases
b. Chromosomal anomalies
c. Renal anomalies
d. Inborn errors of metabolism

Ans. a. Congenital heart diseases

175. An 18 kg child with severe dehydration was admitted to the hospital. The child was treated with boluses of fluids and is in remission. What will be the amount of maintenance fluid for the child?

a. 1500 mL
b. 1800 mL
c. 1400 mL
d. 1160 mL

Ans. c. 1400 mL

176. A term neonate delivered by C-section with mild respiratory distress soon after birth improves spontaneously over hours. The chest X-ray findings in this neonate will be:

a. 'Ground glass haziness'
b. Hyperinflation of lungs
c. Fluids in interlobar fissure
d. Reticulonodular appearance

Ans. c. Fluids in interlobar fissure

177. A child is to be delivered preterm at 32 weeks POG. The dose of antenatal corticosteroid given to the mother will be:

a. Inj. Betamethasone 12 mg 2 doses 24 hours apart IM
b. Inj. Dexamethasone 12 mg 4 doses 12 hours apart IM
c. Inj. Dexamethasone 6 mg 2 doses 12 hours apart IV
d. Inj. Betamethasone 12 mg 2 doses 24 hours apart IV

Ans. a. Inj. Betamethasone 12 mg 2 doses 24 hours apart IM

178. In the following list which is not an example of short limb disproportionate short stature?

a. Rickets
b. Osteogenesis imperfecta
c. Congenital hypothyroidism
d. Hemi vertebra

Ans. d. Hemi vertebra

179. A 3-week-old infant presents with projectile, recurrent nonbilious vomiting, failure to thrive. On per abdominal examination, a palpable olive-shaped mass is felt and USG shows a thickened pylorus. Maternal intake of which drug is responsible for this disease?

a. Doxycycline b. Erythromycin
c. Isoniazid d. Lithium

Ans. b. Erythromycin

180. A child's height increases by 100% by the age of:
a. 1 year b. 2 years
c. 9 months d. 4 years

Ans. d. 4 years

181. Which of the following conditions in a newborn requires a treatment?
a. Erythema toxicun
b. Neonatal pustular melanosis
c. Milia
d. Icthyosis vulgaris

Ans. d. Icthyosis vulgaris

182. All of the following are advantages of delayed cord clamping; except:
a. Lesser risk of neonatal jaundice
b. Lesser risk of intraventricular hemorrhage
c. Lesser need of blood transfusion
d. Higher BP

Ans. a. Lesser risk of neonatal jaundice

183. A neonate is brought to you with poor feeding and hypothermia, with dyspnea, shrill cry and feeding intolerance. The most common organism responsible for this condition in India is:
a. *E. coli*
b. Group B Streptococcus
c. Klebsiella
d. Acinetobacter

Ans. d. Acinetobacter

184. A child with intellectual disability, round face with low set ears, epicanthic fold, gap in the first and second toe, and a flat occiput will have highest risk of which congenital heart disease?
a. Ventricular septal defect
b. Endocardial cushion defect
c. Atrial septal defect
d. Pulmonary stenosis

Ans. b. Endocardial cushion defect

185. Which of the following condition is not an absolute contraindication for breastfeeding?
a. Maternal chemo or radiotherapy
b. Galactosemia in infant
c. Maternal active untreated TB
d. Lactose intolerance in infant

Ans. c. Maternal active untreated TB

186. A mother is suffering from a condition with autosomal recessive inheritance, she delivered a child with microcephaly, blonde hair, blue iris and intellectual disability. All of the following statements are true; except:
a. It is classical case of tyrosinemia
b. Enzyme deficiency is phenylalanine hydroxylase
c. Urine odor is mousy
d. FeC13 test imparts green color to urine

Ans. a. It is classical case of tyrosinemia